Bone's Atlas of *Pulmonary and Critical Care Medicine*

Atlas of

Second Edition

Bone's Atlas of *Pulmonary and Critical Care Medicine*

Second Edition

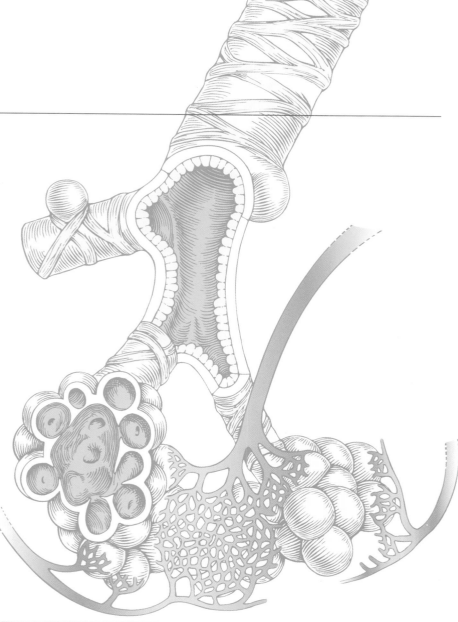

Edited by

G. DOUGLAS CAMPBELL, JR., MD
Professor
Department of Medicine
Division of Pulmonary and Critical Care
Medicine
Louisiana State University Health Sciences
Center
Shreveport, Louisiana

D. KEITH PAYNE, MD
Professor
Department of Medicine
Acting Chief
Division of Pulmonary and Critical Care
Medicine
Louisiana State University Health Sciences
Center
Shreveport, Louisiana

With 45 contributors

Developed by Current Medicine, Inc. Philadelphia, Pennsylvania

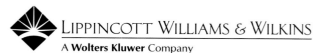

LIPPINCOTT WILLIAMS & WILKINS
A **Wolters Kluwer** Company
Philadelphia • Baltimore • New York • London
Buenos Aires • Hong Kong • Sydney • Tokyo

Current Medicine, Inc.
400 Market Street, Suite 700
Philadelphia, Pennsylvania 19106

Developmental Editor . . . . *June Choe*
Editorial Assistant. . . . . *Annmarie D'Ortona*
Cover Design . . . . *Jennifer Knight*
Layout . . . . *Jennifer Knight and John McCullough*
Illustrator . . . . *Wiesia Langenfeld, Maureen Looney and Kay Elwood*
Assistant Production Manager. . . . . *Simon Dickey*
Indexer . . . . *Susan Thomas*

Bone's atlas of pulmonary & critical care medicine / edited by G.
Douglas Campbell, Jr., D. Keith Payne ; with 45 contributors ; developed
by Current Medicine Inc.--2nd ed.
    p. cm.
    Includes bibliographical references and index.
    ISBN 0-7817-3436-3
    1. Respiratory intensive care—Atlases. 2. Respiratory
organs--Diseases--Atlases.
    [DNLM: 1. Lung Diseases--Atlases. 2. Critical
Care--methods--Atlases. WF 17 B712 2001] 1. Title: Atlas of
pulmonary and critical care medicine. II. Bone, Roger C. III. Campbell,
G. Douglas. IV. Payne, D. Keith. V. Current Medicine, Inc.
    RC735.R48 B66 2001
    616.2'00428--dc21
    for Library of Congress   2001028209

ISBN 0-7817-3436-3

Although every effort has been made to ensure that the drug doses and other information are
presented accurately in this publication, the ultimate responsibility rests with the prescribing
physician. Neither the publishers nor the authors can be held responsible for errors or for any
consequences arising from the use of the information contained herein. Products mentioned in
this publication should be used in accordance with manufacturer's prescribing information. No
claims or endorsements are made for any drug or compound at present under clinical investigation.

Printed
5 4 3 2 1

DISTRIBUTED WORLDWIDE BY Lippincott Williams & Wilkins

PREFACE

This Second Edition of *Bone's Atlas of Pulmonary and Critical Care Medicine* follows in the tradition of the First Edition in trying to help the busy clinician and student of chest disease absorb a large amount of information in a relatively short amount of time. Our atlas format, replete with high-quality images, algorithms, and tables has proven to be an efficient and popular way to convey clinically relevant information. We hope our readers continue to find these "snapshots" of chest diseases helpful in their day-to-day activities.

For the Second Edition, each chapter has been carefully reviewed and updated. Figures and references have been revised to include new advances in diagnosis and therapy. New authors have been recruited and several new chapters have been added, including chapters on sleep disorders, HIV and fungal infections, lower respiratory tract infections, and nutrition.

As its name states, this atlas continues in the memory of one of the true giants in medicine, Dr. Roger Bone. His vision and energy were instrumental in the genesis of the original project and he continues to be a source of inspiration for all of us. We dedicate this book to him.

We wish to thank the many contributors who spent so much time and energy organizing their respective chapters. We thank our students, housestaff, and fellows who serve to inspire us and challenge us to stay current. Finally, we would like to thanks our wives, Drs. Laura Casteel Campbell and Cynthia Black-Payne, for their constant and active support throughout the many evenings and weekends that were necessary to complete the revisions for this edition.

G. Douglas Campbell, MD

D. Keith Payne, MD

CONTRIBUTORS

Muzaffar Ahmad, MD
Chairman
Division of Medicine
Cleveland Clinic Foundation
Cleveland, Ohio

Antonio Anzueto, MD
Associate Professor of Medicine
The University of Texas Health Sciences Center
Chief, Pulmonary Disease Section
South Texas Veterans Healthcare System
San Antonio, Texas

Joseph H. Bates, MD, MS
Professor
Departments of Internal Medicine and
  Microbiology
University of Arkansas for Medical Sciences
Deputy State Health Officer
University of Arkansas for Medical Sciences
  and Veterans Affairs
Little Rock, Arkansas

Robert P. Baughman, MD
Professor
Department of Internal Medicine
University of Cincinnati
Cincinnati, Ohio

Seth Mark Berney, MD
Assistant Professor of Medicine
Center of Excellence for Arthritis and
  Rheumatology
Louisiana State University Health Sciences
  Center
Shreveport, Louisiana

Steven N. Berney, MD
Professor and Section Chief
Department of Rheumatology
Temple University School of Medicine
Philadelphia, Pennsylvania

Robert W. Bradsher, MD
Ebert Professor of Medicine
Department of Medicine
University of Arkansas
Director, Division of Infectious Diseases
Central Arkansas Veterans Administration
Little Rock, Arkansas

G. Douglas Campbell, Jr, MD
Professor
Department of Medicine
Division of Pulmonary and Critical Care
  Medicine
Louisiana State University Health Sciences
  Center
Shreveport, Louisiana

Thomas V. Colby, MD
Professor of Pathology
Mayo Medical School
Scottsdale, Arizona

Nancy Collop, MD
Professor
Department of Medicine
University of Mississippi
Director, Sleep Disorder Laboratory
C.V. (Sonny) Montgomery VA Medical Center
Jackson, Mississippi

Christopher J. Davreux, MD, MSc, FRCS (c)
Assistant Professor
Department of Surgery
McMaster University
Staff Physician
Hamilton Health Sciences Corporation
  (General Campus)
Hamilton, Ontario
Canada

Raed A. Dweik, MD
Staff Physician
Department of Pulmonary Medicine
The Cleveland Clinic Foundation
Cleveland, Ohio

C. Gregory Elliott, MD
Professor
Department of Medicine
Division of Respiratory, Critical Care, and
  Occupational Pulmonary Medicine
University of Utah Health Sciences Center
Pulmonary Division
LDS Hospital
Salt Lake City, Utah

Gary R. Epler, MD
Clinical Associate Professor
Department of Pulmonary and Critical Care
  Medicine
Harvard Medical School
Brigham and Women's Hospital
Boston, Massachusetts

Carol Farver, MD
Staff Pathologist
The Cleveland Clinic Foundation
Cleveland, Ohio

Stanley B. Fiel, MD
Professor
Department of Medicine
Professor and Chief
Department of Pulmonary and Critical Care
  Medicine
MCP Hahnemann University School of
  Medicine
Philadelphia, Pennsylvania

Maureen Heldmann, MD
Assistant Professor
Department of Radiology
Louisiana State University School of Medicine
Shreveport, Louisiana

David W. Hines, MD
Assistant Professor
Department of Internal Medicine
Rush University
Metro Infectious Disease Consultants
Chicago, Illinois

Carlos A. Jimenez, MD
Fellow
Department of Interventional Pulmonary
  Medicine
University of Texas MD Anderson Cancer
  Center
Houston, Texas

Mani S. Kavuru, MD
Director
Pulmonary Function Laboratory
Cleveland Clinic Foundation
Cleveland, Ohio

Sean Keenan, MD
Clinical Scholar
Division of Critical Care Medicine
London Health Sciences Centre
London, Ontario
Canada

Saeed U. Khan, MD
Fellow
Department of Pulmonary and Critical Care
  Medicine
Cleveland Clinic Foundation
Cleveland, Ohio

Ann S. Kirby, MD
Associate Professor
Department of Medicine
University of Western Ontario
Medical Director, ICU
St. Joseph's Health Centre
London, Ontario
Canada

David Leasa, MD, FRCP (c)
Professor
Department of Medicine
University of Western Ontario
Staff Physician
London Health Sciences Center
London, Ontario
Canada

Pyng Lee, MD
Fellow
Department of Pulmonary and Critical Care
  Medicine
Cleveland Clinic Foundation
Cleveland, Ohio

Joseph P. Lynch III, MD
Professor of Internal Medicine
University of Michigan Medical Center
Ann Arbor, Michigan

Boaz A. Markewitz, MD
Assistant Professor
Department of Medicine
University of Utah Health Sciences Center
Salt Lake City, Utah

Claudio Martin, MD, MSc, FRCPC
Associate Professor
Department of Medicine
University of Western Ontario
Attending Physician
London Health Sciences Centre, Critical
  Care/Trauma Center
London, Ontario
Canada

Atul C. Mehta, MD
Professor
Department of Medicine
Head, Section of Bronchology
Vice Chairman of Pulmonary and Critical Care
  Medicine
Cleveland Clinic Foundation
Cleveland, Ohio

Moulay Meziane, MD
Head, Thoracic Imaging Section
Department of Radiology
Cleveland Clinic Foundation
Cleveland, Ohio

John R. Michael, MD
Professor
Department of Medicine
Medical Service
Department of Veterans Affairs Medical Center
Salt Lake City, Utah

Omar A. Minai, MD
Senior Fellow
Department of Pulmonary and Critical Care
  Medicine
Cleveland Clinic Foundation
Cleveland, Ohio

Rodolfo C. Morice, MD
Associate Professor
Department of Interventional Pulmonary
  Medicine
Section Chief
University of Texas MD Anderson Cancer
  Center
Houston, Texas

Jeffrey L. Myers, MD
Professor
Department of Pathology
Mayo Medical School
Consultant
Department of Laboratory Medicine and
  Pathology
Chair, Division of Anatomic Pathology
Mayo Clinic
Rochester, Minnesota

Peter B. O'Donovan, MB, BCh
Staff Radiologist
Cleveland Clinic Foundation
Cleveland, Ohio

Michael W. Owens, MD
Associate Professor
Department of Medicine
Louisiana State University School of Medicine
Chief, Medical Service
Overton Brooks Veterans Affairs Medical
  Center
Shreveport, Louisiana

D. Keith Payne, MD
Professor
Department of Medicine
Acting Chief
Division of Pulmonary and Critical Care
  Medicine
Louisiana State University Health Sciences
  Center
Shreveport, Louisiana

Thomas W. Rice, MD
Head, Section of General Thoracic Surgery
Cleveland Clinic Foundation
Cleveland, Ohio

Richard Robbins, MD
Professor
Department of Medicine
University of Arizona
Chief, Research Service
Southern Arizona VA Healthcare System
Tucson, Arizona

Frank Rutledge, MD
Professor
Department of Medicine
University of Western Ontario
Staff Physician
Program in Critical Care
London Health Sciences Centre—Victoria
  Campus
London, Ontario
Canada

Daniel V. Schidlow, MD
Professor and Chair
Department of Pediatrics
MCP Hahnemann University
Physician-in-Chief
St. Christopher's Hospital for Children
Philadelphia, Pennsylvania

Jennifer A. Sewell, MD
Instructor
Department of Medicine
Louisiana State University Health Sciences
  Center
Shreveport, Louisiana

William J. Sibbald, MD, FRCPC, FCCHSE
Professor of Medicine and Critical Care
University of Toronto
Physician-in-Chief, Department of Medicine
Sunnybrook & Women's College Health
  Sciences Centre
London, Ontario
  Canada

Dessmon Y. H. Tai, MD
Consultant
Department of Respiratory Medicine
Tan Tock Seng Hospital
Singapore

Barbara Tribl, MD
Visiting Fellow
Department of Medicine
Visiting Fellow
Department of Critical Care
Sunnybrook and Women's College Health
  Sciences Center
Toronto, Ontario
Canada

Dona Upson, MD
Staff Physician
Pulmonary Department
VA Medical Center
Albuerque, New Mexico

CONTENTS

SECTION I: PULMONARY OBSTRUCTIVE DISEASES

SECTION II: NEOPLASMS

SECTION III: INFECTIOUS DISEASES

SECTION IV: INTERSTITIAL AND ALVEOLAR INFLAMMATORY DISORDERS

SECTION V: PULMONARY VASCULAR DISEASES

SECTION VI: CRITICAL CARE

SMOKING

*Dona Upson &
Richard Robbins*

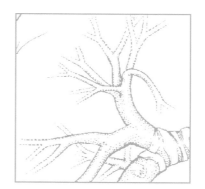
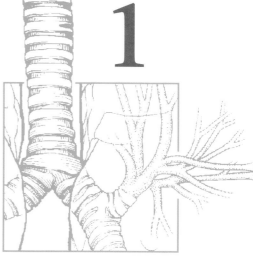
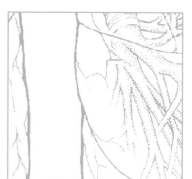

Tobacco use continues to be the leading cause of avoidable illness and death in economically advantaged countries, and is rapidly approaching that status worldwide. In the United States, 50% of continuing smokers will die because of their addiction, and half of them will do so in middle age, losing 20 to 25 years of life. Tobacco use causes the majority of pulmonary disease, is the leading modifiable risk for cardiovascular disease, and causes more than 30% of cancer deaths. Exposure to environmental tobacco smoke (ETS) causes the hospitalization of 20 infants a day because of lower respiratory tract infections and triggers 23 asthma exacerbations per hour in children [1]. Smoking during pregnancy is the main preventable cause of perinatal morbidity and mortality [2]. More than 400,000 people in the United States die prematurely each year from tobacco use, and countless others sustain profound perpetual worry, expense, disability, and pain [3]. Most of these people are not offered the effective treatments available and are unable to quit on their own.

Treatment of tobacco dependence is cost-effective. Smoking cessation decreases the risk of myocardial infarction by 50% within 2 years [4]. After 5 to 15 years, the risk of stroke decreases to that of those who never smoked. This is the only way to slow the decline in lung function associated with emphysema. After 10 years, lung cancer risk is 30% to 50% that of continuing smokers [5]. More than $1 billion/year, or $2 to $4 per pack of cigarettes sold, is spent on smoking-attributable disease in the United States [6,7]. Even otherwise healthy, young adult smokers have greater rates of hospitalization and lost work days than nonsmokers [8]. Health care costs are 40% higher for people who smoke, accounting for 7% to 11% of the national expenditure. Federal and state funds pay 43% of the tab [6]. In the short-term, increases in cessation will reduce costs much more than decreases in initiation. More than 70% of adults and adolescents who smoke are serious about quitting [5], but most clinicians do not receive proper training or support to adequately treat tobacco dependence and many health care programs do not provide coverage.

Public health goals are to increase smoking cessation, decrease initiation, lower exposure to ETS, and eliminate disparities in prevalence and health effects among population groups. Progress has been made in decreasing adult smoking prevalence in the United States, from 42.4% in 1965 to 24.1% in 1998 [9]. However, rates have been level for the past decade, largely because of dramatic increases among youth after aggressive marketing by the tobacco industry. In 1999, 48 million people in the United States smoked cigarettes regularly, with the highest rates seen among those with less education and those with lower incomes. Increases in cigarette excise taxes, with revenues dedicated to comprehensive tobacco control programs, have proven efficacious. All states tax cigarettes, averaging 38.9 cents per pack (from 2.5 cents in Virginia to $1 in Hawaii and Alaska) [10], but many do not allocate the funds for tobacco control. Only 28 states have laws limiting smoking in commercial day care centers [10]. Policy initiatives work, if properly funded and implemented. Services to treat tobacco dependence, high intensity mass media campaigns, bans on tobacco advertising, passage of local ordinances to promote smoke-free indoor environments, school-based prevention and treatment programs, and decreased access to tobacco products by youth act in concert. The tobacco industry has countered with creative marketing and supporting preemptive legislation at state levels, which prevents local jurisdictions from enacting laws more stringent than state law, over which they have more influence. Families also play important roles, by providing messages that encourage or discourage tobacco use [11]. Surveillance will remain crucial in evaluating control programs locally and globally. Hopefully, lessons learned from countries that have borne the brunt of tobacco-related illness over the past several decades will be improved and adopted by the developing world, to stem the impending catastrophic health consequences of the pandemic of tobacco use.

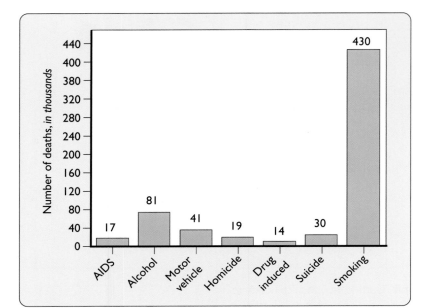

Figure 1-1.
Annual deaths from preventable causes in the United States (comparative causes of annual deaths in the United States). Despite declining consumption, tobacco products continue to play an important role in morbidity and mortality. Approximately half of the 2 million annual deaths in the United States occurs prematurely from preventable causes. Approximately one in five deaths is a result of tobacco use [12]. (*Adapted from* McGinnis and Foege [13].)

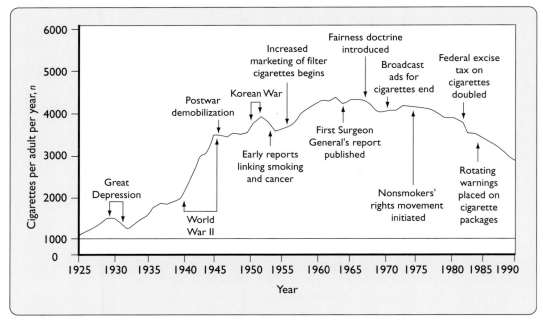

Figure 1-2.
Cigarette consumption among adults. The figure indicates the cigarettes consumed per adult per year in the United States, 1925–1990. Historical events appear to influence consumption rates. A remarkable increase occurred between 1940 and 1945 during WW II, partially due to the free distribution of cigarettes by the US government to military personnel. Equally important is the leveling of consumption between 1960 and 1965, around the time of the Surgeon General's first report on the hazards of tobacco use and the subsequent decline. The gradual decrease since 1975 coincides with significant increases in cost of cigarettes and the placement of warning labels on packages [14]. (*Data from* the Department of Health and Human Services). In the mid-1950s, cigarette manufacturers introduced technical changes that resulted in reduced delivery of tar and nicotine, which was followed by increases in overall consumption. Since 1981, tar delivery has averaged 12.7 to 13 mg, and nicotine delivery at 0.9 mg/cigarette. Manufacturers can manipulate nicotine levels by chemically treating tobacco and by altering the blend of tobaccos in cigarettes. Smokers can control delivery of tar and nicotine by adjusting breathing patterns and by holding their fingers over vent holes in filters [15]. (*Adapted from* Wakeman [16], The Federal Trade Commission [17], *and* RJ Reynolds Tobacco Company [18].)

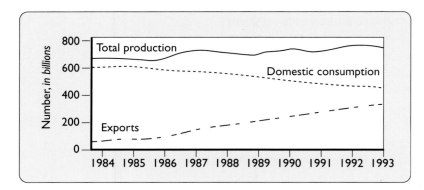

Figure 1-3.
Cigarette production, exports, and domestic consumption—United States, 1984–1993. Although domestic consumption of tobacco has gradually declined, total production has increased, in part due to aggressive marketing of US tobacco products overseas. In 1998, 4 million people died worldwide of tobacco-related illness. That number is expected to increase to 10 million annually by 2030, 70% of them in poor countries. Currently, 80% of the world's 1.1 billion smokers live in low income and middle income countries, where there is little knowledge regarding the risks of smoking and efforts to prevent and treat tobacco dependence are insufficient [19]. Consumption has decreased in the United States because fewer people are smoking and because consumption by individual smokers has declined. In 1999, 81.2% of smokers consumed 1 to 20 cigarettes/day, 17.1% smoked 21 to 40 per day, and 1.5% more than 40. Cigarette consumption among smokers appears to be higher among men, whites, people aged 35 to 65 years, and those with lower levels of education. Although prevalence of smoking is higher among those in lower socioeconomic levels, income is not associated with differences in consumption among those who smoke. (*Data from* the BRFSS 1999.)

A. ODDS RATIOS FOR THE COVERAGE OF THE RISKS OF SMOKING BY MAGAZINES WITH ANY CIGARETTE ADVERTISEMENTS, AS COMPARED WITH MAGAZINES WITH NO CIGARETTE ADVERTISEMENTS

Magazines	Magazine-years,* n	Probability of coverage, %	Odds ratio (95% CI)	
			Without adjustment	With adjustment†
All magazines				
No cigarette advertising	403	11.9	0.88 (0.60–1.03)	0.73 (0.42–1.30)
Any cigarette advertising	900	8.3		
Women's magazines				
No cigarette advertising	104	11.7	0.22 (0.05–0.90)	0.13 (0.02–0.69)
Any cigarette advertising	212	5.0		

*A magazine-year is defined as a single magazine in a single year.
†We adjusted for the following covariates: the number of subscriptions for each magazine in each year; the number of articles on nine health risk factors published in each magazine in each year and the square of this value; whether or not a magazine was a newsmagazine (for all magazines only); whether or not a magazine was a women's magazine (for all magazines only); an interaction term between women's magazine and the measure of cigarettes advertising (for all magazines only); and the time-period variables for 1964, the 1970s, and the 1980s.

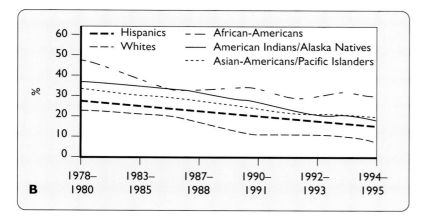

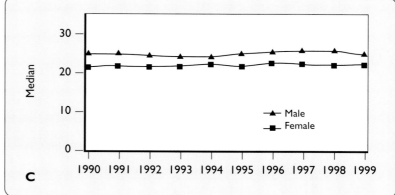

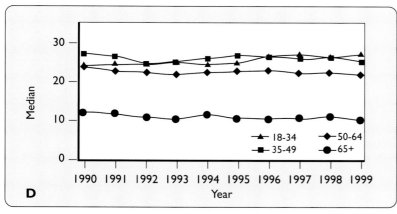

Figure 1-4.
Trends in the prevalence of cigarette smoking in the United States. Smoking prevalence declined dramatically in the mid-1960s to the mid-1980s. The greatest decrease was seen among men, whose rate decreased from 52% to 31.7% (panel A). The smoking rate among women, which was not as high initially, fell modestly [15]. However, for most racial and ethnic groups (panel B) and between genders (panel C), rates were level throughout the 1990s, largely because increases in smoking by younger adults more than compensated for those who were able to quit smoking or had died (panel D). In 1998, 24.1% of all adults in the United States were smokers, which included 27.5% of those 18 to 24 years of age. The lowest prevalence (11.3%) was in adults with 16 or more years of education [20], although between 1993 and 1997 the prevalence of cigarette smoking increased 28% among US college students to 28.5%, and cigar smoking rose to 8.5% [20]. American Indians and Alaska Natives demonstrated the highest levels of smoking in 1998 (40%), followed by whites (25%) and African-Americans (24.7%) [20]. African-Americans suffer disproportionately from chronic and preventable disease, including lung cancer and stroke [21]; approximately 45,000 die annually from a smoking-related disease [21]. African-American smokers have higher levels of serum cotinine (metabolized nicotine) than white or Mexican-American smokers for the same number of cigarettes [22], which may be related to a preference for mentholated brands [21]. (Panels B, C, and D *adapted from* CDC [23].)

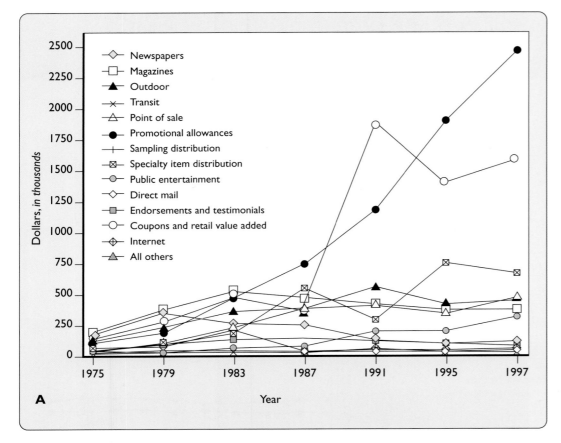

A

Figure 1-5.
A, Domestic cigarette advertising and promotional expenditures—United States, 1975–1997. Tobacco industry documents indicate that concerns about declining smoking prevalence and market share resulted in markedly enhanced advertising and promotional efforts, beginning in the 1970s. Expenditures for many advertising venues remained stable, partially due to increased legal restrictions, while promotional activities skyrocketed. **B**, Comparison of advertising to brand preference in adolescents and adults, 1993. A study done in 1996 revealed that one third of students in grades 6 to 12 owned at least one cigarette promotional item and that there was a causal relationship between the number of items owned and smoking behavior [24]. Adolescents are more likely than adults to be influenced by advertising, with brand preferences mirroring expenditures in advertising and promotion. In 1993, 86% of teen smokers purchased one of the three most heavily advertised brands [25]. Cigar consumption increased by 50% from 1993 to 1998 after a dramatic increase in promotional activities [20]. (Panel A *adapted from* American College of Chest Physicians [26]. Panel B *adapted from* CDC [27].)

B. COMPARISON OF ADVERTISING TO BRAND PREFERENCE* IN ADOLESCENTS AND ADULTS, 1993

Advertising, *millions*	Adolescent brand preference, %	Adult brand† preference, %
Marlboro, $75	Marlboro, 60.0	Marlboro, 23.5
Camel, $43	Camel, 13.3	Winston, 6.7
Newport, $35	Newport, 12.7	Newport, 4.8
Kool, $21	Kool, 1.2	Camel, 3.9
Winston, $17	Winston, 1.2	Salem, 3.9
Benson & Hedges, $4	Salem, 1.0	Kool, 3.0
Salem, $3	Benson & Hedges, 0.3%	Benson & Hedges, 2.5

*Among name brands from 1983 TAPS.
†Overall market share used as estimate.

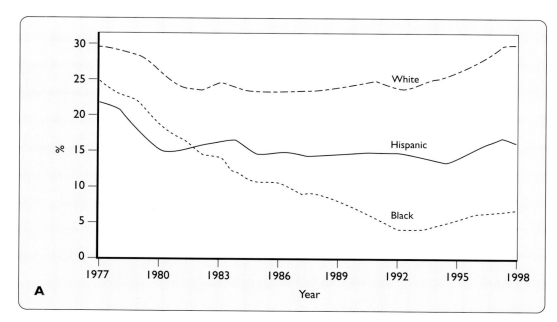

A

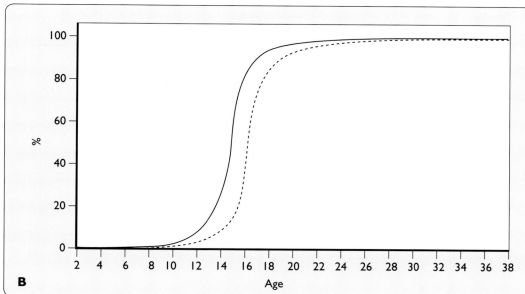

B

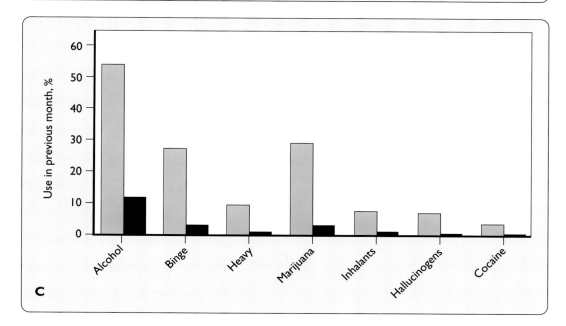

C

Figure 1-6.

A, Trends in daily cigarette smoking by high school seniors by race/ethnic group—United States, 1977–1997. Smoking prevalence among adolescents increased by 32% between 1991 and 1997 [20]. In 1999, smoking (one or more cigarettes during the previous 30 days) was highest among white students (38.6%), followed by rates for Hispanic students (32.7%) and African-American students (19.7%). Overall, prevalence was similar for young men (34.7%) and women (34.3%), although African-American and Hispanic males were more likely than their female counterparts to smoke. Higher rates have been found among adolescents who left school without graduating. In addition, there has been an increase in non-cigarette tobacco use, including cigars, spit tobacco, kreteks (clove cigarettes), bidis, and pipes, in declining order of prevalence.

B, Cumulative age of initiation of cigarette smoking—United States, 1991 [19]. Most people who become daily smokers (one or more cigarettes per day during the previous 30 days) do so by age 18. The younger people are when they begin smoking, the more likely they are to become heavily addicted to nicotine and the more difficult it will be for them to quit. Seventy-five percent of young smokers state that they continue to smoke because they are addicted to nicotine. Smoking during youth can impair lung growth and diminish the level of maximum lung function. More than 3000 adolescents become daily smokers every day, a 73% increase since 1988 [21].

C, Use of illicit drugs and alcohol by 12- to 17-year-old smokers and nonsmokers, 1995. Smokers are much more likely to have used other substances, including alcohol, marijuana, and cocaine. Tobacco serves as an entry drug and generally precedes use of other substances. In this figure, marijuana and cocaine use indicates more than 10 times each. (Panel A *adapted from* CDC [28]. Panels B and C *adapted from* CDC [29].)

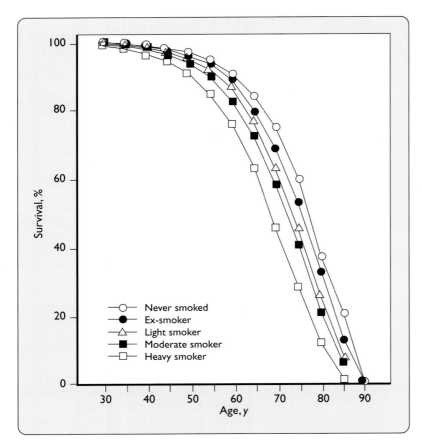

Figure 1-7.
Survival by smoking habit. On average, smokers die 7 years earlier than people who never smoked [Centers for Disease Control and Prevention. Office on Smoking and Health, unpublished data, 1994]. In this figure, the median survival for British male doctors who never smoked was 77 years, versus 69 years for heavy smokers. The numbers for women were 81 years for those who never smoked and 76 years for heavy smokers. There is a clear dose-response relationship between smoking and life span that, when compared with the median life span of men who never smoked, suggests a loss of 1 year for ex-smokers, 3 years for light smokers, 5 years for moderate smokers, and 8 years for heavy smokers. If one looks at age 65, the survival rate is 85% for those who never smoked compared with 65% for heavy smokers. To view these data another way, any cancer treatment that increased the survival rate from 65% to 85% would be considered remarkable [30]. (*Adapted from* West [30].)

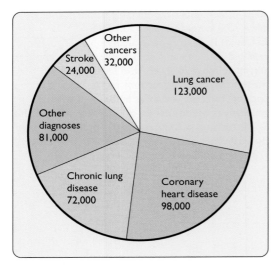

Figure 1-8.
Annual deaths attributable to cigarette smoking—United States, 1990–1994. Between 1990 and 1994, 430,000 deaths each year were attributable to cigarette smoking. Since the Surgeon General's first report in 1964 on the risks of tobacco use, there have been 10 million deaths in the United States attributable to smoking, 2 million of those due to lung cancer [Centers for Disease Control and Prevention. Office on Smoking and Health, unpublished data, 1994]. On average, there is a 22-fold increase in mortality rate from lung cancer among men who smoke, and a 12-fold increase among women. The risk of dying from chronic obstructive pulmonary disorder (COPD) is 10 times greater in smokers of both genders. Deaths from cardiovascular disease are tripled by smoking among middle-aged men and women [31]. (*Adapted from* CDC [3].)

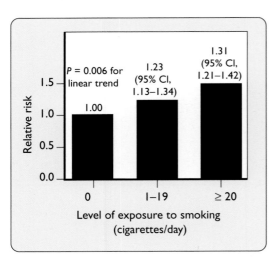

Figure 1-9.
Risk of coronary heart disease as a result of environmental tobacco smoke. Smoking is a major modifiable risk for the development and progression of cardiovascular disease because of the effects on atherosclerosis and hemostasis. In a dose-dependent relationship, exposure to environmental tobacco smoke (ETS) increases the average relative risk of coronary heart disease to 1.25 [32] and of progression of atherosclerosis to 1.20 [33]. Given that cardiovascular disease is the leading cause of death in the United States and that approximately 40% of nonsmoking children and adults are regularly exposed to ETS, these numbers represent a significant public health burden [34]. In addition, every year, 3000 people in the United States die of ETS caused by lung cancer [35]. (*Adapted from* He et al. [32].)

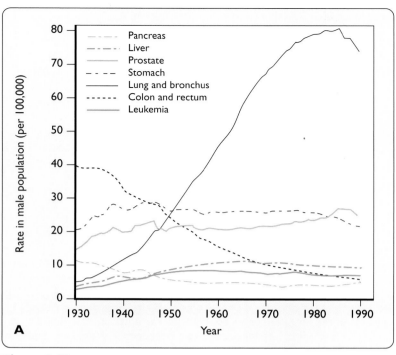

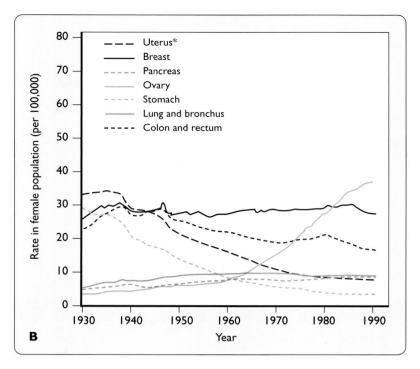

Figure 1-10.

Age-adjusted cancer death rates in the United States, 1930–1995. Tobacco use causes more than 30% of all cancer deaths in the United States [National Cancer Institute; Tobacco Research Implementation Plan, 11/98]. The mortality rate from lung cancer began to decline among men in 1991, reflecting their decreased prevalence of smoking since the mid-1960s. Lung cancer among women increased by more than 500% between 1950 and 1995, surpassing breast cancer in the mid-1980s as the leading cause of cancer-related deaths,

and continues to increase [36] [National Cancer Institute/National Institutes of Health; Press Release 5/14/00]. In 1999, 68,000 women died of lung cancer in the United States [37]. A recent study in the United Kingdom revealed that the cumulative risk of death by age 75 in men who smoke was 16%, which dropped to 10%, 6%, 3%, and 2% among those who had quit at ages 60, 50, 40, and 30, respectively. Cessation before middle age eliminated more than 90% of the risk attributable to tobacco [38]. (*Adapted from* Clinics in Chest Medicine [39].)

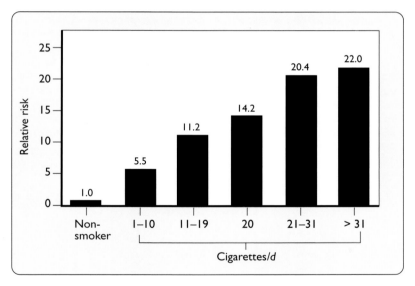

Figure 1-11.

Risk of lung cancer death among women. Data from the Cancer Prevention Study II revealed a dose-dependent increased risk of lung cancer among women who smoke. Cigarette smoking accounts for nearly 90% of all lung cancers, and is the leading cause of all four major types (squamous cell, adenocarcinoma, small cell, and large cell).

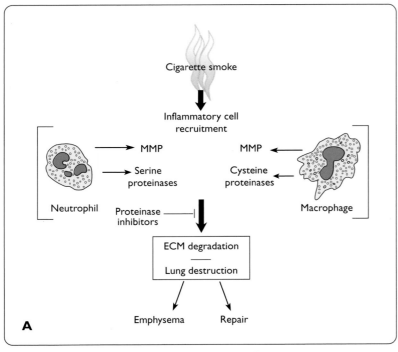

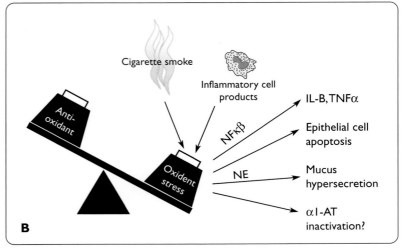

B

proteinases. Normally, these enzymes are in balance with their inhibitors and lung destruction does not occur. Tobacco smoke incurs an excess amount of proteinases, enhances their effects, and inactivates proteinase inhibitors. In addition, cigarette smoke and inflammatory cells increase the number of oxidants in the lung, leading to epithelial cell production of IL-8 and TNF-α, before apoptosis. Mucus secretion occurs via an oxidant-mediated signal transduction pathway using neutrophil elastase (NE). It is hypothesized that oxidant-mediated inactivation of α-1 antitrypsin (α-AT) occurs, thus further shifting the balance. The net effect of proteinase and oxidant activities is destruction of the extracellular matrix (ECM). (*Adapted from* Shapiro [40].)

Figure 1-12.
Pathogenesis of emphysema. Proposed mechanism of injury by cigarette smoke leading to emphysema. Chronic exposure to cigarette smoke causes recruitment of inflammatory cells to the lungs, where they release

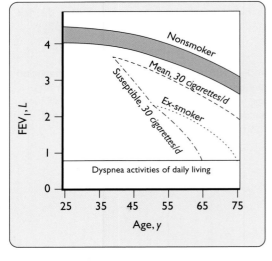

Figure 1-13.
Decline of lung function due to smoking. Relationship of FEV_1, age, and smoking. Nonsmokers lose FEV_1 at an accelerated rate with age; the average loss is approximately 30 mL/year. People who smoke 30 cigarettes/day average a slightly greater rate of decline and have FEV_1 values slightly below average when first observed at age 40 years. A small proportion of susceptible smokers (approximately 15%) lose function much more rapidly, approximately 150 mL/year, with FEV_1 of 0.8 L by age 65, a level so low that they experience dyspnea in the course of ordinary daily living. Susceptible smokers who stop smoking at age 50 do not regain lost function or regain only a little, but they subsequently lose function at the same rate as people who never smoked; dyspnea with ordinary activity will not develop until the mid-70s. The Lung Health Study found that cessation of cigarette smoking was the only intervention that slowed the rate of decline in lung function in chronic obstructive pulmonary disorder (COPD), with an average loss of 14.4 mL/year in sustained quitters, versus 60.2 mL/year in continuing smokers. In most cases, if a person quits smoking by age 40, there will be no significant difference in lung function compared with those who never smoked [41]. (*Adapted from* Snider [42].)

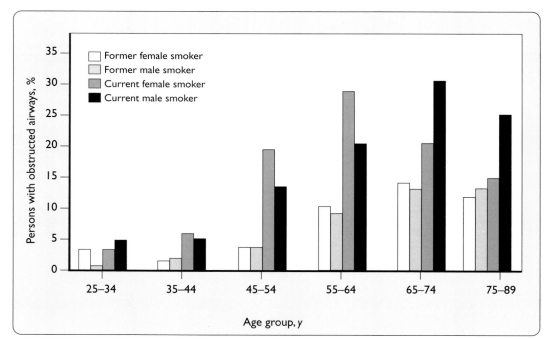

Figure 1-14.
Prevalence of airways obstruction. The prevalence of airways obstruction (FEV_1 and FEV_1/FEV_6 below the LLN) in the NHANES III sample of the US adult population (the abnormality rate in those who never smoked was less than 3.5%). Tobacco use accounts for 80% to 90% of COPD in the United States. Death rates for COPD among men increased in the 1960s to the mid-1970s and have since remained stable. Rates for women have continued to increase since 1960, with the most recent data for 1998. (*Adapted from* Enright and Crapo [43] and CDC [44].)

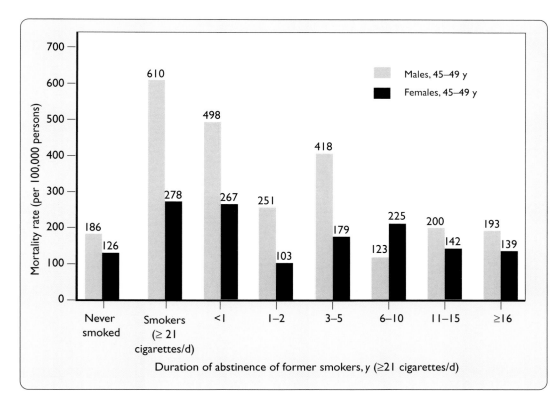

Figure 1-15.
Benefits of smoking cessation on mortality. The benefits of smoking cessation begin immediately and at all ages, to the point where, after 15 years of abstinence, all-cause mortality is nearly that of people who never smoked. In this figure, mortality rates are depicted for ages 45 to 49 years. The burden of non-lethal events and illness are not shown. Some of the mortality seen in the first few years after quitting represent deaths as a result of conditions that prompted individuals to stop smoking. People who quit before age 50 have half the risk of dying in the next 15 years compared with continuing smokers. (*Data from* DHHS [45].)

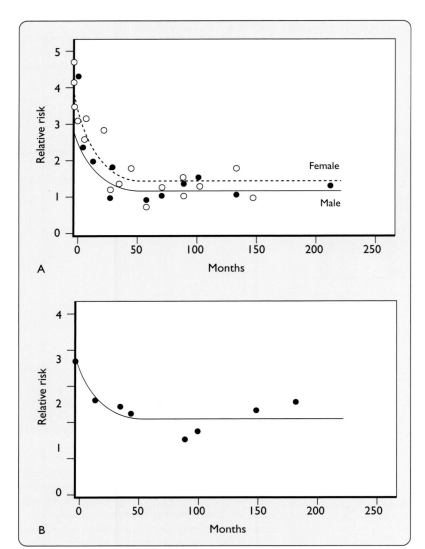

A

B

Figure 1-16.

Decline in cardiovascular deaths after smoking cessation. **A,** Acute myocardial infarction. **B,** Stroke. Estimated decline in relative risk for acute myocardial infarction and stroke over time with smoking cessation. The cardiovascular effects of tobacco use are the most amenable to improvement after cessation. The increased risk of a myocardial infarction or stroke decreases by 50% within 2 years, approaching that of those who never smoked, 4 years after quitting. When counseling smokers, it is important to highlight the short-term benefits of cessation. It has been estimated that an annual 1% reduction in smoking prevalence would result in 98,000 fewer hospitalizations and save $2.7 billion during the next 7 years due to decreased cardiovascular mortality alone; for each person in the United States who is treated successfully for tobacco dependence, $853 will be saved over 7 years. (*Adapted from* Lightwood and Glantz [4].)

Tobacco dependence is a chronic condition that often requires repeated intervention.

Effective treatments are available.

Every patient who uses tobacco should be offered at least one of these treatments.

Patients willing to try to quit tobacco use should be provided treatments identified as effective.

Patients unwilling to try to quit tobacco use should be provided a brief intervention designed to increase their motivation to quit.

It is essential that clinicians and health care delivery systems (including administrators, insurers, and purchasers) institutionalize the consistent identification, documentation, and treatment of every tobacco user seen in a health care setting.

Brief tobacco dependence treatment is effective; every patient who uses tobacco should be offered at least brief treatment.

There is a strong dose-response relationship between the intensity of tobacco dependence counseling and its effectiveness.

Treatments involving person-to-person contact (via individual, group, or proactive telephone counseling) are consistently effective, and their effectiveness increases with treatment intensity (*eg,* minutes of contact).

Three types of counseling and behavioral therapies were found to be especially effective and should be used with all patients attempting tobacco cessation:

Provision of practical counseling (problem solving/skills training).

Provision of social support as part of treatment.

Help in securing social support outside of treatment.

Numerous effective pharmacotherapies for smoking cessation exist. Except in the presence of contraindications, they should be used with all patients attempting to quit smoking.

First-line pharmacotherapies are bupropion SR and nicotine replacement products (patch, gum, nasal spray, inhaler).

Second-line pharmacotherapies are nortriptyline and clonidine.

Tobacco dependence treatments are clinically effective and cost-effective relative to other medical and disease prevention interventions.

All insurance plans should include as a reimbursed benefit the counseling and pharmacotherapeutic treatments identified as effective.

Clinicians should be reimbursed for providing tobacco dependence treatment as they are for treating other chronic conditions.

Figure 1-17.

Treating tobacco use and dependence—a clinical practice guideline. In 2000, the Surgeon General's office published the clinical practice guideline, *Treating Tobacco Use and Dependence, an Update of the 1996 Smoking Cessation, Clinical Practice Guideline No. 18* that was sponsored by the Agency for Health Care Policy and Research. Seventy percent of smokers seriously want to stop smoking, but are thwarted by nicotine addiction. In 1999, 51% of smokers quit smoking for at least one day; most relapsed [data from Behavioral Risk Factor Surveillance System]. For most patients, treatment of tobacco dependence is the most important intervention clinicians can perform to improve health. Even 3 minutes of discussion is associated with a 2% to 3% increase in permanent quit rates (OR 1.7) [46]. Given the many smokers who visit a clinician each year, the potential public health impact of universal advice to quit smoking is substantial [47].

META-ANALYSIS OF EFFICACY (ESTIMATED ODDS RATIO AND ABSTINENCE RATES) FOR SEVEN PHARMACOTHERAPIES USED IN TOBACCO DEPENDENCE TREATMENT

Pharmacotherapy (number of studies)	Number of study groups	Estimated odds ratio (95% CI)	Estimated abstinence rate (95% CI)
Bupropion SR (*n* = 2)			
Placebo	2	1.0	17.3
Bupropion SR	4	2.1 (1.5, 3.0)	30.5 (23.2, 37.8)
Nicotine gum, 2 mg (*n* = 13)			
Placebo	16	1.0	17.1
Nicotine gum	18	1.5 (1.3, 1.8)	23.7 (20.6, 26.7)
Nicotine inhaler (*n* = 4)			
Placebo	4	1.0	10.5
Nicotine inhaler	4	2.5 (1.7, 3.6)	22.8 (16.4, 29.2)
Nicotine nasal spray (*n*=3)			
Placebo	3	1.0	13.9
Nicotine spray	3	2.7 (1.8, 4.1)	30.5 (21.8, 39.2)
Transdermal nicotine (patch) (*n* = 27)			
Placebo	28	1.0	10.0
Transdermal nicotine	32	1.9 (1.7, 2.2)	17.7 (16.0, 19.5)
Clonidine (*n* = 5)			
Placebo	6	1.0	13.9
Clonidine	8	2.1 (1.4, 3.2)	25.6 (17.7, 33.6)
Nortriptyline (*n* = 2)			
Placebo	3	1.0	11.7
Nortriptyline	3	3.2 (1.8, 5.7)	30.1 (18.1, 41.6)

Figure 1-18.

Efficacy of pharmacotherapies used in tobacco dependence treatment. Meta-analyses of efficacy (estimated odds ratios and abstinence rates) for seven pharmacotherapies used in the treatment of tobacco dependence. Pharmacologic adjuncts double or triple success rates for smoking cessation, with baselines set by patient selection and intensity and quality of psychosocial support. Combinations of medications or modalities may further improve rates. Behavioral components work best if there are multiples sessions (at least 20 minutes each) of problem-solving and social support counseling over several weeks. Nicotine replacement therapy (NRT) helps establish and sustain remission long enough to develop preventive strategies for long-term success. Non-nicotine medications appear to work via dopaminergic and noradrenergic pathways. Anxiolytics are ineffective. A patient's experience and preferences are the best guides to choosing the type of treatment. CI—confidence interval; SR—sustained release. (*Adapted from* Fiore *et al.* [48].)

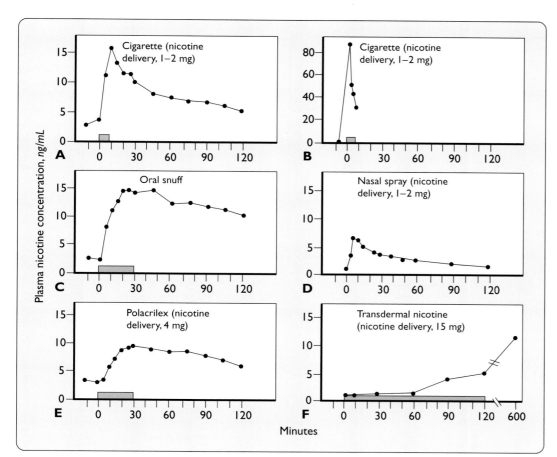

Figure 1-19.
Nicotine replacement therapy. Plasma nicotine concentrations before and after the administration of a single dose of nicotine, using different modalities. In contrast to smoking, which causes rapid absorption, nicotine medications provide slower, lower, and less variable concentrations. The shaded bars indicate periods of nicotine delivery. *Panel B* is based on arterial blood; the rest are venous. Patches provide a constant level of nicotine, but morning values may be uncomfortably low. Skin irritation is common but self-limited, and tolerance usually occurs within a week. Other modalities offer more flexibility. Gum is best when chewed on a regular schedule, with adjustments. The nicotine is absorbed by the oral mucosa; swallowing nicotine may cause esophageal spasm, gastric reflux, and hiccups. The nasal spray is absorbed by the nasal mucosa; it is not meant to be inhaled. Inhalers provide a very low dose of nicotine but mimic the action of smoking.

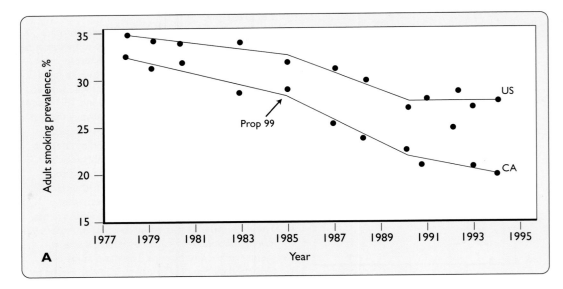

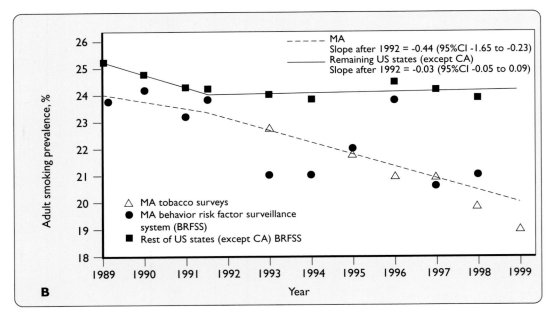

Figure 1-20.

Smoking prevalence response to increased taxes and tobacco control programs. **A,** Increasing taxes is the most effective way to reduce demand for tobacco, with an estimated 4% decrease in smoking per 10% cost increase [8]. Lower income, minority, and younger populations are the most likely to reduce smoking in response to price [49]. If the proceeds are dedicated to tobacco control efforts, further improvements are seen. Voters in California (CA) were the first to approve a comprehensive program funded by increases in cigarette taxes designed to reduce tobacco use (Proposition 99). After the implementation of the program in 1989, decline in smoking prevalence accelerated compared to the rest of the country [50]. **B,** Massachusetts (MA) voters approved ballot initiative "Question 1" in November, 1992, raising the cigarette tax an extra $0.25/pack. From 1988 to 1992, the 3% to 4% annual decline in per capita consumption was similar to comparison states. From 1992 to 1993, there was a 12% decrease in Massachusetts caused by the tax, versus 4% elsewhere. In the subsequent years, a consistent 4% annual decline in Massachusetts compared favorably with a less than 1% decrease in other states. After 1992, smoking prevalence in Massachusetts dropped 0.43% annually versus a 0.03% increase in comparison states (*panel B*). Forty percent of cigarette taxes were spent on services (treatment programs such as telephone counseling, youth leadership, educational materials), 30% on mass media, especially television, and 12% to 19% to promote local policies to improve tobacco control ordinances. Nationally, at $6.50/person, Massachusetts has the highest per capita expenditure for tobacco control, meeting the CDC recommendation of $6 to $20/person. In 1998, only five other states significantly funded tobacco programs, spending $0.24-$4.91/person [51]. Oregon increased cigarette taxes an extra $0.30/pack in 1996 and initiated a comprehensive tobacco prevention program; in the subsequent 2 years, consumption decreased 11% and smoking prevalence 6.4% [52]. It has been estimated that $600/person/year is spent on tobacco-related health care in Massachusetts, and that the decline in smoking has saved $85 million annually [51]. (Panel A *adapted from* Siegal *et al.* [50]. Panel B *adapted from* Biener *et al.* [51].)

REFERENCES

1. Centers for Disease Control and Prevention: Tobacco Information and Prevention Source. www.cdc.gov/tobacco/overview/30yrs2t.htm. Accessed February 14, 2001.

2. US Department of Health and Human Services: The health benefits of smoking cessation. Atlanta, Georgia: US Department of Health and Human Services, Public Health Service, CDC; 1990: DHHS publication no. 90-8416.

3. Centers for Disease Control and Prevention: MMWR Morb Mortal Wkly Rep 1997, 46:448–451.

4. Lightwood JM, Glantz SA: Short-term economic and health benefits of smoking cessation. Circulation 1997, 96:1089–1096.

5. Centers for Disease Control and Prevention: Great American Smokeout Day. Fact sheet. www.cdc.gov/tobacco/research_data/99gasofacts.htm. Accessed February 14, 2001.

6. Centers for Disease Control and Prevention: Medical care expenditures attributable to cigarette smoking—United States, 1993. MMWR Morb Mortal Wkly Rep 1994, 43(26);469–472.

7. American Cancer Society: Cancer facts & figures—1999. Tobacco Use 1999:25–28.

8. Robbins AS, Fonseca VP, Chao SY, Coil GA, Bell NS, Amoroso PJ: Short term effects of cigarette smoking on hospitalisation and associated lost workdays in a young healthy population. Tob Control 2000, 9:389–396.

9. Centers for Disease Control and Prevention: Cigarette smoking among adults—United States, 1998. MMWR Morb Mortal Wkly Rep 2000:10/6.

10. Centers for Disease Control and Prevention: State laws on tobacco control—United States, 1998. Fact sheet. www.cdc.gov/tobacco/research_data/legal_policy/mmwr699fs.htm. Accessed February 14, 2001.

11. Mermlstein and the Tobacco Control network Writing Group: Explanations of ethnic and gender differences in youth smoking: a mulyi-site, qualitative investigation. Nicotine Tobac Res 1999, 1: S91–S98.

12. Centers for Disease Control and Prevention: Smoking: attributable mortality and years of potential life lost—United States, 1990. MMWR Morb Mortal Wkly Rep 1993, 42(33):645–648.

13. McGinnis JM, Foege WH: Actual cases of deaths in the United States. JAMA 1993, 270:2207–2212.

14. Bartecchi CE, MacKenzie TD, Schrier RW: The human cost of tobacco use. N Engl J Med 1994, 330:975–980.

15. US Department of Health and Human Services: Reducing the Health Consequences of Smoking: 25 Years of Progress. A Report of the Surgeon General. Washington, DC: US Department of Health and Human Services, Public Health Service, Centers for Disease Control, Centers for Chronic Disease Prevention and Health Promotion, Office on Smoking and Health. DHHS Publication No. (CDC) 89-8411; 1989.

16. Wakeham H: Sales weighted average "tar" and nicotine deliveries of U.S. cigarettes from 1957 to present. In Lung Cancer, UICC Technical Report Series, vol 25. Edited by Wynder E, Hecht S. Geneva: International Union Against Cancer; 1976:151–152.

17. Federal Trade Commission: Report to Congress Pursuant to the Federal Cigarette Labeling and Advertising Act for the Year 1981. Federal Trade Commission; July 1984.

18. RJ Reynolds Tobacco Company: Chemical and Biological Studies on New Cigarette Prototypes that Heat Instead of Burn Tobacco. Winston-Salem, NC: RJ Reynolds Tobacco Co; 1988.

19. Jha P, Chaloupka FJ: The economics of global tobacco control. BMJ 2000, 321:358–361.

20. Rigotti NA, Lee JE, Wechsler H: US college students' use of tobacco products. JAMA 2000, 284:699–705.

21. Centers for Disease Control and Prevention, National Center for Health Statistics: National Health Interview Surveys, public use data tapes, 1978–1993.

22. US Department of Health and Human Services: Tobacco use among US racial/ethnic minority groups: African Americans, American Indians and Alaska Natives, Asian Americans and Pacific Islanders, and Hispanics. A report of the Surgeon General. Atlanta: DHHS, CDC, 1998.

23. Caraballo R: Racial and ethnic differences in serum cotinine levels of cigarette smokers. Third National Heath and Nutrition Examination Survey, 1988–1991. JAMA 1998, 280(2):135–139.

24. Sargent JD, Dalton M: Exposure to cigarette promotions and smoking uptake in adolescents: evidence of a dose-response relation. Tob Control 2000, 9:163–168.

25. Centers for Disease Control and Prevention: Changes in the cigarette brand preferences of adolescent smokers. MMWR Morb Mortal Wkly Rep 1994, 43(32);577–581.

26. Federal Trade Commission: Report to Congress for 1997 Pursuant to the Federal Cigarette Labeling and Advertising Act. Issued 1999.

27. Centers for Disease Control and Prevention: 1993 TAPS II. The Maxwell Consumer Report 1994. Ad & Summary, 1993.

28. Centers for Disease Control and Prevention: Institute for Social Research, University of Michigan, Monitoring the Future Project.

29. Centers for Disease Control and Prevention: National Household Survey on Drug Abuse.

30. West RR: Smoking: its influence on survival and cause of death. J Royal Coll Phys London 1992, 26:357–366.

31. Centers for Disease Control and Prevention: Smoking-attributable mortality and years of potential life lost—United States, 1990. MMWR Morb Mortal Wkly Rep 1993, 42(33):645–648.

32. He J, Vupputuri S, Allen K, Prerost MR, Hughes J, Whelton PK: Passive smoking and the risk of coronary heart disease: a meta-analysis of epidemiologic studies. N Engl J Med 1999, 340:920–926.

33. Howard G, Wagenknecht LE, Burke GL, et al.: Cigarette smoking and progression of atherosclerosis. JAMA 1998, 279:119-24.

34. Pirkle JL, Flegal KM, Bernert JT, Brody DJ, Etzel RA, Maurer KR: Exposure of the US population to environmental tobacco smoke: the Third National Health and Nutrition Examination Survey, 1988 to 1991. JAMA 1996, 275:1233-40.

35. US Environmental Protection Agency: Respiratory health effects of passive smoking: lung cancer and other disorders. Washington, DC: US Environmental Protection Agency, Office of Health and Environmental Assessment, Office of Research and Development. EPA/600/6-90/006F. December 1992.

36. Centers for Disease Control and Prevention: Mortality trends for selected smoking-related and breast cancer—United States, 1950–1990. MMWR Morb Mortal Wkly Rep 1993, 42(44):857, 863–866.

37. Landis SH, Murray T, Bolden S, et al.: Cancer statistics. CA Cancer Clin 1999, 49:8–31.

38. Peto R, Darby S, Deo H, Silcocks P, Whitley E, Doll R: Smoking, smoking cessation, and lung cancer in the UK since 1950: combination of national statistics with two case-control studies. BMJ 2000:321–329.

39. Clinics in Chest Medicine: Smoking and Pulmonary and Cardiovascular Diseases, March 2000:52–54.

40. Shapiro SD: Evolving concepts in the pathogenesis of chronic obstructive pulmonary disease. In Clinics in Chest Medicine. Edited by Rochester CL. Philadelphia: WB Saunders; 2000:622, 629.

41. Anthonisen NR, Connett JE, Kiley JP, et al.: Effects of smoking intervention and the use of inhaled anti-cholinergic bronchodilator on the rate of decline in FEV_1: the lung health study. JAMA 1994, 272:1497–1505.

42. Snider GL, Faling LJ, Rennard SI: Chronic bronchitis and emphysema. In Textbook of Respiratory Medicine. Edited by Murray JF, Nadel JA. Philadelphia: WB Saunders; 1994:1342.

43. Enright PL, Crapo RO: Controversies in the use of spirometry for early recognition and diagnosis of chronic obstructive pulmonary disease in cigarette smokers. In Clinics in Chest Medicine. Edited by Rochester CL. Philadelphia: WB Saunders; 2000:649.

44. Centers for Disease Control and Prevention: www.cdc.gov/tobacco/SGR/SGR.2000/chap 4.pdf. Accessed February 8, 2001.

45. US Department of Health and Human Services: The Health Benefits of Smoking Cessation. A Report of the Surgeon General. Rockville, MD: US Government Printing Office, 1990.

46. Lancaster T, Stead L, Silagy C, Sowden A: Effectiveness of interventions to help people stop smoking: findings from the Cochrane Library. BMJ 2000, 321:355–358.

47. Surgeon General: http://www.surgeongeneral.gov/tobacco/smokesum.htm. Accessed February 8, 2001.

48. Fiore MC: Surgeon General's Report 2000:114.

49. Centers for Disease Control and Prevention: Response to increases in cigarette prices by race/ethnicity, income, and age groups—United States, 1976–1993. MMWR Morb Mortal Wkly Rep 1998:7/31.

50. Siegal M, Mowery PD, Pechacek TP, et al.: Trends in adult cigarette smoking in California compared with the rest of the United States, 1978–1994. Am J Public Health 2000, 90:372–379.

51. Biener L, Harris JE, Hamilton W: Impact of the Massachusetts tobacco control programme: population based trend analysis. BMJ 2000, 321:351–354.

52. Centers for Disease Control and Prevention: Decline in cigarette consumption following implementation of a comprehensive tobacco prevention and education program—Oregon, 1996–1998. MMWR Morb Mortal Wkly Rep 1999, 2/26.

ASTHMA

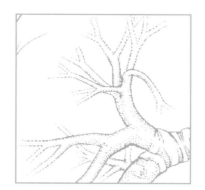
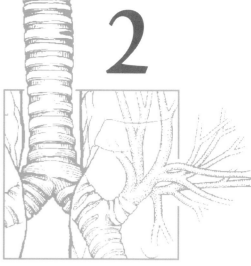

Jennifer A. Sewell &
D. Keith Payne

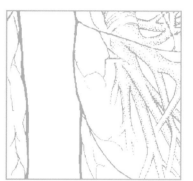

Asthma is a chronic inflammatory disease confined to the airways of the lung, resulting in episodic airflow obstruction, which is usually reversible (spontaneously or as a result of treatment), and in increased airway responsiveness to a variety of stimuli. An understanding of the disease is important for several reasons. Asthma is extremely common in many industrialized countries, with a prevalence of 3% to 7%. In the United States, about 5.5% of the population has asthma; that is, 14 to 15 million people [1]. For reasons that are not well understood, the prevalence and severity of asthma appear to be increasing in the United States and in many other countries. In the United States, between 1982 and 1992, the overall, annual, age-adjusted prevalence of self-reported asthma increased 42% [2]. From 1982 to 1991, the overall age-adjusted death rate from asthma increased 40%. These increased morbidity and mortality rates have been most striking among minority populations. Finally, the economic burdens inflicted on society by asthma are enormous. In the United States alone, annual asthma-related expenditures amount to more than $6.2 billion in direct and indirect costs [3].

Over the past 15 years, research efforts by various clinicians and scientists have resulted in a paradigmatic shift in the way we view asthma. Rather than perceiving asthma as a disease consisting primarily of bronchospasm with resultant airway obstruction, we understand it to be an airway disorder resulting from a complex inflammatory process involving many cells, cytokines, and other mediators. Therefore, optimal medical management of asthma has been changed from regimens that relied almost exclusively on bronchodilators for control of symptoms to protocols emphasizing the importance of the use of anti-inflammatory agents in all patients except those with the mildest case of asthma.

A more comprehensive strategy for the treatment of asthma has emerged, based on four critical components of therapy as outlined by the National Asthma Education Program. They include the use of 1) objective measures of lung function to assess the severity of asthma and to monitor the course of therapy, 2) pharmacologic therapy designed to reverse and prevent airway inflammation and to treat airway narrowing, 3) control measures to avoid or eliminate environmental trigger factors, and 4) patient education to encourage the development of a partnership between the patient, his or her family, and the clinician. The concept of step therapy for asthma has been introduced, by which asthma is classified as mild intermittent, mild persistent, moderate persistent, or severe persistent, based on the frequency and severity of symptoms. Pharmacologic therapy then proceeds in steps, beginning with β_2-agonists as needed and progressing to the addition of potent anti-inflammatory agents and other drugs.

Despite advances in our understanding of asthma, the pathophysiology of this disease remains poorly understood and is the subject of intense research efforts in clinics and laboratories around the world. New insights in this area will have a major impact on asthma therapy. Methods are needed to detect the early onset of chronic inflammation and to assess its resolution after appropriate therapy. Additional anti-inflammatory agents are required to prevent and control cellular infiltration and cytokine release at an early stage. Experimental drugs in development include adhesion molecule antagonists, cytokine antagonists, and anti-IgE monoclonal antibodies. New delivery systems will make use of the available medications easier for patients.

Although clinical and basic science research on asthma appears to hold promise for the future, we must maintain our perspective. Facilitating access to medical care and emphasizing well-designed patient education programs may be the most cost-effective ways to improve asthma outcomes.

EPIDEMIOLOGY AND IMPACT

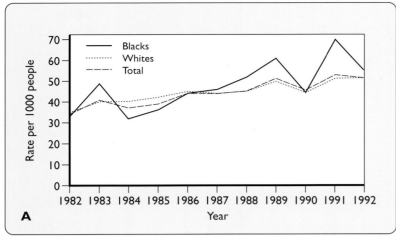

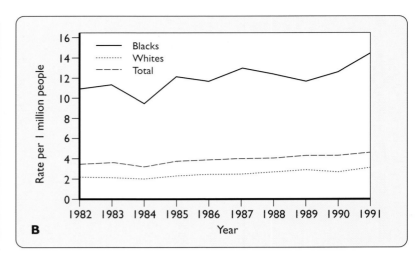

Figure 2-1.
A, Age-adjusted prevalence rate of self-reported asthma for persons aged 5 to 34 years, by race and year. During the period shown, the prevalence increased 52% from 34.6 per 1000 people to 52.6 per 1000 people. **B,** Age-adjusted death rate for asthma for persons aged 5 to 34 years, by race and year. In the period shown, the death rate increased 42% from 3.4 per million people to 4.9 per million people. Death rates were consistently higher for blacks than for whites. (*Adapted from* the Centers for Disease Control and Prevention [2].)

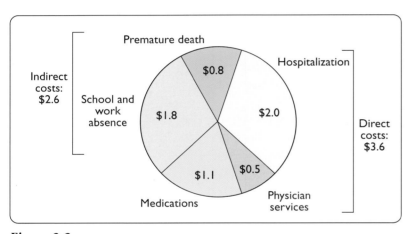

Figure 2-2.
Economic cost of asthma for 1 year in the United States. Figures (expressed in 1990 dollars) amount to $6.2 billion. Hospitalization costs represent the largest single direct medical expenditure. Reduced productivity at work and absence from school represent the largest indirect cost [3].

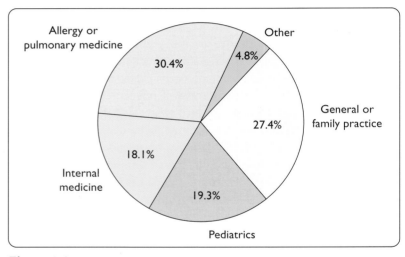

Figure 2-3.
Asthma-related visits to physicians' offices according to specialty. Two thirds of the asthma cases in the United States are treated by primary care physicians. To be successful, policies aimed at improving asthma care must recruit these health care providers [3].

PATHOPHYSIOLOGY

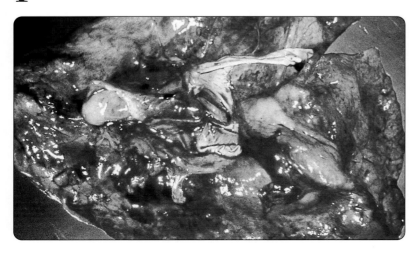

Figure 2-4.
Lung taken at autopsy from a patient who died of asthma. Note that the lung is still expanded because of the presence of trapped air. Extensive plugging of airways by mucus is evident throughout the specimen. (*See* Color Plate.) (*Courtesy of* Webb Waring Institute, Denver, CO.)

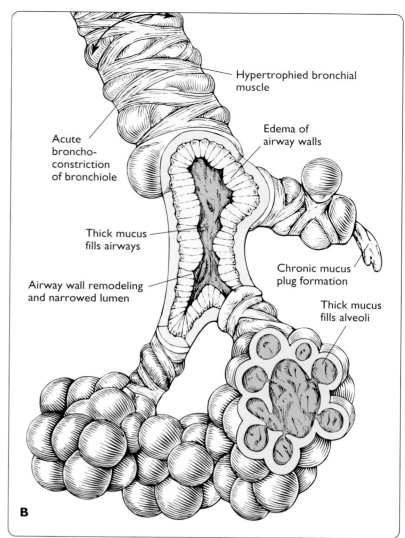

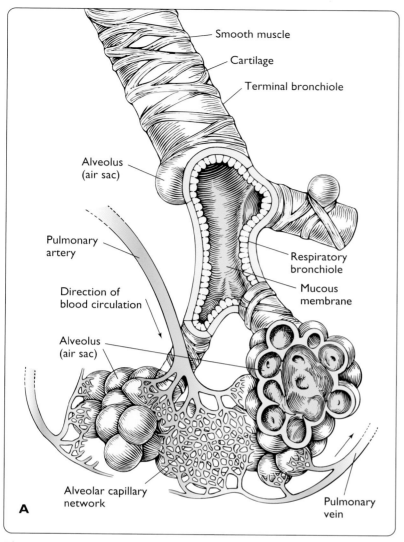

A, labels: Smooth muscle, Cartilage, Terminal bronchiole, Alveolus (air sac), Pulmonary artery, Direction of blood circulation, Alveolus (air sac), Alveolar capillary network, Respiratory bronchiole, Mucous membrane, Pulmonary vein

B, labels: Hypertrophied bronchial muscle, Acute broncho-constriction of bronchiole, Edema of airway walls, Thick mucus fills airways, Airway wall remodeling and narrowed lumen, Chronic mucus plug formation, Thick mucus fills alveoli

Figure 2-5.
A, Normal anatomy of lung near the terminal bronchiole demonstrating the efficiency with which normal gas exchange occurs. **B,** Same region during acute asthmatic episode, demonstrating airflow obstruction in asthma. Smooth muscle along airway walls is constricted and hypertrophied. Along with extensive plugging of the airways by mucus, airway walls are thickened and edematous as a result of inflammatory changes. Eventually, airway walls may be remodeled, leading to fixed obstruction in some patients. Unchecked airway inflammation resulting in such extensive pathologic changes may cause severe hypoxemia from ventilation-perfusion mismatches and even intrapulmonary shunting.

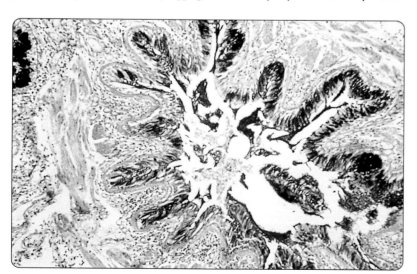

Figure 2-6.
Photomicrograph of patient who died of asthma, demonstrating extensive bronchial smooth muscle constriction with resultant airway narrowing. There is extensive sloughing of bronchial epithelium, along with mucous and inflammatory cells partially occluding the airway lumen. (See Color Plate.) (*From* Fanta [4]; with permission.)

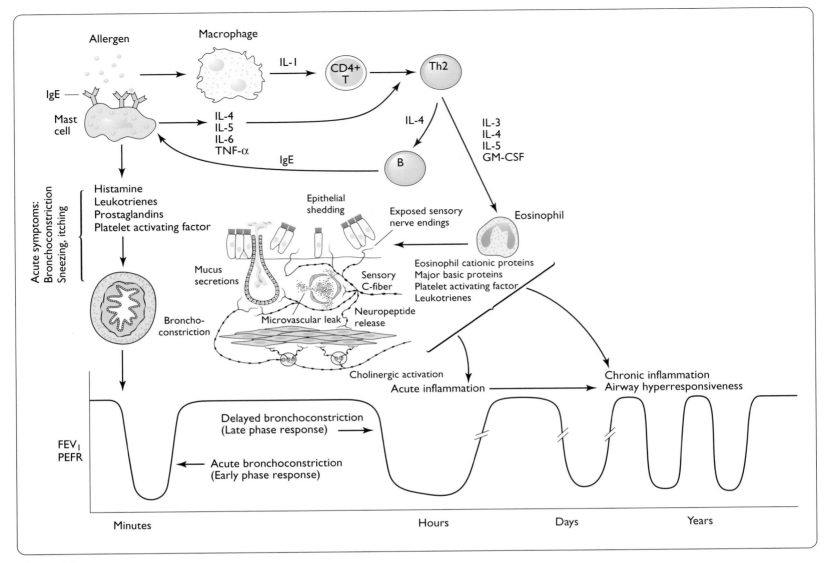

Figure 2-7.

Mechanisms of airway inflammation in asthma. Allergen exposure initiates a complex, self-amplifying interplay among cells, cytokines, and neurogenic components resulting in chronic, symptomatic inflammation with bronchial hyperresponsiveness. Mast cells in the bronchial lumen and epithelium and within the bronchial wall may become activated by allergen exposure, releasing a variety of mediators. These mediators initiate an acute phase reaction (within minutes), including bronchospasm, thus resulting in airflow obstruction. Quiescent CD4+ T-helper (Th2) lymphocytes may also become activated by cytokines secreted by allergen-stimulated cells such as macrophages, initiating a more chronic inflammatory process. Activated Th2 lymphocytes secrete various cytokines that attract other cells,

such as eosinophils, which in turn release potent epithelial-disrupting agents. Exposed epithelial sensory nerve endings may contribute to ongoing inflammation by releasing neuropeptides and by initiating reflex arcs involving cholinergic pathways. Th2-secreted interleukin-4 (IL-4) initiates B-lymphocyte IgE release, which in turn amplifies mast cell–mediated events. Some evidence exists that mast cells also produce cytokines, such as IL-4, which may be important in chronic inflammation [5–7]. FEV_1—forced expiratory volume in 1 second; GM-CSF—granulocyte-macrophage colony-stimulating factor; PEFR—peak expiratory flow rate; TNF—tumor necrosis factor. (*Adapted from* Barnes [7] and Freitag and Newhouse [8].)

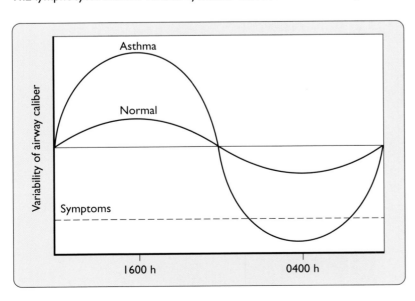

Figure 2-8.

Circadian rhythms in bronchomotor tone. The normal diurnal variability in airway caliber is exaggerated in many patients with asthma and may be important in the pathogenesis of nocturnal symptoms. Circadian variations in cholinergic tone, endogenous neurohormones (such as cortisol and epinephrine), and histamine may contribute. In addition, bronchoalveolar lavage in patients with asthma in the early morning hours has demonstrated increased numbers of inflammatory cells, including eosinophils and T lymphocytes [9,10]. (*Adapted from* Barnes [9].)

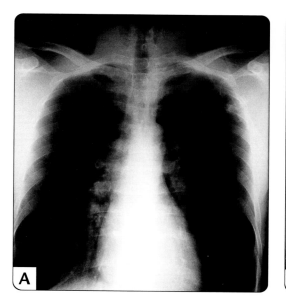 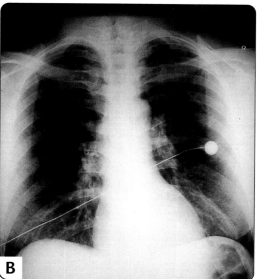

Figure 2-9.
A, Chest radiograph of patient during acute asthma episode. The lungs are hyperexpanded from trapped air with flattened diaphragms and black lung fields. **B,** Same patient after 24 hours of effective treatment. Note the overall decrease in lung size with return of normal lung markings and normal diaphragm shape.

DIAGNOSIS

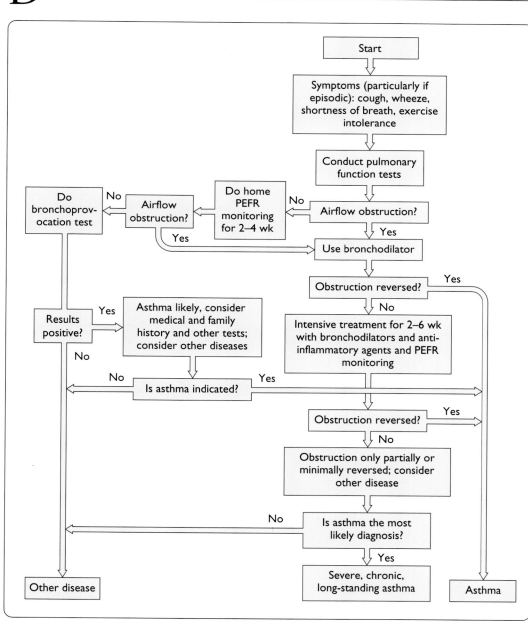

```
                          Start
                            │
                            ▼
              Symptoms (particularly if
              episodic): cough, wheeze,
             shortness of breath, exercise
                      intolerance
                            │
                            ▼
                  Contuct pulmonary
                   function tests
                            │
                            ▼
   Do           No    Do home                No
bronchoprov- ◄─── Airflow ◄─── PEFR     ◄─── Airflow obstruction?
 ocation test    obstruction?  monitoring
                    │          for 2–4 wk         │ Yes
                    │ Yes                         ▼
                    └──────────────────►  Use bronchodilator
                                                  │
                                                  ▼                    Yes
                                         Obstruction reversed? ──────────►
   Results    Yes   Asthma likely, consider       │ No
   positive? ────►  medical and family    Intensive treatment for 2–6 wk
                    history and other tests;  with bronchodilators and anti-
      │ No          consider other diseases  inflammatory agents and PEFR
                            │                      monitoring
              No            ▼              Yes        │
         ◄──────── Is asthma indicated? ──────        ▼
                                         Obstruction reversed? ──────► Yes
                                                  │ No
                                         Obstruction only partially or
                                         minimally reversed; consider
                                               other disease
                                                  │
                         No                       ▼
         ◄──────────────────────  Is asthma the most
                                   likely diagnosis?
                                                  │ Yes
                                                  ▼
   Other disease              Severe, chronic,           Asthma
                              long-standing asthma
```

Figure 2-10.
Algorithm for the diagnosis of asthma. This diagnosis may be relatively simple, or it may be complicated by other diseases. Symptomatic patients may be tested for the presence of reversible airway obstruction. If none is present on initial testing, repeated testing or the use of home peak flow meters may increase the likelihood of documenting an obstructive episode. In symptomatic patients with no obstruction, bronchoprovocation testing may be useful. In a few patients, long-standing airway inflammation may result in minimally reversible airflow obstruction. If compatible symptoms are present and no other explanation is likely, a diagnosis of asthma may be made. PEFR—peak expiratory flow rate. (*Adapted from* the National Asthma Education Program [11].)

DIFFERENTIAL DIAGNOSIS OF ASTHMA

Chronic bronchitis
Emphysema
Cystic fibrosis
Viral bronchiolitis
Bronchial stenosis
Mechanical airway obstruction
  Aspirated foreign body
  Endobronchial tumor
  Superior vena cava syndrome
  Substernal thyroid

Vocal cord dysfunction
Congestive heart failure
Pulmonary embolism
Eosinophilic pneumonia
Drug-induced cough
  β-Blockers
  Angiotensin-converting enzyme inhibitors
Systemic vasculitis
Carcinoid syndrome
Allergic bronchopulmonary aspergillosis

Figure 2-11.
The differential diagnosis of asthma in adults may include several of the more common pulmonary disorders, such as chronic bronchitis, cystic fibrosis, and congestive heart failure. Psychogenic vocal cord dysfunction mimicking exercise-induced asthma has been described [12].

THERAPY

GOALS OF ASTHMA THERAPY

Maintain (near) normal pulmonary function
Maintain normal activity levels
Prevent chronic and troublesome symptoms
Prevent recurrent exacerbations of asthma
Avoid adverse effects of asthma medications
Satisfy patient's and family's expectations for asthma care

Figure 2-12.
Goals of asthma therapy. Because asthma is a chronic disease with episodic exacerbations, the patient and physician must recognize the importance of adhering to general principles of therapy. The National Asthma Education Program Expert Panel Report II set forth six distinct goals for the effective, long-term treatment of asthma [13].

Measurement of Lung Function

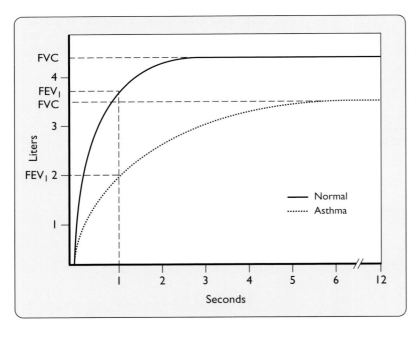

Figure 2-13.
Normal spirogram compared with spirogram obtained during asthma attack. Asthma exacerbations produce an obstructive pattern on spirometry with a ratio of forced expiratory volume in 1 second (FEV_1) to forced vital capacity (FVC) of less than 75%. Note that the FVC is also reduced because of air trapping, which decreases the volume of air that can be forcibly expelled. Also, expiration is delayed, as shown by the "tail" on the asthma FVC curve. The FEV_1 is a reproducible measurement and is useful for evaluating response to bronchodilation therapy.

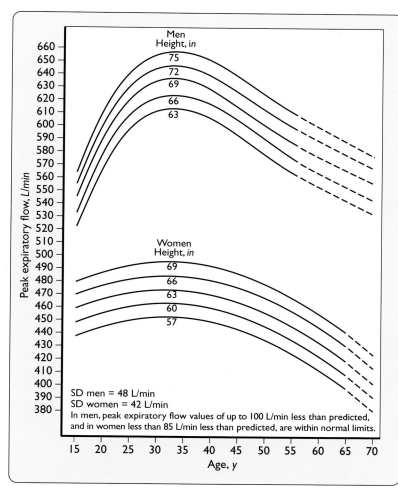

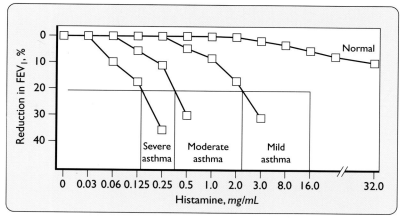

Figure 2-15.

Measurement of bronchial hyperreactivity to histamine challenge. Bronchoprovocation testing with histamine or methacholine may be helpful in the diagnosis of asthma if the history, physical examination, and standard pulmonary function testing are nondiagnostic [15–17]. For patients complaining of exercise-induced symptoms, testing may also be accomplished using exercise as a provocative stimulus. A 20% decrease in forced expiratory volume in 1 second (FEV_1) is the provocative concentration (PC), or PC 20, of histamine or methacholine. Patients with severe asthma tend to have a lower PC 20 than those with milder forms, although exceptions may be seen. Airway hyperresponsiveness may also be seen in other patients with conditions such as allergic rhinitis, cystic fibrosis, and chronic obstructive pulmonary disease, and in otherwise normal people after viral infections or oxidant exposure. (*Adapted from* Cockcroft *et al.* [15].)

Figure 2-14.

Peak expiratory flow rate nomogram. Peak flow meters provide a quick, accurate assessment of airflow in patients with asthma. Relatively inexpensive, they are useful in hospital, office, and home settings and should be used by all patients with moderate to severe persistent asthma. Peak flow rates are usually measured twice daily, at approximately the same time each day. The best of three separate efforts is recorded. As the nomogram indicates, substantial variability from predicted values may occur. Frequently, the establishment of a "personal best" value provides a useful guide for judging the severity of airflow obstruction during exacerbations and the effectiveness of therapy. (*Adapted from* Nunn and Gregg [14].)

Pharmacologic Therapy

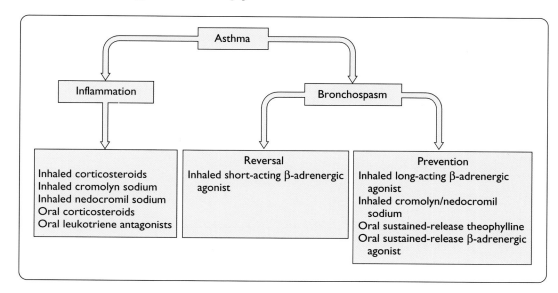

Figure 2-16.

Drug treatment for asthma. Overall pharmacologic therapy for asthma consists of drugs to control inflammation and bronchospasm. Drugs used to control bronchospasm may be subdivided into short-acting agents designed to reverse bronchospasm (rescue therapy) and agents designed to prevent bronchospasm. Anti-inflammatory agents such as cromolyn and nedocromil sodium may also be used to prevent exercise-induced bronchospasm. (*Adapted from* Kamada and Szefler [18].)

β-ADRENERGIC AGONISTS

Short-acting, short-duration
Epinephrine (Primatene Mist and others)
Isoetharine (Bronkosol)
Isoproterenol (Isuprel)

Short-acting, intermediate-duration
Metaproterenol (Alupent, Metaprel)
Terbutaline (Brethaire, Bricanyl)
Albuterol (Proventil, Ventolin)
Pirbuterol (Maxair)
Bitolterol (Tornalate)
Fenoterol*

Long-duration
Salmeterol (Serevent)
Formoterol*

Not available in the United States.

Figure 2-17.
β-Adrenergic agonists. These drugs interact with β_2 receptors in the lung, resulting in bronchodilation [19,20]. Popular over-the-counter inhalers containing epinephrine provide moderate but short-acting, short-duration relief and are β-nonspecific. Short-acting, intermediate-duration β-agonists are much more β_2-specific. They provide symptomatic relief for 3 to 6 hours and are rapidly effective (ie, less than 5 minutes), making them the drugs of choice for relief of acute asthma symptoms. They are best used on an as-needed basis. More frequent use may be an indication that additional anti-inflammatory medication is needed. Salmeterol is the only long-duration β-adrenergic agonist available in the United States. Its duration of action may be as long as 12 hours, although its onset of action is relatively slower compared with short-acting β-adrenergic drugs. It is a maintenance drug for use twice daily and should never be used as needed. It is probably best reserved for patients with moderate to severe asthma who are already receiving significant doses of anti-inflammatory medication. Its long duration of action may be particularly effective for nocturnal symptoms.

INHALED GLUCOCORTICOIDS

Steroid	Trade names	Binding affinity	Topical potency	Dose, μg/puff
Beclomethasone diproprionate	Beclovent, Vanceril	0.4	600	42
Triamcinolone acetonide	Azmacort	3.6	330	100
Flunisolide	Aerobid	1.8	330	250
Budesonide		9.4	980	200
Fluticasone proprionate	Flovent	18.0	1200	44, 110, 220

Figure 2-18.
Inhaled glucocorticoids. The term *binding affinity* refers to affinity for the glucocorticoid receptor [21,22]. The term *topical potency* refers to vasoconstrictive properties in human skin blanching systems. Although clinicians frequently equate beclomethasone dipropionate (BDP), triamcinolone, and flunisolide on a microgram-per-microgram basis, it is difficult to compare their clinical potency because of a paucity of relevant clinical data. Newer inhaled corticosteroids, such as fluticasone propionate and budesonide, are thought to be more potent, but clinical experience with these agents in the United States has been limited. Threshold doses for significant adverse effects (eg, bone loss, immunosuppression, adrenal suppression) are unknown. Effects such as these appear to be rare with BDP equivalent doses of up to 800 μg/day in adults and up to 400 μg/day in children.

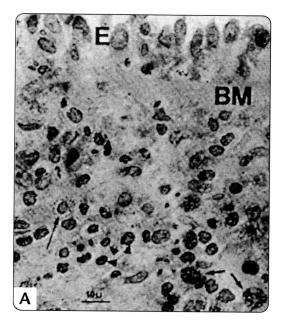
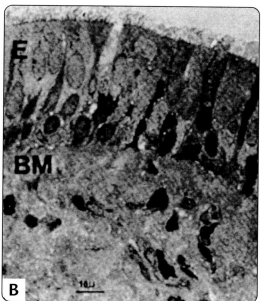

Figure 2-19.

A and **B,** Electron microscopic views of a bronchial biopsy of airway wall in a patient with asthma before *(panel A)* and after *(panel B)* 3 months of therapy with an inhaled corticosteroid [22]. Airway epithelium (E) is disrupted in *panel A* with infiltration of inflammatory cells *(arrows)* below basement membrane (BM). *Panel B* shows marked improvement in inflammatory infiltrate with re-establishment of the airway epithelium. In this 3-month study, AM and PM peak flow rates improved more significantly in patients treated with inhaled corticosteroids alone than in patients treated with β_2-agonists alone. (*From* Laitinen *et al.* [23]; with permission.)

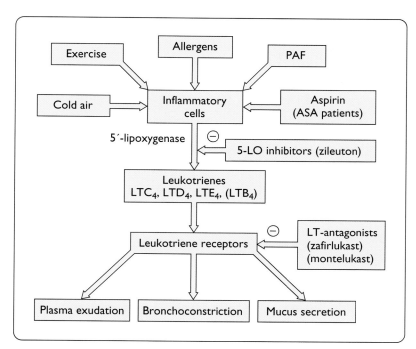

Figure 2-20.

Effects of leukotriene inhibitors. Leukotrienes produced by activated airway eosinophils and mast cells may produce marked airway inflammation. Available antileukotriene drugs work by two different mechanisms. Zileuton decreases the formation of leukotrienes by inhibiting the action of 5-lipoxygenase. Zafirlukast and montelukast inhibit the action of LTD_4 at the receptor site. In many patients with asthma, these agents may increase forced expiratory volume in 1 second (FEV_1) by 10% to 15%, and decrease asthmatic symptoms and the need for rescue beta-2 agonists [24,25]. These drugs may be particularly effective for patients with aspirin-sensitive asthma and in patients with exercise-induced asthma [7]. Leukotriene inhibitors are recommended as an effective alternative to inhaled steroids in patients with mild persistent asthma (*see* Fig. 2-21). The use of these drugs in moderate to severe asthma is being studied. There is some evidence that they may be effective as adjuvant therapy in selected patients already being treated with higher doses of inhaled steroids [26,27].

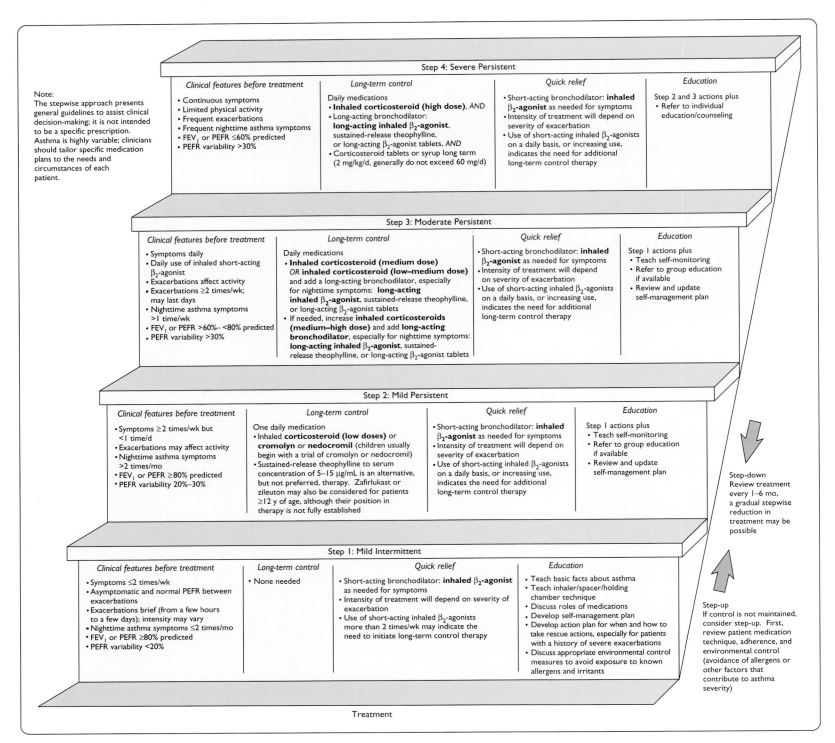

Figure 2-21.

Stepwise approach for managing asthma in adults and children older than 5 years of age. The presence of one of the features of severity is sufficient to place a patient in that category. An individual should be assigned to the most severe grade in which any feature occurs. The characteristics noted in this figure are general and may overlap because asthma is highly variable; further-more, an individual's classification may change over time. Patients at any level of severity can have mild, moderate, or severe exacerbations. Some patients with intermittent asthma experience severe and life-threatening exacerbations separated by long periods of normal lung function and no symptoms. The physician should gain control as quickly as possible, then decrease treatment to the least medication necessary to maintain control. Gaining control may be accomplished by either starting treatment at the step most appropriate to the initial severity of the condition or starting at a higher level of therapy. A rescue course of systemic corticosteroids may be needed at any time and at any step. At each step, patients should control their environment to avoid or control factors that make their asthma worse (*eg*, allergens, irritants); this requires specific diagnosis and education. Referral to an asthma specialist for consultation or comanagement is recommended if there are difficulties achieving or maintaining control of asthma or if the patient requires step 4 care. Referral may be considered if the patient requires step 3 care. Preferred treatments are in bold print. FEV$_1$—forced expiratory volume in 1 second; PEFR—peak expiratory flow rate. (*Adapted from* the National Heart, Lung, and Blood Institute [13].)

Patient Education

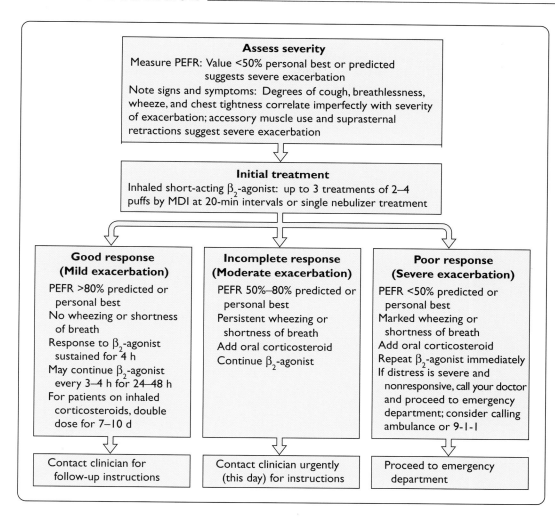

Assess severity

Measure PEFR: Value <50% personal best or predicted suggests severe exacerbation

Note signs and symptoms: Degrees of cough, breathlessness, wheeze, and chest tightness correlate imperfectly with severity of exacerbation; accessory muscle use and suprasternal retractions suggest severe exacerbation

Initial treatment

Inhaled short-acting β_2-agonist: up to 3 treatments of 2–4 puffs by MDI at 20-min intervals or single nebulizer treatment

Good response (Mild exacerbation)

PEFR >80% predicted or personal best
No wheezing or shortness of breath
Response to β_2-agonist sustained for 4 h
May continue β_2-agonist every 3–4 h for 24–48 h
For patients on inhaled corticosteroids, double dose for 7–10 d

Contact clinician for follow-up instructions

Incomplete response (Moderate exacerbation)

PEFR 50%–80% predicted or personal best
Persistent wheezing or shortness of breath
Add oral corticosteroid
Continue β_2-agonist

Contact clinician urgently (this day) for instructions

Poor response (Severe exacerbation)

PEFR <50% predicted or personal best
Marked wheezing or shortness of breath
Add oral corticosteroid
Repeat β_2-agonist immediately
If distress is severe and nonresponsive, call your doctor and proceed to emergency department; consider calling ambulance or 9-1-1

Proceed to emergency department

Figure 2-22.
Home management of asthma exacerbations based on symptoms and peak expiratory flow rate (PEFR). Therapy of asthma exacerbations should begin at home. This home treatment avoids needless delays, prevents exacerbations from becoming severe, and involves the patient directly in the treatment process. This generalized home management plan may need to be tailored for specific patients based on the patient's abilities, prior pattern of asthma exacerbations, and accessibility of emergency care. MDI—metered-dose inhaler. (*Adapted from* the National Heart, Lung, and Blood Institute [13].)

Special Considerations in Asthma Management

COMMON AGENTS THAT MAY CAUSE OCCUPATIONAL ASTHMA

Agent	Workers at risk
High-molecular weight agents	
Cereals	Bakers, millers
Animal-derived allergens	Animal handlers
Enzymes	Detergent users, pharmaceutical workers, bakers
Gums	Carpet makers, pharmaceutical workers
Latex	Health professionals
Seafoods	Seafood processors
Low-molecular weight agents	
Isocyanates	Spray painters; insulation installers; manufacturers of plastics, rubbers, foam
Wood dusts	Forest workers, carpenters, cabinetmakers
Anhydrides	Users of plastics, epoxy resins
Amines	Shellac and lacquer handlers, solderers
Fluxes	Electronics workers
Chloramine-T	Janitors, cleaners
Dyes	Textile workers
Persulfate	Hairdressers
Formaldehyde, glutaraldehyde	Hospital staff
Acrylate	Adhesives handlers
Metals	Solderers, refiners
Drugs	Pharmaceutical workers, health care professionals

Figure 2-23.
Common agents that may cause occupational asthma. It is estimated that up to 15% of newly diagnosed cases of asthma may be caused by occupational exposures [28]. Because about 250 agents are known to cause occupational asthma, details of current and past employment should be obtained in the evaluation of patients with asthma. High-molecular weight agents are frequently associated with IgE antibodies, whereas many low–molecular weight agents are not. Removal from exposure is essential in the therapy of these patients. (*Adapted from* Chan-Yeung and Malo [28].)

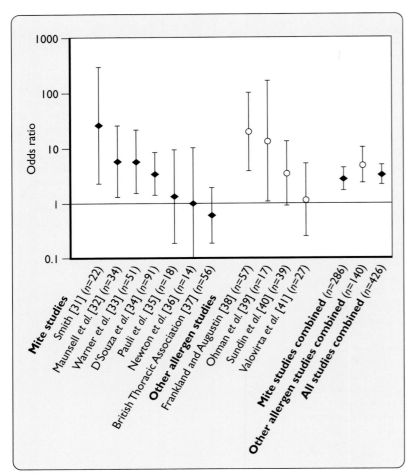

Figure 2-24.
Studies of effectiveness of immunotherapy with mites and other allergens. Immunotherapy for asthma remains controversial with conflicting reports from studies concerning its effectiveness [29]. A recently published meta-analysis demonstrates the odds ratios and 95% CI for improvement in asthma symptoms after allergen immunotherapy [30]. In this meta-analysis, an improvement in asthma symptoms was demonstrated for mites and other allergens, although CIs for several individual studies were large. Allergen immunotherapy is probably best used in a minority of younger patients with mild to moderate seasonal asthma who are unable to avoid known allergen triggers when appropriate medications fail to control symptoms adequately. Immunotherapy for asthma should not be used when forced expiratory volume in 1 second (FEV_1) is less than 70% of predicted value, because the risk of serious adverse reactions may be increased during asthma exacerbations. If symptoms improve, treatment is usually continued for 3 to 5 years. If symptoms do not improve after maintenance levels have been achieved for two allergy seasons, immunotherapy should be discontinued. (*Adapted from* Abramson *et al.* [30].)

Future Therapies

FUTURE DIRECTIONS OF ASTHMA THERAPY

Understanding pathogenesis
    Role of inflammatory cells and mediators
    Environmental vs hereditary factors
    Genetic control of inflammatory mediators
Detecting airway inflammation
Improving drugs and delivery systems
    New formulations of drugs
    Easier-to-use delivery devices
    New anti-inflammatory agents
Enhancing patient educational efforts

Figure 2-25.
Future directions of asthma therapy. Major advances in our understanding of the pathogenesis of asthma and the true nature of airway inflammation will lead to better therapies. Improved drug delivery systems and automated monitoring devices to record the date and time of medication and peak flow meter use may improve patient compliance. Widespread, culturally sensitive asthma education programs and improved access to health care in general may also be useful in improving asthma outcomes.

REFERENCES

1. Adams PF, Marano MA: Current estimates from the National Health Interview Survey, 1994. *Vital Health Stat* 1995, 10:94.

2. Centers for Disease Control and Prevention: Asthma—United States, 1982–1992. *MMWR* 1995, 43:952–955.

3. Weiss KB, Gergen PJ, Hodgson TA: An economic evaluation of asthma in the United States. *N Engl J Med* 1992, 326:862–866.

4. Fanta C: *Current Views in Allergy and Immunology.* Augusta, GA: Medical College of Georgia; 1985.

5. Shelhamer JH, Levine SJ, Wu T, *et al.*: Airway inflammation. *Ann Intern Med* 1995, 123:288–304.

6. Horwitz RJ, Busse, WW: Inflammation and asthma. In *Clinics in Chest Medicine.* Edited by Martin RJ. Philadelphia: WB Saunders; 1995: 583–602.

7. Barnes PJ: Inflammatory mediators and neural mechanisms in severe asthma. In *Severe Asthma: Pathogenesis and Clinical Management.* Edited by Szefler SJ, Leung DYM. New York: Marcel Dekker; 1996:129–163.

8. Freitag A, Newhouse MT: Management of asthma in the 1990s. *Curr Pulmonol* 1994, 15:19–74.

9. Barnes PJ: Circadian variation in airway function. *Am J Med* 1980, 79:5–9.

10. Pincus DJ, Beam WR, Martin RJ: Chronobiology and chronotherapy of asthma. In *Clinics in Chest Medicine.* Edited by Martin RJ. Philadelphia: WB Saunders; 1995: 699–713.

11. National Asthma Education Program: *Guidelines for the Diagnosis and Management of Asthma: Expert Panel Report.* Bethesda, MD: National Heart, Lung, and Blood Institute; 1991. [DHHS publication no. (PHS) 91-3042A.]

12. McFadden ER, Zawadski DK: Vocal cord dysfunction masquerading as exercise-induced asthma. *Am J Respir Crit Care Med* 1996, 153:942–947.

13. National Heart, Lung, and Blood Institute: *Expert Panel Report II: Guidelines for the Diagnosis and Management of Asthma.* Bethesda, MD: National Institutes of Health; 1997. [NIH publication no. 97-4051.]

14. Nunn AJ, Gregg I: New regression equations for predicting peak expiratory flow in adults. *Br Med J* 1989, 298:1068–1070.

15. Cockcroft DW, Killian DN, Mellon JJA, *et al.*: Bronchial reactivity to inhaled histamine: a method and clinical survey. *Clin Allergy* 1977, 7:235–243.

16. Chatham M, Bleecker E, Smith PL, *et al.*: A comparison of histamine, methacholine, and exercise airway reactivity in normal and asthmatic subjects. *Am Rev Respir Dis* 1982, 126:235–240.

17. Chatham M, Bleecker ER, Norman P, *et al.*: A screening test for airways reactivity: an abbreviated methacholine inhalation challenge. *Chest* 1982, 82:15–18.

18. Kamada AK, Szefler SJ: Pharmacological management of severe asthma. In *Severe Asthma: Pathogenesis and Clinical Management.* Edited by Szefler SJ, Leung DYM. New York: Marcel Dekker; 1996:165–205.

19. Busse WW: Long- and short-acting β_2-adrenergic agonists. *Arch Intern Med* 1996, 156:1514–1520.

20. Nelson HS: β-Adrenergic bronchodilators. *N Engl J Med* 1995, 333:499–506.

21. Kamada AK, Szefler SJ, Martin RJ, *et al.*: Pulmonary perspective: issues in the use of inhaled glucocorticoids. *Am J Respir Crit Care Med* 1996, 153:1739–1748.

22. Barnes PJ: Inhaled glucocorticoids for asthma. *N Engl J Med* 1995, 332:868–874.

23. Laitinen LA, Laitinen A, Haahtela T: A comparative study of the effects of an inhaled corticosteroid, budesonide, and a β_2-agonist, terbutaline, on airway inflammation in newly diagnosed asthma: a randomized, double-blind, parallel-group controlled trial. *J Allergy Clin Immunol* 1992, 90:32–42.

24. Reiss TF, Chervinsky P, Dockhorn RJ, Shingo S, Seidenberg B, Edwards TB: Montelukast, a once-daily leukotriene receptor antagonist, in the treatment of chronic asthma: a multi-center, randomized, double-blind trial. Montelukast Clinical Research Study Group. *Arch Intern Med* 1998, 158:1213–1220.

25. Israel E, Rubin P, Kemp JP, *et al.*: The effect of inhibition of 5-lipoxygenase by zileuton in mild-to-moderate asthma. *Ann Intern Med* 1993, 119:1059–1066.

26. Lofdahl CG, Reiss TF, Leff JA, *et al.*: Randomised, placebo controlled trial of effect of a leukotriene receptor antagonist, montelukast, on tapering inhaled corticosteroids in asthmatic patients. *BMJ* 1999, 319:87–90.

27. Laviolette M, Malmstrom K, Lu S, *et al.*: Montelukast added to inhaled beclomethasone in treatment of asthma. Montelukast/Beclomethasone Additivity Group. *Am J Respir Crit Care Med* 1999, 160:1862–1868.

28. Chan-Yeung M, Malo J: Occupational asthma. *N Engl J Med* 1995, 333:107–112.

29. Creticos PS, Reed CE, Norman PS, *et al.*: Ragweed immunotherapy in adult asthma. *N Engl J Med* 1996, 334:501–506.

30. Abramson MJ, Puy RM, Weiner JM: Is allergen immunotherapy effective in asthma? *Am J Respir Crit Care Med* 1995, 151:969–974.

31. Smith AP: Hyposensitisation with *Dermatophagoides pteronyssinus* antigen trial in asthma induced by house dust. *Br Med J* 1971, 4:204–206.

32. Maunsell K, Wraith DG, Hughes AM: Hyposensitisation in mite asthma. *Lancet* 1971, 1:967–968.

33. Warner JO, Price JF, Soothill JF, *et al.*: Controlled trial of hyposensitisation to *Dermatophagoides pteronyssinus* in children with asthma. *Lancet* 1978, 2:912–915.

34. D'Souza MF, Pepys J, Wells ID, *et al.*: Hyposensitisation with *Dermatophagoides pteronyssinus* in house dust allergy: a controlled study of clinical and immunological effects. *Clin Allergy* 1973, 3:177–193.

35. Pauli G, Bessot JC, Bigot H, *et al.*: Clinical and immunologic evaluation of tyrosine adsorbed *Dermatophagoides pteronyssinus* extract: a double-blind placebo-controlled trial. *J Allergy Clin Immunol* 1984, 74:524–535.

36. Newton DAG, Maberly DJ, Wilson R: House dust mite hyposensitisation. *Br J Dis Chest* 1978, 72:21–28.

37. British Thoracic Association: A trial of house dust mite extract in bronchial asthma. *Br J Dis Chest* 1979, 73:260–270.

38. Frankland AW, Augustin R: Prophylaxis of summer hayfever and asthma. *Lancet* 1954, 1:1055–1057.

39. Ohman JL, Findlay SR, Leitermann KM: Immunotherapy in cat-induced asthma: double-blind trial with evaluation of in vivo and in vitro responses. *J Allergy Clin Immunol* 1984, 74:230–239.

40. Sundin B, Lilja G, Graff-Lonnevig V, *et al.*: Immunotherapy with partially purified and standardised animal dander extracts: I. Clinical results from a double-blind study on patients with animal dander asthma. *J Allergy Clin Immunol* 1986, 77:478–487.

41. Valovirta E, Koivikko A, Vanto T, *et al.*: Immunotherapy in allergy to dog: a double-blind clinical study. *Ann Allergy* 1984, 53:85–88.

CHRONIC OBSTRUCTIVE PULMONARY DISEASE

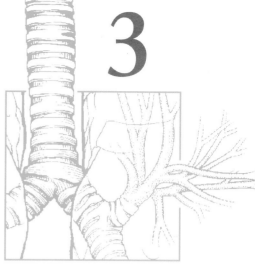

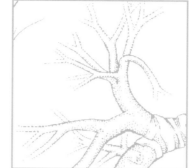

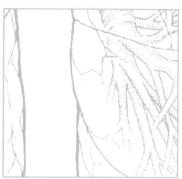

3

Michael W. Owens &
G. Douglas Campbell, Jr

Chronic obstructive pulmonary disease (COPD) is defined by the American Thoracic Society (ATS) as a disorder characterized by abnormal forced expiratory air flow, of a structural or functional nature, that does not change markedly over several months. Clinicians use the term *COPD* to describe a group of clinical and pathologic findings that often produces disability of a chronic and unremitting nature and sometimes results in death. The diagnosis is usually based on the presence of chronic bronchitis associated with varying degrees of emphysema, with or without bronchospasm.

More than 14 million Americans are afflicted with COPD [1]. Although chronic bronchitis is the most common component, most patients with COPD also have emphysematous involvement and may have episodes of bronchospasm. The incidence of chronic bronchitis has risen dramatically over the past 30 years, whereas emphysema appears to be increasing slightly in prevalence [1]. COPD and related conditions (*eg*, asthma, bronchiectasis, hypersensitivity pneumonitis) rank as the fourth most frequent cause of death in the United States. In 1997, COPD accounted for 4.5% of all deaths (a total of 110,600), with an age-adjusted mortality rate of 21.4 per 100,000 people [2]. Of even greater significance is the chronic, progressive nature of the disease, which may result in severe, prolonged disability. As a consequence of the severe morbidity and mortality rate of COPD, its treatment and prevention has become an increasingly important public health issue.

It is useful to address the three major components of the disease—chronic bronchitis, emphysema, and bronchospasm—because their manifestations, treatment requirements, and prognoses differ somewhat. The ATS defines chronic bronchitis as the persistence of cough and excessive mucus secretion on most days over a 3-month period for at least 2 successive years. The closest pathologic correlate to this syndrome is mucous gland hypertrophy, based on the "Reid Index," which is the ratio of the width of the mucous glands to the thickness of the bronchial walls. Most patients with chronic bronchitis do not have airflow obstruction; however, about 10% to 15% of smokers develop an abnormally rapid decline in airflow with aging, resulting in COPD [3]. Patients who do not develop airflow obstruction have simple chronic bronchitis; those who have a progressive decline in airflow have chronic obstructive bronchitis, and constitute the majority of patients with COPD [3].

Emphysema is pathologic, rather than clinical, and can be diagnosed in vivo based on its clinical characteristics. The ATS defines emphysema as permanent enlargement of air spaces distal to the terminal bronchiole and destruction of the alveolar wall, in the absence of fibrosis. The classic subtype of emphysema associated with cigarette smoking is centrilobular emphysema, which involves destruction of the central portions of the acinus and affects primarily the apices and periphery of the lungs. Marked hyperinflation and airflow obstruction are characteristics of patients with advanced emphysema. They have abnormal values for diffusing capacity of the lung for carbon monoxide ($D_{L}CO$), exhibit fixed obstruction, and respond poorly to bronchodilator therapy.

Although marked variability of airflow obstruction is a characteristic of asthma rather than COPD, some patients with typical signs of chronic bronchitis (about 10% in one study) have significant changes in airflow after bronchodilator administration, comparable to those seen in patients with asthma [4]. This reversible component of COPD represents the "opposite" of emphysema (*ie*, reversible versus fixed obstruction) and has been labeled asthmatic bronchitis. In contrast to patients with emphysema, those with asthmatic bronchitis have little alteration of $D_{L}CO$, exhibit wheezing on physical examination and eosinophils in the blood and sputum, and may have a family history of atopy. These patients appear to respond well to long-term therapy with bronchodilators and corticosteroids [5].

CHARACTERISTICS OF EMPHYSEMA AND CHRONIC BRONCHITIS

CLINICAL CHARACTERISTICS OF EMPHYSEMA AND CHRONIC BRONCHITIS

Feature	"Pink puffer" (emphysematous)	"Blue bloater" (bronchitic)
Onset	Age 40–50 y	Age 30–40 y; disability in middle age
Etiology	Smoking; genetic predisposition; unknown factors; air pollution	Smoking; unknown factors; air pollution
Sputum	Minimal	Copious
Dyspnea	Relatively early onset	Relatively late onset
$\dot{V}/\dot{Q}$ ratio	Minimal imbalance	Marked imbalance
Anteroposterior diameter of chest	"Barrel chest" common	Not increased
Pathologic lung anatomy	Centrilobular emphysema	Mucus gland hypertrophy
Pulmonary function tests	Low FEV_1, marked increase in total lung capacity and residual volume, low D_{LCO}	Low FEV_1; moderate increase in residual volume, normal D_{LCO}
Pa_{CO_2}	Normal or low	Elevated
Sa_{O_2}	Normal	Decreased
Hematocrit	Normal	Elevated
Cyanosis	Rare	Common
Cor pulmonale	Rare, except terminally	Frequent

D_{LCO}—*diffusing capacity of lung for carbon monoxide;* FEV_1—*forced expiratory volume in 1 s;* $\dot{V}/\dot{Q}$—*ventilation-perfusion.*

Figure 3-1.

Characteristics of emphysema and chronic bronchitis. Differences between the clinical findings in emphysema and chronic obstructive bronchitis were first recognized many years ago by clinicians who noted that some patients with chronic obstructive pulmonary disease (COPD) were "pink puffers" (emphysematous), whereas others were "blue bloaters" (chronic bronchitic). These represent the extremes of a wide clinical spectrum. Most patients with COPD fall somewhere between these two extremes and demonstrate some characteristics of both. Although emphysema and chronic bronchitis are characterized by an imbalance between ventilation and perfusion, chronic bronchitis results in more shunting of arterial blood through unventilated alveoli and therefore results in more severe hypoxemia and cor pulmonale. However, emphysema is associated with more air-trapping, hyperinflation, and dyspnea than would be expected for a given degree of hypoxemia. (*Adapted from* Owens [6].)

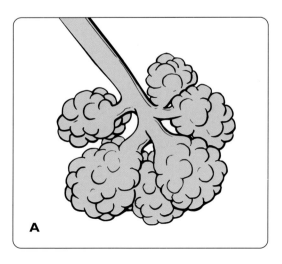

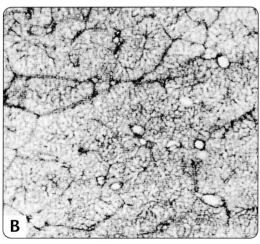

Figure 3-2.

Diagrams and macrosections showing normal lung, centrolobular emphysema, and panlobular emphysema. **A** and **B**, Normal secondary lobule, *ie,* the area supplied by a terminal bronchiole (approximately 0.5 cm in diameter). *Panel A* shows the terminal bronchiole, respiratory bronchioles, and respiratory cavities. In *panel B,* the secondary lobule is bounded by thin septa.

(*Continued on next page*)

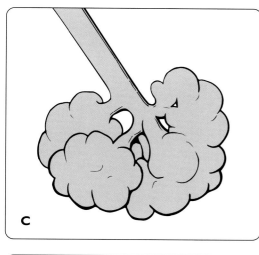

C

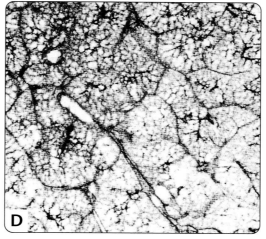

D

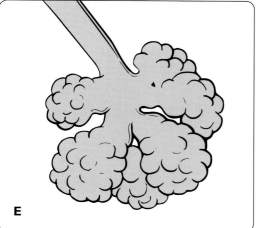

E

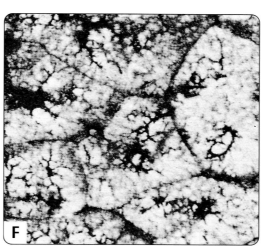

F

Figure 3-2. (*Continued*)
C and **D**, Findings in panlobular emphysema, which affects the entire secondary lobule. This type of emphysema is associated with α_1 antitrypsin deficiency. In *panel C*, the bronchioles are normal, but respiratory cavities are enlarged and confluent. The process appears uniform through the lobule in *panel D*. **E** and **F**, Findings in centrilobular emphysema, the most common type, which is associated with cigarette smoking. The respiratory bronchioles are dilated in *panel E*. Destruction is central in *panel D* and tends to coincide with pigment deposits. (*From* Morris *et al.* [7]; with permission.)

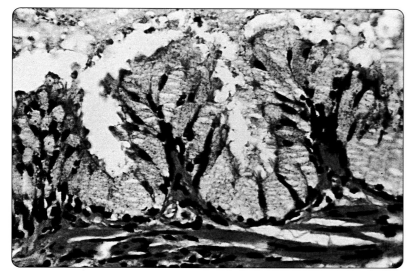

Figure 3-3.
Goblet cell hyperplasia in a patient with chronic bronchitis. Mucus hypersecretion is a major cause of airflow limitation in patients with chronic obstructive pulmonary disease. (*See* Color Plate.)

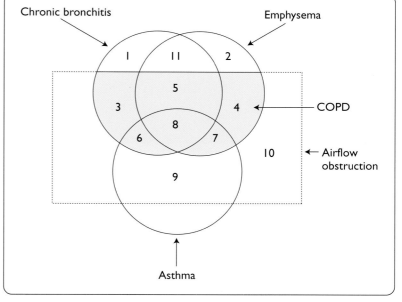

Figure 3-4.
Nonproportional Venn diagram showing subsets of patients with bronchitis, emphysema, asthma, and combinations of these components of chronic obstructive pulmonary disease (COPD). The subsets comprising COPD are *shaded*. Patients with reversible asthma (subset 9) do not have COPD, whereas patients with emphysema and/or bronchitis (subsets 6, 7, and 8) are considered to have "asthmatic bronchitis." Most patients with COPD have chronic bronchitis and emphysema (subset 5). (*Adapted from* Celli *et al.* [8].)

RISK FACTORS FOR CHRONIC OBSTRUCTIVE PULMONARY DISEASE

Environmental factors
   Cigarette smoking
   Passive smoking
   Ambient air pollution
   Occupational factors
   Recurrent infections
     "The British hypothesis"
   Socioeconomic status
Genetic factors
   Hyperresponsive airways
     "The Dutch hypothesis"
   Familial factors
     α_1 Antitrypsin deficiency
     Other (familial)
   Gender
   Race

Figure 3-5.

Risk factors for chronic obstructive pulmonary disease (COPD). Risk factors may be divided into environmental irritants or genetic predisposing factors. Among the environmental irritants, by far the most important is cigarette smoking (active and passive). More than 85% of COPD cases are related to cigarette smoking. Other factors that have been associated with the development of COPD include ambient air pollution and occupational exposure. Recurrent respiratory infections usually result in a temporary decrease in airflow rate; however, the "British hypothesis" proposes that chronic airway inflammation may, over time, result in permanent airflow obstruction. Lower socioeconomic status has been associated with an increased incidence of airway obstruction, possibly due to increased exposure to pollutants or to more common airway infections. Among the inherited factors associated with an increase in COPD incidence is a deficiency in protease inhibitors. The lack of α_1 protease inhibitors permits the destruction of alveolar walls by proteolytic enzymes released into lung tissue. The "Dutch hypothesis" proposes that there is a gradual spectrum of obstructive airway diseases, which includes hyperresponsive airways. The presence of eosinophils in sputum, bronchial hyperreactivity, and wheezing have been related to a rapid decline in forced expiratory volume in 1 second in some studies. Other genetic factors that may be associated with emphysema include male gender and Caucasian race. In some families, the increased incidence of COPD is idiopathic.

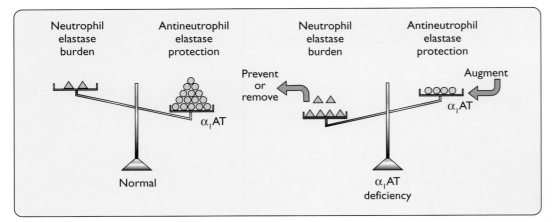

Figure 3-6.

α_1 Antitrypsin deficiency (α_1AT). Normal subjects have a mild but chronic burden of elastase in the lower respiratory tract, which is balanced by an excess of α_1AT, which protects the alveoli. Lung destruction in α_1AT deficiency results from an increase in the elastase burden in the presence of a marked reduction in α_1AT levels. (*Adapted from* Hubbard and Crystal [9].)

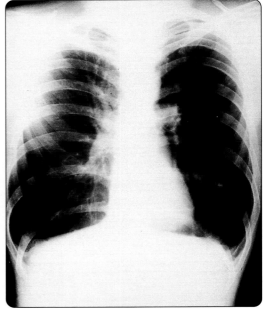

Figure 3-7.

Chest radiograph of a patient with α_1 antitrypsin deficiency. Note evidence of bilateral hyperinflation and the presence of bullous disease, especially in the bases of the lungs.

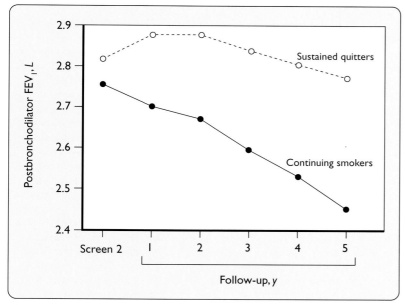

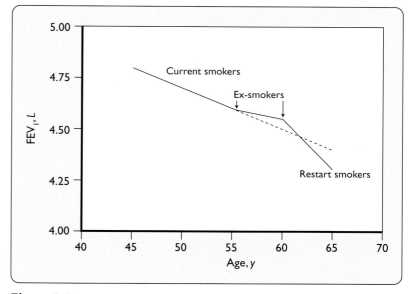

Figure 3-8.
Mean forced expiratory volume in 1 second (FEV_1) over a 5-year period in sustained quitters and continuing cigarette smokers in the Lung Health Study. The two curves diverge sharply from the start. Smoking cessation is the only intervention that has been shown to have a beneficial effect on the rate of FEV_1 decline. (*Adapted from* Anthonisen *et al.* [10].)

Figure 3-9.
Effect of smoking resumption on the forced expiratory volume in 1 second (FEV_1). The figure represents expected changes in FEV_1 in male smokers who quit smoking at age 55 years, then resumed smoking at age 60. The resumption of cigarette smoking after 5 years of cessation resulted in a greater than expected rate of decline in FEV_1. (*Adapted from* Sherill *et al.* [11].)

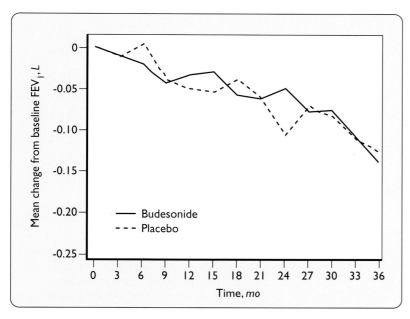

Figure 3-10.
The crude rates of decline in the forced expiratory volume in 1 second (FEV_1) in patients with chronic obstructive pulmonary disease (COPD) who received placebo or budesonide for 36 months (800 μg in the morning plus 400 μg in the evening for 6 months and then 400 μg twice daily for 30 months). All patients had a FEV_1, that showed no response (<15% change) to 1 mg terbutaline or prednisolone 37.5 mg orally once daily for 10 days. The estimated rates of decline did not differ significantly between the two groups (placebo group 49.1 mL/year, budesonide group 45.1 mL/year; $P = 0.7$). Inhaled budesonide also had no effect on respiratory symptoms. This long-term single-center study was unable to demonstrate an effect of budesonide on the rate of decline in lung function in patients with irreversible COPD [12].

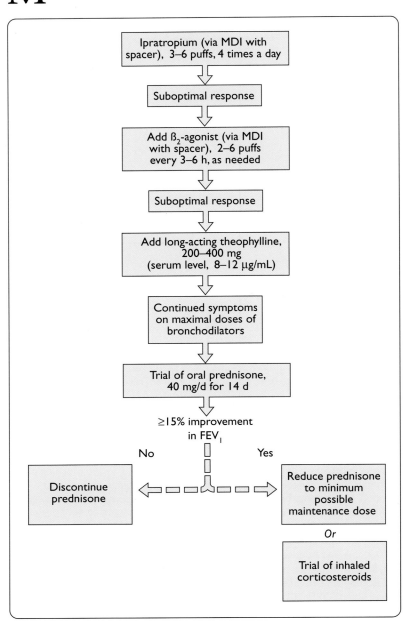

Figure 3-11.

Proposed algorithm for the pharmacologic management of stable chronic obstructive pulmonary disease. Inhaled ipratropium bromide is recommended as first-line bronchodilator therapy because of its relatively long duration of action and lack of side effects. The package insert recommends a dose of two puffs four times daily via metered-dose inhaler (MDI); however, some experts recommend much higher doses, up to a total dosage of 24 puffs per day. If patients complain of bouts of dyspnea during ipratropium therapy, an inhaled β_2-agonist should be added at 3- to 6-hour intervals as needed. The as-needed administration of a β-agonist decreases the likelihood of tolerance, and the number of puffs required may be used as a measure of symptoms. If patients are still symptomatic, long-acting oral theophylline may be administered at bedtime, with dosage adjusted to maintain a peak serum level of 8 to 12 µg/mL. Alternatively, for nocturnal dyspnea, a very long-acting β-agonist, such as salmeterol, may be administered at bedtime. If symptoms persist on maximum bronchodilator therapy, a trial of oral prednisone is justified. An improvement of 15% or more in forced expiratory volume in 1 second (FEV_1) on corticosteroid therapy is an indication for long-term maintenance, preferably via inhaled corticosteroids. Long-term, low-dose oral prednisone is an alternative to inhaled corticosteroid therapy; however, it is associated with a marked increase in side effects. (*Adapted from* Ferguson and Cherniack [13].)

CHARACTERISTICS OF β-ADRENERGIC AGONISTS

| Drug | Dose/puff, *mg* | β-Receptor activity | | Time of effect, *min* | | |
		β_1	β_2	Onset	Peak	Duration
Isoproterenol	0.08	+++	+++	3–5	5–10	60–90
Isoetharine	0.34	++	++	3–5	5–20	60–150
Metaproterenol	0.65	+	+++	5–15	10–60	60–180
Terbutaline	0.20	+	++++	5–30	60–120	180–360
Albuterol	0.09	+	++++	5–15	60–90	240–360
Bitolterol	0.37	+	++++	5–10	60–90	300–480
Pirbuterol	0.20	+	+++	5–10	30–60	240–480
Salmeterol	0.025	+	++++	10–20	~180	600–720

Figure 3-12.

Characteristics of β-agonists. Isoproterenol and isoetharine are short-acting agents with mixed, β_1 and β_2 activity. Metaproterenol is more β_2 specific and has an intermediate duration of action. Terbutaline, albuterol, bitolterol, and pirbuterol are β_2-specific drugs with a relatively long duration of action. Salmeterol is a β_2-specific agent with a very long duration of action, up to 12 hours. Selection of a relatively long-acting agent is made on the basis of patient preference, available dose forms, and cost. (*Adapted from* Ferguson and Cherniack [13].)

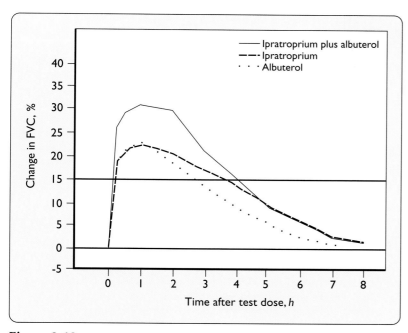

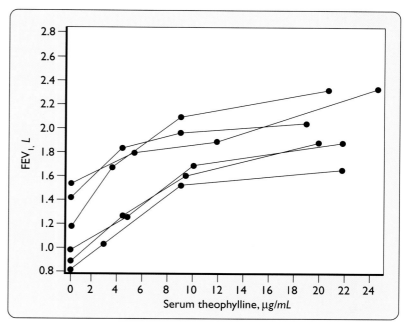

Figure 3-13.

Changes in mean forced vital capacity (FVC) after administration of albuterol, ipratropium, and ipratropium plus albuterol. Albuterol produces a rapid increase in FVC, which decreases over the subsequent 5 to 6 hours. Ipratropium produces a similar increase with a more prolonged duration of 7 to 8 hours. The combination produces a higher peak with a duration of action similar to ipratropium. The combination is more effective than either drug alone. (*Adapted from* the Combivent Inhalation Aerosol Study Group [14].)

Figure 3-14.

Relationship between serum theophylline levels and improvement in forced expiratory volume in 1 second (FEV_1) in six patients with asthma. The amount of improvement in FEV_1 with increasing serum levels of theophylline decreases above 8 to 12 μg/mL [15,16]. (*Adapted from* Rogers et al. [15].)

ACUTE EXACERBATIONS

INDICATIONS FOR HOSPITALIZATION OF PATIENTS WITH CHRONIC OBSTRUCTIVE PULMONARY DISEASE

Acute exacerbation (increased dyspnea, cough, or sputum production), plus one or more of the following:

Inadequate response to outpatient management

In a patient previously mobile, inability to ambulate due to dyspnea

Inability to eat or sleep due to dyspnea

Inadequate home care resources

Serious co-morbid condition

Prolonged progressive symptoms before emergency visit

Altered mentation

Worsening hypoxemia

New or worsening hypercapnia

New or worsening cor pulmonale unresponsive to outpatient management

Planned invasive surgical or diagnostic procedure requiring analgesics or sedatives that may worsen pulmonary function

Co-morbid condition, *eg*, severe steroid myopathy or acute vertebral compression fractures, that has worsened pulmonary function

Figure 3-15.

Indications for hospitalization of patients with chronic obstructive pulmonary disease (COPD). The indications for hospitalization are recommended by a panel of experts experienced in the management of patients with COPD. They are based on an observed decline in the patient's clinical status, the need for a procedure requiring analgesia or sedation, or the presence of a complication of therapy. (*Adapted from* Celli et al. [8].)

INDICATIONS FOR INTENSIVE CARE UNIT ADMISSION OF PATIENTS WITH ACUTE EXACERBATION OF CHRONIC OBSTRUCTIVE PULMONARY DISEASE

Severe dyspnea that responds inadequately to initial emergency therapy

Confusion or lethargy

Respiratory muscle fatigue (especially paradoxic diaphragmatic motion)

Persistent or worsening hypoxemia despite supplemental oxygen or severe/worsening respiratory acidosis (pH <7.30)

Need for noninvasive or invasive assisted mechanical ventilation

Figure 3-16.

Indications for intensive care unit admission of patients with acute exacerbations of chronic obstructive pulmonary disease. Patients should be considered for intensive care if ventilatory function declines, if they are unable to clear their airways, or if persistent hypoxemia or respiratory acidosis does not respond to nasal or mask oxygen. Additional indications for intensive care include trauma, hemoptysis, or pneumothorax, which results in a decline in ventilation or gas transfer. (*Adapted from* Celli *et al.* [8].)

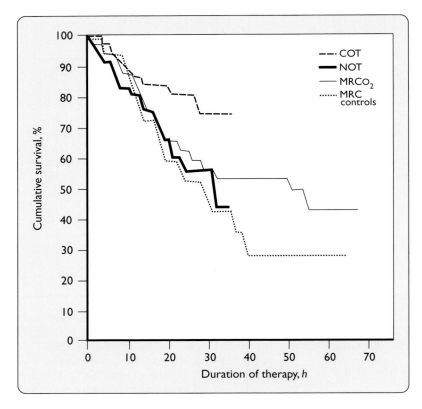

Figure 3-17.

Survival of men younger than 70 years of age with hypoxemic chronic obstructive pulmonary disease receiving long-term oxygen therapy versus survival of control subjects who did not receive oxygen. The data summarized in the figure was obtained from the Medical Research Council (MRC; limited oxygen therapy) and the Nocturnal Oxygen Therapy (NOT) trials, whose subjects received varying amounts of oxygen throughout the day. Survival of men in the control group who received no oxygen was the worst, but survival of men in the NOT group who received oxygen for 12 hours per 24-hour day was similar to that of men in the MRC group who received 15 hours of oxygen per day ($MRCo_2$). The best survival was in the continuous oxygen therapy (COT) group, whose members received oxygen for more than 19 hours per day. (*Adapted from* Flenley [17].)

Measure	Time	Mild	Moderate	Severe	P value
Six-minute walk, *ft*	Baseline	1639.4 ± 26.9	1465.8 ± 67.0	1485.4 ± 87.1	
	Follow-up	1839.0 ± 30.1	1704.0 ± 67.0	1591.4 ± 72.1	
	Difference	200.5 (165.4, 235.7)	238.3 (143.3, 333.3)	112.1 (34.6, 189.6)	0.08
	P value	< 0.01	< 0.0001	<0.01	
Overhead task, *s*	Baseline	24.8 ±0.5	26.6 ± 1.1	24.3 ± 1.1	
	Follow-up	23.9 ± 0.5	25.2 ± 1.2	23.6 ± 0.7	
	Difference	0.91 (1.72, 0.11)	1.39 (2.66, 0.13)	1.06 (3.16, -1.05)	0.78
	P value	0.03	0.03	0.48	
Stair climb, *s*	Baseline	11.5 ± 0.3	12.5 ± 0.6	14.3 ± 1.1	
	Follow-up	11.0 ± 0.3	12.7 ± 0.7	13.5 ± 0.8	
	Difference	0.57 (0.96, 0.18)	-0.23 (0.57, -1.02)	1.14 (2.60, -0.32)	0.14
	P value	< 0.01	0.56	0.28	
Treadmill time, *min*	Baseline	7.5 ± 0.2	6.0 ± 0.5	6.2 ± 0.6	
	Follow-up	7.9 ± 0.2	6.6 ± 0.4	6.6 ± 0.6	
	Difference	0.42 (0.20, 0.64)	0.64 (0.14, 1.14)	0.41 (-0.30, 1.11)	0.63
	P value	< 0.01	0.01	0.24	

Figure 3-18.

Effects of a 12-week exercise training program on physical performance in a group of 151 patients with mild (99), moderate (36), or severe (16) chronic obstructive pulmonary disease (COPD). Physical performance was evaluated by 6-minute walk test, treadmill time, time to perform an overhead task, and a stair climb. Six-minute walk distance increased significantly in all three groups. Treadmill time increased significantly in patients with mild and moderate disease. There was a significant decrease in the time to complete the overhead task in participants with mild and moderate COPD. These results demonstrate that an exercise program improves physical performance in all patients with COPD, not just those with moderate and severe disease. All values are mean ± SEM. The difference values are absolute difference from baseline to follow-up and include 95% confidence intervals. The P value in row 4 of each measure indicates whether the difference from baseline to follow-up is significant. The P values in column 6 indicate whether the differences among the three groups are significant. (*Adapted from* Berry [18].)

REHABILITATION

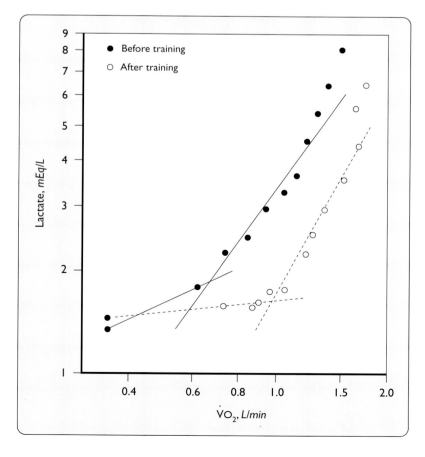

Figure 3-19.

Effect of exercise training on blood lactate levels during exercise. The figure indicates changes in blood lactate concentrations in one patient enrolled in a high work rate training program. Arterial lactate is plotted against oxygen uptake on a log scale. Before training, blood lactate rose very early in exercise. After training, elevation in blood lactate is delayed, and the lactate threshold occurs at a considerably higher oxygen consumption ($\dot{V}o_2$), indicating that a physiologic training response has occurred. (*Adapted from* Casaburi et al. [19].)

COMPARISON OF OUTCOMES DURING 6 MONTHS' USE OF NASAL AND TRANSTRACHEAL OXYGEN DELIVERY

Variable	Nasal cannula		Transtracheal	
	Mean	SD	Mean	SD
Oxygen, $L/min*$				
Rest[†]	2.7	0.9	1.5	0.6
Exercise[‡]	3.3	1.2	2.0	0.8
Oxygen used, $lb/mo*$[§]	316.0	85.0	272.0	64.0
12-min walk, ft[¶]	687.0	347.0	982.0	414.0
Spirometry				
FVC, L	2.31	0.89	2.34	0.89
FEV_1, L	0.86	0.51	0.78	0.46
FEV_1/FVC, %	37.0	12.0	35.0	12.0
Arterial blood gases				
pH	7.41	0.04	7.4	0.03
Pao_2, $mm\ Hg$	69.0	11.0	73.0	11.0
$Paco_2$, $mm\ HG$	48.0	10.0	49.0	12.0
HCO_3, mEq/L	30.0	3.0	31.0	5.0
Sao_2, %	93.0	3.0	92.0	3.0

*Excludes subjects (n = 2) with refractory hypoxemia during nasal delivery.
[†]t = 9.96, P < 0.0001.
[‡]t = 9.27, P < 0.0001.
[§]t = 5.01, P < 0.0001.
[¶]t = -6.81, P < 0.0001.
FEV₁—forced expiratory volume in 1 s; FVC—forced vital capacity.

Figure 3-20.
Comparison of outcomes during 6 months of therapy with nasal and transtracheal oxygen delivery devices. Transtracheal oxygen delivery was associated with increased arterial oxygen levels, and improved exercise tolerance was associated with a significant decrease in the amount of oxygen required. The catheter is inserted into the distal trachea, which acts as an oxygen reservoir. Carbon dioxide is washed out of the trachea, leading to a decrease in anatomic dead space. Disadvantages of transtracheal oxygen include drying of tracheal mucus with formation of mucus balls on the catheter tip, and increased cost of catheter insertion. (*Adapted from* Hoffman et al. [20].)

VOLUME REDUCTION THERAPY

	Preoperative	Postoperative	Change, %	P value
FEV_1, L (% predicted)	0.77 (25)	1.4 (44)	+82	<0.001
FVC, L (% predicted)	2.2 (56)	2.8 (73)	+27	<0.05
TLC, L (% predicted)	8.5 (140)	6.6 (100)	-22	<0.001
RV, L (% predicted)	5.9 (288)	3.6 (177)	-39	<0.001
Trapped gas, L	2.4	1.2	-50	<0.001
Pao_2 (room air)	64.0*	70.0	—	<0.05
$Paco_2$ (room air)	40.0*	39.0	—	NS

*Two patients receiving oxygen excluded.
FEV₁—forced expiratory volume in 1 s; FVC—forced vital capacity; NS—not significant; RV—residual volume; TLC—total lung capacity.

Figure 3-21.
Pre- and postoperative physiologic measurements in patients undergoing bilateral pneumectomy (volume reduction) for chronic obstructive pulmonary disease. A total of 20 patients with severe emphysema has studied immediately before and between 1 to 15 months (mean, 6.4 months) after surgery. There was a marked increase in forced expiratory volume in 1 second and forced vital capacity, with a decrease in total lung capacity and residual volume. Room-air arterial oxygen improved slightly, but significantly. (*Adapted from* Cooper et al. [21].)

Variables	Baseline data (n = 26)	Predicted or normal value, %	Short-term responders Died (n = 10) Before-LVRS	Responders (n = 9) Before LVRS	>3 y after LVRS[†]
VC, L	2.4 ± 0.7	$67 \pm 6\%$	$59 \pm 5\%$[*]	$73 \pm 13\%$	$85 \pm 14\%$
FVC, L	2.1 ± 0.6	$58 \pm 14\%$	$52 \pm 4\%$[*]	$64 \pm 12\%$	$79 \pm 13\%$
FEV$_1$, L	0.7 ± 0.2	$29 \pm 10\%$	$24 \pm 9\%$	$33 \pm 10\%$	$47 \pm 15\%$
TLC, L	8.6 ± 1.8	$147 \pm 17\%$	$150 \pm 15\%$	$146 \pm 16\%$	$128 \pm 18\%$
RV, L	6.0 ± 1.4	$268 \pm 46\%$	$275 \pm 40\%$	$254 \pm 34\%$	$186 \pm 42\%$
RV/TLC, %	71 ± 6	$176 \pm 21\%$	$185 \pm 19\%$	$170 \pm 17\%$	$141 \pm 19\%$
DL/VA, mL/min/mm Hg/L	1.1 ± 0.5	$29 \pm 15\%$	$26 \pm 4\%$	$30 \pm 21\%$	$51 \pm 23\%$
Pst at TLC, cm H$_2$O	11 ± 1.7	25 ± 7	10.8 ± 0.5	10.9 ± 1.9	12.9 ± 1.8
Raw, cm H$_2$O/L/s	5.1 ± 1.9	<2.5	5.7 ± 0.6	5.1 ± 2.0	3.6 ± 1
SGaw, L/s/cm H$_2$O/L	0.032 ± 0.01	$13 \pm 6\%$	$11 \pm 2\%$	$17 \pm 10\%$	$25 \pm 9\%$
Coefficient retraction Pst at TLC/TLC, cm H$_2$O/L	1.3 ± 0.4	>3.10	1.2 ± 0.3	1.2 ± 0.7	2.0 ± 0.6
Gs, L/s/cm H$_2$O	0.20 ± 0.10	0.6 ± 0.1	0.18 ± 0.04	0.20 ± 0.11	0.31 ± 0.08
VO$_2$max, mL/kg/min	6.7 ± 3.8	>18	5.0 ± 2.0	4.5 ± 1.5	9.5 ± 1.4
Dyspnea score	3.2 ± 0.05	0	3.3 ± 0.05	3.2 ± 0.05	2.2 ± 0.05

Data are presented as mean ± SD unless otherwise indicated.

*Statistical difference (P < 0.01) at baseline before LVRS in 10 short-term responders who died within 4 years of LVRS when compared to nine patient responders. The short-term responders showed physiologic improvement ± 2 years after LVRS.

†P < 0.05 comparing results before and >3 years after LVRS in nine responders (FEV$_1$ ≥ 0.2 L, FVC ≥ 0.4 L, or both ≥ 3 years from baseline).

DL/VA—diffusing capacity/L of alveolar volume; Pst—static lung elastic recoil pressure; RAW—airway resistance; SGaw—specific airway conductance; VO$_2$max—maximum oxygen consumption.

Figure 3-22.

Bilateral upper lobe lung volume reduction surgery using a video thorascopic technique was performed in 26 patients with severe emphysema. All patients had heterogenous distribution of the emphysema demonstrated by lung computed tomography (CT) scans. A variety of lung function studies was performed on the patients before surgery and afterward for up to 4 years or until the patient died. Baseline data demonstrate that the patients had severe emphysema with a severe expiratory airflow limitation, hyperinflation at TLC, severely reduced DLCO, decreased elastic lung recoil at TLC, increased airway resistance, and severe reduction in maximum oxygen consumption. The mortality rate 1, 2, 3, and 4 years after surgery was 4%, 9%, 31%, and 46%, respectively. An increase above baseline for FEV$_1$ (>200 mL) and FVC (>400 mL) 1, 2, 3, and 4 years after surgery was 73%, 46%, 35%, and 27% of patients, respectively. Nine of the 26 patients had an improvement in the clinical and physiologic parameters that lasted longer than 3 years. This was primarily due to increases in the elastic lung recoil and small airway caliber and decreases in the degree of hyperinflation. The long-term responders had a higher VC and FVC at baseline when compared to 10 short-term (> 2 years) responders [22]. DLCO—diffusing capacity for carbon monoxide; Gs—conductance of the small airway S segment; RV—residual volume; TLC—total lung capacity; VC—vital capacity.

GENERAL GUIDELINES FOR RECIPIENT SELECTION FOR LUNG TRANSPLANTATION IN COPD

Indications
Life expectancy < 18 mos
Severe dyspnea with significant disruption of daily activities
Psychosocial stability
FEV_1 < 25% of predicted
Pa_{O_2} < 55 mm Hg at rest
Rapid decline in FEV_1
Body mass index < 20 kg/m^2

Absolute contraindications
Clinically significant cardiac, liver, renal, or central nervous system disease
HIV-associated diseases
Incurable malignancy
Tracheostomy/ventilator dependency
Drug or alcohol dependency
Profound wasting
Secondary pulmonary hypertension
Chronic high-dose corticosteroid therapy (>15 mg/d prednisone)

Relative contraindications
Severe psychosocial problems
Noncompliance with medical regimen
Age > 60 y
Severe diabetes mellitus
Presence of *Aspergillus* species in sputum
Colonization of airways with resistant flora
Previous thoracic surgery or pleurodesis

Figure 3-23.
Appropriate recipient selection is extremely important for an acceptable outcome after lung transplantation. Indications and contraindications for lung transplantation are listed in this figure. In general, the more medical problems the patient has the lower the likelihood is for a successful outcome. While patients should ideally be younger than 60 years of age, physiologic age is a more important determinant of patient outcome. Immunosuppressive therapy can have a profound effect on patients with pre-existing systemic diseases, making careful scrutiny before enrollment a necessity. High-dose corticosteroid use is a contraindication to lung transplantation because it is associated with poor wound healing and potentially serious infections. The patient should be ambulatory and have some potential for physical rehabilitation after surgery. Contraindications to lung transplantation are constantly evolving and vary from center to center [23,24].

SURGERY

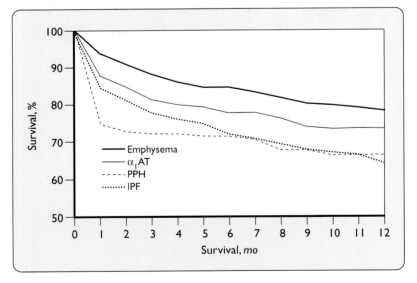

Figure 3-24.
Actuarial survival after single lung transplantation for patients with emphysema, idiopathic pulmonary fibrosis (IPF), primary pulmonary hypertension (PPH), and α_1 antitrypsin deficiency (α_1AT). Mean survival is longest after transplantation for severe emphysema. (*Adapted from* Hosenpud et al. [25].)

PROGNOSIS

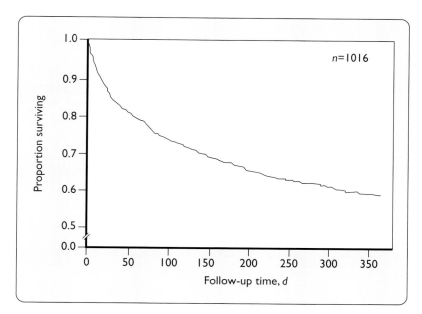

Figure 3-25.

One-year survival after an acute exacerbation of chronic obstructive pulmonary disease in 1016 patients. Although hospital mortality was low (11%), long-term survival was poor: 57% at 1 year and 51% at 2 years. The median length of hospital stay for acute respiratory failure was 9 days, and the median cost per hospital stay was $7100. Six months after hospitalization, only one of four patients reported a good quality of life. (*Adapted from* Conners *et al.* [26].)

REFERENCES

1. Adam PF, Benson V: Current estimates from the National Health Interview Survey, 1991. *Vital Health Stat [10]* 1992, 184:1–232.

2. Stastical Abstract of the United States Department of Commerce 1999 ed. 119. pp99-100

3. Fletcher EC, Peto R: The natural history of chronic airflow obstruction. *Br Med J* 1997, 1:1645–1648.

4. Anthonisen NR, Wright EC: IPPB Trial Group: Bronchodilator response in chronic obstructive pulmonary disease. *Am Rev Respir Dis* 1986, 133:814–819.

5. Mandella LA, Manfreda J, Warren CPW, Anthonisen NR: Steroid response in stable chronic obstructive pulmonary disease. *Ann Intern Med* 1982, 96:17–21.

6. Owens GR: Chronic obstructive pulmonary disease: asthma, emphysema, chronic bronchitis, bronchiectasis, and related conditions. In *Pulmonary and Critical Care Medicine.* Edited by Bone RC, Dantzker DR, George RB, *et al.* St. Louis: Mosby; 1993:G3–G5.

7. Morris J, Edwards M, Haas H, *et al.*: *Chronic Obstruction Pulmonary Disease.* New York: American Lung Association; 1977:11–19.

8. Celli BR, Snider GL, Heffner J, *et al.*, for the American Thoracic Society: Standards for the diagnosis and care of patients with chronic obstructive pulmonary disease. *Am J Respir Crit Care Med* 1995, 152:S77–S121.

9. Hubbard RC, Crystal RG: Alpha-1-antitrypsin augmentation therapy for alpha-1-antitrypsin deficiency. *Am J Med* 1988, 84(suppl 6A):52–62.

10. Anthonisen NR, Connett JE, Kiley JP, *et al.*: Effects of smoking intervention and the use of an inhaled anticholinergic bronchodilator on the rate of decline of FEV1. *JAMA* 1994, 272:1497–1505.

11. Sherrill DL, Enright P, Cline M, *et al.*: Rates of decline in lung function among subjects who restart cigarette smoking. *Chest* 1996, 109:1001–1005.

12. Vestbo J, Sorensen T, Lange P, Brix A, Torre P, Viskum K: Long-term effect of inhaled budesonide in mild and moderate chronic obstructive pulmonary disease: a randomised controlled trial. *Lancet* 1999, 353:1819–1823.

13. Ferguson GT, Cherniack RM: Management of chronic obstructive pulmonary disease. *N Engl J Med* 1993, 328:1017–1022.

14. Combivent Inhalation Aerosol Study Group: In chronic obstructive pulmonary disease, a combination of ipratropium and albuterol is more effective than either agent alone: an 85-day multicenter trial. *Chest* 1994, 105:1411–1419.

15. Rogers RM, Owens GR, Pennock BE: The pendulum swings again: toward a rational use of theophylline. *Chest* 1985, 87:280–282.

16. Mitenko PA, Ogilvie RI: Rational intravenous doses of theophylline. *N Engl J Med* 1973, 289:600–603.

17. Flenley DC: Oxygen therapy in the treatment of COPD. In *Chronic Obstructive Pulmonary Disease*, edn 1. Edited by Cherniack NS. Philadelphia: WB Saunders; 1991:468–476.

18. Berry MJ, Rejeski WJ, Adair NE, Zaccaro D: Exercise rehabilitation and chronic obstructive pulmonary disease stage. *Am J Respir Crit Care Med* 1999, 160:1248–1253.

19. Casaburi R, Patessio A, Ioli F, *et al.*: Reductions in exercise lactic acidosis and ventilation as a result of exercise training in patients with obstructive lung disease. *Am Rev Respir Dis* 1991, 143:9–18.

20. Hoffman LA, Wesmiller SW, Sciurba FC, *et al.*: Nasal cannula and transtracheal oxygen delivery: a comparison of patient response after 6 months of each technique. *Am Rev Respir Dis* 1992, 145:827–831.

21. Cooper JD, Trulock EP, Triantofillou AN, *et al.*: Bilateral pneumectomy (volume reduction) for chronic obstructive pulmonary disease. *J Thorac Cardiovasc Surg* 1995, 109:106–119.

22. Gelb AF, McKenna RJ, Brenner M, Schein MJ, Zamel N, Fischel R: Lung function 4 years after lung volume reduction surgery for emphysema. *Chest* 1999, 116:1608–1615.

23. Heritier F, Madden B, Hodson ME, Yacoub M: Lung allograft transplantation: indications, preoperative assessment and postoperative management. *Eur Respir J* 1992, 5:1262–1278.

24. Davis RD, Pasque MK: Pulmonary transplantation. Ann Surg 1995, 221:14–28.22. Elmes PC, King TKC, Langlands JHM, et al.: Value of ampicillin in the hospital treatment of exacerbations of chronic bronchitis. BMJ 1965, 2:904–908.

25. Hosenpud JD, Novick RJ, Breen TJ, Daily OP: The Registry of the International Society for Heart and Lung Transplantation: eleventh official report—1994. *J Heart Lung Transplant* 1994, 13:561–570.

26. Conners AF, Dawson NV, Thomas C, *et al.*, for the SUPPORT Investigators: Acute exacerbations of COPD. *Am J Respir Crit Care Med* 1996, 154:959–967.

CYSTIC FIBROSIS

4

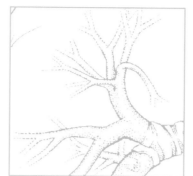
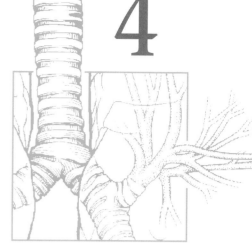
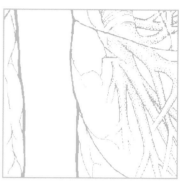

Stanley B. Fiel &
Daniel V. Schidlow

"Woe to that child which when kissed on the forehead tastes salty.
He is bewitched and soon must die."
—Adage from northern European folklore referring to the salty sweat that characterizes cystic fibrosis,
    circa 1705.

Cystic fibrosis (CF) is the most common life-threatening genetic disease of the white population in the United States [1]. Approximately 1000 new cases are diagnosed each year, and some 30,000 Americans live with the disease [2,3].

The diverse manifestations of CF, including the salty brow to which the adage refers, are caused by mutations in the gene that encodes the cystic fibrosis transmembrane conductance regulator (CFTR) protein. The CFTR protein is a chloride channel that plays an essential role in regulating the movement of electrolytes across epithelial membranes and maintaining the appropriate balance of intracellular and extracellular fluids. Defective electrolyte transport changes the ionic composition of the airway surface fluid, thus reducing its water content and dehydrating the mucus. Ultimately, viscous secretions accumulate, occluding the airways and impairing pulmonary function. Consequently, respiratory disease is the primary cause of death among patients with CF.

The lungs and sweat glands are not the only tissues affected by CF. Chloride channel dysfunction affects exocrine glands throughout the body and contributes to pancreatic insufficiency (in 80% to 90% of patients) and biliary tract disease. Prenatal ductal obstruction may also inhibit development of the Wolffian ducts, leading to congenital bilateral absence of the vas deferens (CBAVD), which causes infertility in almost all men.

Reported cases of steatorrhea and pancreatic insufficiency date to the mid-17th century [4]; however, the first description of CF as a clinical entity did not appear until the 1930s, when the disease was characterized as a genetic disorder of the pancreas and lung [5–8]. By 1953, an elevated concentration of chloride in sweat had been established as a diagnostic feature of the disease [9]. This advance led to the development of the sweat test [10], which is still one of the cornerstones of diagnosis. The reason for abnormal electrolyte concentrations in sweat remained obscure for 30 more years, until investigators identified a defect in chloride conductance in the epithelial cells of sweat glands [11] and airways [12]. It is now clear that the defect in chloride conductance occurs in secretory epithelial cells throughout the body and plays a key role in the clinical manifestations of CF. CFTR dysfunction produces a change in the electrical potential of ion transport in all epithelial cells, including the cells lining the nose. Increasing proficiency in the measurement of this change using nasal potential difference (NPD) suggests that this test can serve as another diagnostic tool for CF. In the future, NPD may also be used to measure the level of correction in chloride transport obtained in the course of clinical trials of new CF treatments.

A cure for this complex disease is not imminent, but therapeutic strides throughout the last half of the 20th century have improved the quality of life for thousands of patients and extended their lives by several decades. The pace at which new therapeutic strategies for CF are introduced into clinical medicine has quickened in the past decade, as new data on the pathophysiology of CF have emerged to serve as a blueprint for clinical investigators.

EPIDEMIOLOGY

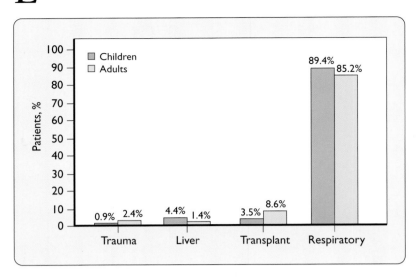

Figure 4-1.
Primary cause of death in adult and pediatric cystic fibrosis populations, 1994. Although the manifestations of cystic fibrosis can be widespread, the primary cause of morbidity and mortality in patients with cystic fibrosis is lung disease. Respiratory disease—bronchiectasis and obstructive pulmonary disease—accounts for nearly 90% of deaths in children and adults. (*Adapted from* the New Insights Editorial Board [13].)

EPIDEMIOLOGY OF CYSTIC FIBROSIS—1994

Whites	1 in 3000*
Blacks	1 in 17,000
Asians	1 in 90,000
Native Americans	1 in 80,000

*Per live births.

Figure 4-2.
Incidence of cystic fibrosis. Cystic fibrosis, also known as "mucoviscidosis" (especially in some European countries), occurs equally in both sexes. Although it appears in virtually every race, it is most common among whites.

GENETICS

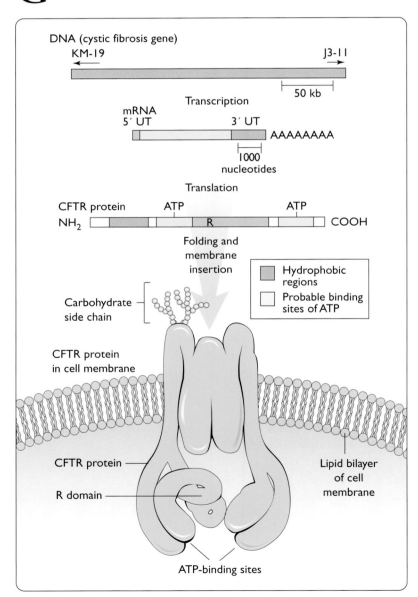

Figure 4-3.
Predicting the structure of the cystic fibrosis transmembrane conductance regulator (CFTR) protein. The *CFTR* gene, located on chromosome 7, was first cloned and sequenced in 1989 [14–16]. The gene contains 27 exons and is flanked by genetic markers KM-19 and J3-11. The messenger RNA (mRNA) is 6129 bp in length, including two hydrophobic transmembrane domains, two nucleotide-binding sites, and a highly charged regulatory (R) domain. The diagram of protein folding is hypothetical. The CFTR protein plays a critical role in electrolyte transport, serving not only as a chloride channel [17], but also as a "switch" that regulates other transepithelial ion channels [18]. (*Adapted from* Ramsey [19].)

A. EXAMPLES OF CFTR MUTATIONS ORGANIZED BY CLASSIFICATION OF THE DEFECT IN CFTR BIOSYNTHESIS

Type	Genotype	Phenotype	Defect	Drugs that may improve phenotype
Class I	G542X 621 + 1 G → T 3905insT W1282X R553X 1717-1 G → A	PI	No CFTR protein No cell surface chloride transport	Gentamicin G418
Class II	ΔF508 N1303K (P574H)* (A455E)*	PI	Defective CFTR processing Defective CFTR trafficking No cell surface chloride transport	Chemical chaperones CPX Phenylbutyrate Deoxyspergualin
Class III	G551D G551S	PI	Defective chloride channel regulation Reduced or absent cell surface Chloride transport	Genistein Pyrophosphate
Class IV	R117H R334W G314E R347P (ΔF508)* P574H	PS	Reduced chloride conductance Reduced levels of cell surface Chloride transport	Genistein Milrinone Phenylbutyrate
Class V	3849 + 10 kb C → T 2789 + 5 G → A 3272 - 26 A → G A455E 3120 + 1 G → A 1811 + 1.6 kb A → G 5T†	PS	Normal CFTR channels Fewer normal CFTR Reduced cell surface chloride transport	Genistein Milrinone

Phenylbutyrate

*Some mutants have features of more than one class of defect.
†5T is an intron variant that is not considered bona fide mutation but renders different levels of expression of normal CFTR.

Figure 4-4.

Mutations that disrupt cystic fibrosis transmembrane conductance regulator (CFTR) function. **A,** Thus far, investigators have described the mechanisms by which five classes of cystic fibrosis mutations disrupt protein function. Recently, investigators [21,22] have proposed that identified mutants that impair regulation of other types of ion channels should be labeled as class VI. Others [23] have suggested that C-terminal truncations in CFTR, which lead to accelerated degradation of CFTR, should comprise class VI mutations. The mechanisms for these five classes are described in *panels A* and *B*.

(Continued on next page)

B. CLASSES OF CYSTIC FIBROSIS MUTATIONS

Class I

Mutations produce premature termination signals and result in defective production of CFTR before the protein reaches the endoplasmic reticulum for posttranslational processing. This category includes nonsense, splice-site, and frameshift mutations, all of which are predicted to eliminate channel function. These mutations are associated with severe disease.

Class II

Mutations result in failure to traffic the protein to the correct cellular location. In the well-known case of ΔF508, the CFTR protein does not meet the apical membrane and is localized largely in the endoplasmic reticulum. These mutations are associated with severe disease.

Class III

Mutations impair protein regulation, resulting in a net decrease in Cl⁻ channel activity. Most, but not all, mutations in this class are associated with severe disease.

Class IV

Mutations impair conduction of Cl⁻ through the CFTR channel pores. At least three mutations in this class are associated with mild disease. R117H is associated with two different phenotypes. Some men with the R117H genotype have CBAVD and pulmonary disease, whereas others have only CBAVD. This anomaly is the focus of some attention.

Class V

Defined by defects in splicing and production of the full-length normal CFTR, these mutations lead to a deficit of normal CFTR and a reduction in cell surface chloride transport, despite the presence of normal CFTR channels. Researchers concur that 10% wild-type CFTR expression represents the critical point for disease. Commonly, these patients will be pancreatic sufficient. Several genotypes are associated with this class, including $3849 + 10$ kb C $\rightarrow$ T; $2789 + 5$ G $\rightarrow$ A; 3272-26 A $\rightarrow$ G; A455E, and others. In addition, there is controversy regarding the inclusion of an intron variant, 5T, which renders different levels of expression of a normal CFTR [21].

CBAVD—congenital bilateral absence of the vas deferens; CFTR—cystic fibrosis transmembrane conductance regulator.

Figure 4-4. (*Continued*)
B, The relationship between specific *CFTR* gene mutations and clinical manifestations of the disease are much more complex than was previously thought [20,21]. In general, classes I, II, and III are associated with the more severe phenotypic expression of the *CFTR* gene and classes IV and V associated with less severe clinical consequences. Although most of the reported mutations in CFTR are rare and unclassified, it may be possible to use genotype-phenotype correlations to determine the best approach. (*Adapted from* Zeitlin [21].)

TYPES OF NON-ΔF508 MUTATIONS

Mutation	Example	Description
Missense	G551D	Substitution of glycine (G) at codon 551 by aspartic acid (D)
Nonsense	G542X	Substitution of glycine (G) at codon 542 by a stop signal (X)
Frameshift	3095 insT	Insertion of thymine (T) after nucleotide 3905 in exon 20
Splice-site	621+1G→T	Substitution of thymine (T) for guanine (G) immediately after nucleotide 621 (last base in exon 4)

Figure 4-5.
Four major types of non-ΔF508 mutations. More than 1000 mutations have been identified. The most common of them, carried by more than 70% of the affected chromosomes worldwide, is known as ΔF508.

This mutation is the result of the deletion of three nucleotides, which leads to the loss of phenylalanine at position 508 of the gene product [3]. This mutation may have appeared first in Europe more than 50,000 years ago [24]. Examples of four other common mutations types are provided in the figure. Many of the mutations reported to date are rare, appearing in only one family. Others are concentrated in a particular ethnic group. For example, the stop codon mutation W12182X (not shown here), which constitutes only 2% of all cystic fibrosis mutations worldwide, is carried by 50% of the cystic fibrosis chromosomes in Ashkenazi Jews, by contrast, the frequency of ΔF508 is relatively low (40%) in this population [24].

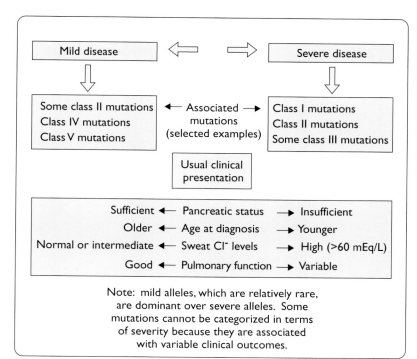

Note: mild alleles, which are relatively rare, are dominant over severe alleles. Some mutations cannot be categorized in terms of severity because they are associated with variable clinical outcomes.

Figure 4-6.

Genotype-phenotype relationships. Phenotypic severity bears some relationship to genotype [20,27]. However, the relationship between genotype and clinical expression is complicated and remains poorly understood. Investigators have studied the impact of genotype on the severity of pancreatic and pulmonary disease and the occurrence of congenital bilateral absence of the vas deferens (CBAVD). The incidence of CBVAD among men with cystic fibrosis is less than 95%, but the condition also occurs in men with few or no other manifestations of the disease. CBAVD is unrelated to severity. Although the relationship is not invariant, pancreatic status is linked to particular classes of mutations, and cystic fibrosis phenotypes have traditionally been classified as "mild" or "severe" on the basis of pancreatic function. Many mutations, including ΔF508, are associated with pancreatic insufficiency (ie, dependence on pancreatic enzymes), whereas a much smaller number is associated with pancreatic sufficiency. The severity and course of pulmonary disease are predicted less reliably by genotype; some mutations are common among patients with "mild" lung disease, but variability is high among patients with "severe" mutations [28,29]. Variability in pulmonary disease may be due, in part, to environmental factors.

PATHOPHYSIOLOGY

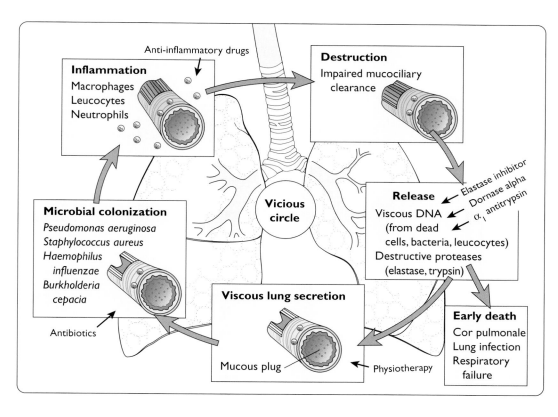

Figure 4-7.

The "vicious circle" of lung disease in cystic fibrosis. Pulmonary disease associated with cystic fibrosis is characterized by a "vicious circle" of obstruction, infection, and inflammation that impairs local host-defense mechanisms, produces progressive bronchiectasis and, ultimately, causes respiratory failure. Although much has been learned about the effect of CFTR on the cell, investigators are still trying to understand how defective transepithelial electrolyte transport leads to the devastating consequences seen throughout the airways. The pathophysiology of airway obstruction, infection, and inflammation is being actively studied.

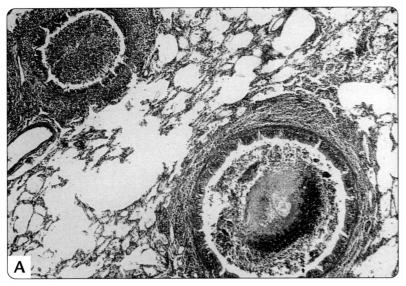 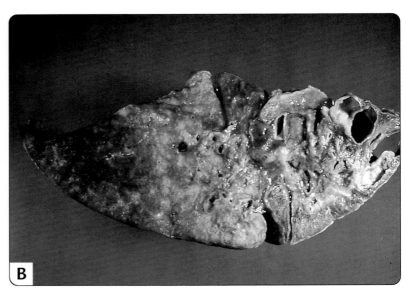

Figure 4-8.

Airway obstruction. Airway obstruction is rooted, in part, in *CFTR* dysfunction. Defective electrolyte transport depletes the airway surface fluid of water, thus compromising the viscoelasticity of mucus and impairing its ability to clear microorganisms from the respiratory tract [30]. DNA deposited by neutrophils that flood cystic fibrotic airways further increases the viscosity of airway secretions. **A,** Pathology of early lung

disease. Thickening and sloughing of the peribronchial mucosa lead to occlusion of the lumen with viscous secretions and cellular debris in an infant 5 months of age. (*See* Color Plate.) **B,** Advanced lung disease. The disease has spread from the small airways to larger airways. Bronchiectasis, cystic changes, diffuse mucus plugging, and fibrosis are visible. (*See* Color Plate.)

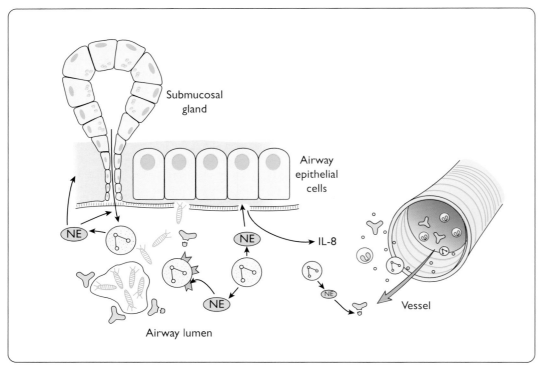

Figure 4-9.

Airway inflammation mediated by neutrophils and neutrophil products. The inflammatory response in cystic fibrosis is dominated by polymorphonuclear neutrophils and their destructive products, which

perpetuate and amplify lung damage. Once recruited to the site of inflammation and primed by interleukin-8 (IL-8) and other cytokines [31], neutrophils release an arsenal of proteases, oxidative radicals (including H_2O_2), and other inflammatory mediators that stimulate mucus hypersecretion and exacerbate the pathologic process [32–36]. The most damaging of the products to flood the cystic airways is neutrophil elastase (NE), which has been called an "omnivorous" serine protease. Under normal circumstances, NE is complex and inactivated by α_1 antitrypsin and secretory leukoprotease inhibitor. In cystic fibrosis, however, the lungs' normal defenses against this proteolytic enzyme are overwhelmed [37]. Unopposed in its action, NE contributes to progressive pulmonary damage by 1) directly injuring the cellular and matrix components of the airways, 2) impairing antibody- and complement-mediated opsonophagocytosis, 3) stimulating mucus secretion, 4) reducing ciliary beat frequency, and 5) inducing epithelial cell production of IL-8. Chronic neutrophil-dominated inflammation and impaired antineutrophil elastase defense have been reported in children with cystic fibrosis as young as 1 year [31–38]. Decaying neutrophils release DNA into the airways, where it accumulates, further increasing the viscosity and adhesiveness of mucus. (*Adapted from* Marshall [30].)

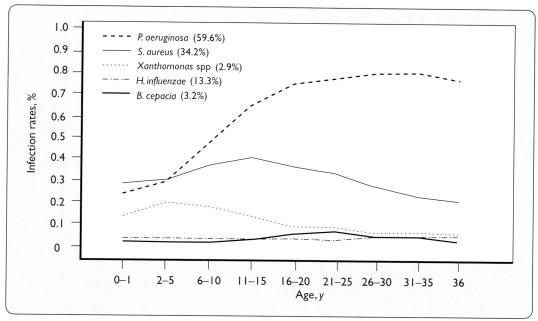

Figure 4-10.

Age-specific frequencies of five common airway pathogens. Chronic airway inflammation and/or infection from early infancy may also be rooted in the *CFTR* defect. The concentration of chloride in the airway surface fluid of patients with cystic fibrosis (CF) may be abnormally high; this property may compromise the bactericidal capacity of the airway surface fluid, thereby impairing the lungs' natural defenses and predisposing them to chronic infection [32]. *Pseudomonas aeruginosa* supersedes *Staphylococcus aureus* to become the predominant pathogen by the end of the first decade of life. Once established in CF airways, *P. aeruginosa* is difficult or impossible to eradicate. Initial infection is usually with nonmucoid, piliated organisms; however, the nonmucoid form often switches to a mucoid variant in the airway. Alginate gel produced by mucoid organisms protects them against host defenses and manufactures a broad range of virulent proteases, toxins, and antigenic agents. Patients with CF lack alginate-specific opsonic antibodies [39]. *Pseudomonas* pili appear to bind avidly to asialylated CF cells, perhaps explaining in part the puzzling affinity of this pathogen for CF airways [40]. The high prevalence of *P. aeruginosa* in this population may also be a consequence of selection associated with increased life expectancy and aggressive antibiotic treatment [19,33–41,43]. Selection may also result in an increased incidence of newer pathogens and resistant strains (eg, methicillin-resistant *S. aureus*). The new pathogen of greatest concern is *Burkholderia cepacia*, which is transmissible by close person-to-person contact. Infection with *B. cepacia* can be associated with slowly declining lung function; however, some colonized patients succumb to an accelerated and fatal deterioration and others show no change in clinical status. Pulmonary colonization by *B. cepacia* can occur 2 years before it is detectable by routine culturing [44]. Seven genomovars of the *B. cepacia* complex, known to be present in patients with CF in the United States, have been identified [44]. In addition, multiple novel species have been identified for bioremediation, but no human isolates have been observed thus far. As scientists continue to examine the epidemiology of these strains, analysis suggests that the *B. cepacia* complex may be comprised approximately as follows: 50% genomovar III (G III); 35% *B. multivorans* (G II); 5% *B. vietnamiensis* (G V); 10% included genomovars I, VI, and VII (*B. stabilis* [G IV], recA group C [G VII]). These efforts to confirm species identification will hopefully be informative regarding infection transmissibility and virulence, leading to infection control consensus. The clinical significance of *Stenotrophomonas (Xanthomonas) maltophilia*, nontuberculosis mycobacteria, *Alcaligenes xylosoxidans*, and *Aspergillus* species in patients with CF is not yet clear. There is evidence to suggest that colonization with *S. (Xanthomonas) maltophilia* does not alter the course of CF but is associated with an increased use of antibiotics [46]. Improved surveillance may account for some of the apparent increase in prevalence of these pathogens [45]. *Mycobacterium tuberculosis*, although rare in patients with CF [46], can be associated with an increase in disease progression. Data shown here are based on cultures obtained at CF care centers in the United States.

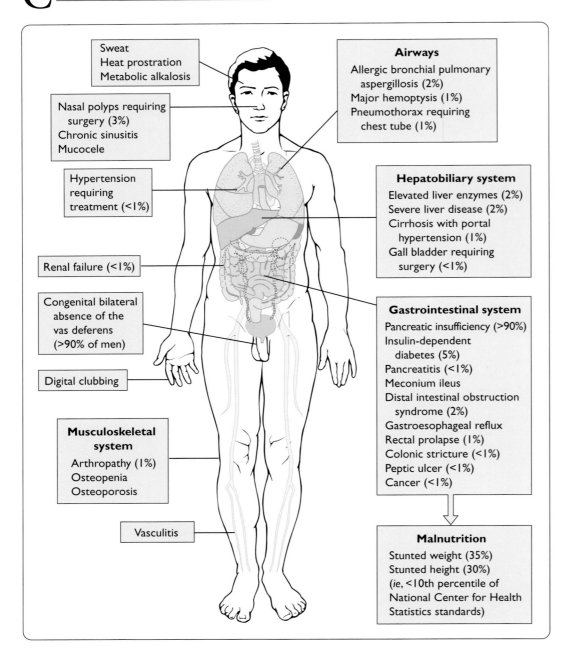

Sweat
Heat prostration
Metabolic alkalosis

Nasal polyps requiring surgery (3%)
Chronic sinusitis
Mucocele

Hypertension requiring treatment (<1%)

Renal failure (<1%)

Congenital bilateral absence of the vas deferens (>90% of men)

Digital clubbing

Musculoskeletal system
Arthropathy (1%)
Osteopenia
Osteoporosis

Vasculitis

Airways
Allergic bronchial pulmonary aspergillosis (2%)
Major hemoptysis (1%)
Pneumothorax requiring chest tube (1%)

Hepatobiliary system
Elevated liver enzymes (2%)
Severe liver disease (2%)
Cirrhosis with portal hypertension (1%)
Gall bladder requiring surgery (<1%)

Gastrointestinal system
Pancreatic insufficiency (>90%)
Insulin-dependent diabetes (5%)
Pancreatitis (<1%)
Meconium ileus
Distal intestinal obstruction syndrome (2%)
Gastroesophageal reflux
Rectal prolapse (1%)
Colonic stricture (<1%)
Peptic ulcer (<1%)
Cancer (<1%)

Malnutrition
Stunted weight (35%)
Stunted height (30%)
(ie, <10th percentile of National Center for Health Statistics standards)

Figure 4-11.

Clinical manifestations and co-morbidity of cystic fibrosis. Cystic fibrosis is associated with numerous complications and co-morbid conditions. As indicated in the figure, almost every patient with cystic fibrosis who lives long enough will eventually develop pulmonary symptoms. However, the age of onset, the rate at which cystic fibrosis progresses, and the incidence of co-morbid conditions are extremely variable. The 1999 incidence of some of these manifestations and co-morbid conditions, obtained from the Cystic Fibrosis Foundation Registry, are provided in parentheses. It is important to note that the incidence of most of these conditions increases significantly with age and disease progression. Thus, the prevalence of some conditions (eg, liver disease and diabetes mellitus) in a clinical setting that includes adolescents and young adults can be significantly higher than these figures suggest.

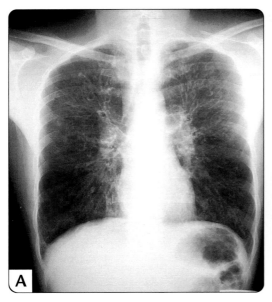

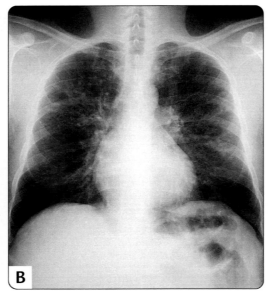

Figure 4-12.

Advanced respiratory disease and pulmonary complications. Recurrent pulmonary infections are the principal causes of morbidity in patients with cystic fibrosis. Respiratory failure, defined by hypoxemia and hypercapnia, is the usual cause of death. Complications associated with advanced disease include pneumothorax, experienced by 16% to 20% of patients older than age 18 years, and major hemoptysis. Guidelines on the management of pulmonary complications have been published [47,48]. **A,** Radiograph showing bronchiectasis in a man aged 29 years with advanced cystic fibrosis. Ring shadows and tram-tracking present in both upper lobes are secondary to bronchial thickening and dilation. Hyperaeration is also seen. **B,** Radiograph showing mucus plugging in a 38-year-old man with advanced cystic fibrosis. Branching tubular and nodular densities in the right upper lobe correspond to mucus impaction within the bronchial tree.

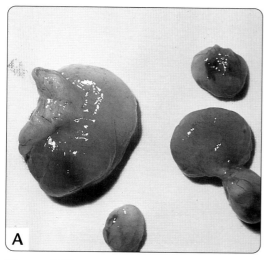

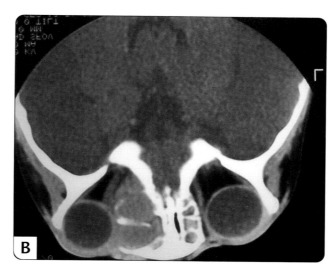

Figure 4-13.

Other respiratory tract complications and manifestations in cystic fibrosis (CF). These complications and manifestations include persistent productive cough (a hallmark of CF pulmonary disease from infancy); infectious exacerbations, which punctuate periods of clinical stability and are defined by increased cough, weight loss, increased sputum volume, and decrements in pulmonary function [49]; and treatment-resistant sinus disease, which occurs in more than 90% of patients with CF and is associated with a high frequency of local complications [50]. Although some children are asymptomatic, a history of headache, postnasal drip, and nasal obstruction can often be elicited. There is considerable variation in the degree and type of sinus disease in patients with CF, but there does not seem to be a strong correlation between the severity of lung disease and the symptoms of sinus disease [50]. Thickening of the mucosal lining of the paranasal sinuses, fluid accumulation, and recurrent sinusitis are common. Opacification on sinus radiographs is so characteristic of CF that normal sinus radiographs should cast doubt on the diagnosis [51]. **A,** Nasal polyps, which originate in the paranasal sinuses, are present in up to 40% of patients with CF and tend to recur after resection. (*See* Color Plate.) **B,** This computerized axial tomography shows a large mucocele arising from the ethmoid sinus causing a mass effect into the right orbit. Mucoceles are slow-growing cysts that fill with mucoid secretions when sinus drainage is obstructed by inflammatory processes or other causes. The expanding mass can erode bone and compress adjacent structures [52]. Clinical manifestations of paranasal mucoceles include headache, eyelid ptosis, and limitation of eye movement. In children, paranasal sinus mucoceles are rare and occur almost exclusively in patients with CF [52]. Mucoceles are thought to be extremely rare. However, routine imaging of the paranasal sinuses of patients with CF is not usual practice; thus, prevalence of paranasal mucoceles may be higher than expected [51]. Treatment involves resection of the mucocele.

DIAGNOSIS

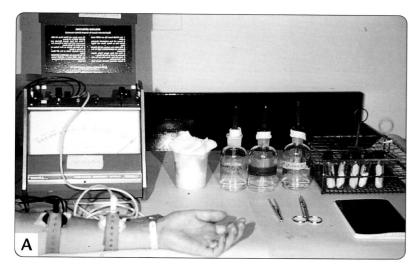

Figure 4-14.

The sweat test. Sweat testing, genotyping, and measurement of nasal potential difference (nasal PD) are available to confirm or exclude the diagnosis of cystic fibrosis [54]. Other specialized diagnostic capabilities include electron microscopic examination of bronchial biopsies for the immotile cilia syndromes and immunologic evaluation for various immune deficiencies that predispose patients to respiratory infections. The sweat test remains one of the cornerstones of the diagnosis and characterization of the cystic fibrosis (CF) syndrome, and it is helpful in confirming the diagnosis in patients with a suspicious clinical picture. Quantitative determinations of chloride in sweat obtained by the Gibson and Cooke iontophoresis method [10] are highly reliable; errors are usually a consequence of sample contamination and technical inexperience. Subcutaneous edema and severe malnutrition can cause false-negative results. False-negative results are associated with hypothyroidism, hypoparathyroidism, and other rare metabolic disorders. **A,** Sweat test administration. Indications for a sweat test include a history of CF in the immediate family, chronic pulmonary disease, or pancreatic insufficiency. Other indicators include nasal polyposis, cirrhosis in childhood, and clinical signs or symptoms suggesting a diagnosis. (*Continued on next page*)

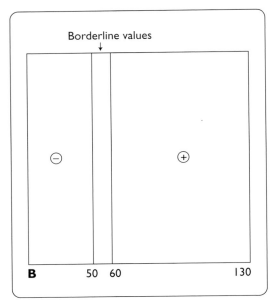

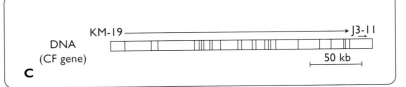

Figure 4-14. (Continued) **B**, Borderline sweat chloride values (50 to 60 mmol/L). More than 98% of patients have abnormal chloride concentrations (ie, >60 mmol/L); however, some individuals present with borderline or normal values, which are usually associated with less common mutations of the CF gene and occur most frequently in adult patients. **C**, CF mutation is

located on the long arm of chromosome 7. When test values are borderline (ie, 50 to 60 mmol/L) and the clinical picture is unclear, genetic testing can be useful in confirming the diagnosis. Commercially available genetic tests can identify up to 60 mutations of the CF gene, which account for approximately 85% of patients. Therefore, approximately 15% of cases are not identified by these tests. Patients with unusual presentations still pose a significant diagnostic challenge. In patients with clinical evidence of CF but normal or borderline sweat chloride concentrations, it is difficult to make the diagnosis of CF. Conventional genetic analysis identifies only a few of the more common CF mutations. In addition, the extension of the analysis to rare mutations is often not practicable. The characteristic differences in nasal PD values from normal subjects and patients with CF can determine if a patient has CF, in cases in which the sweat electrolyte test and genotyping tests are inconclusive [54]. As Na^+ and Cl^- ions move across airway cells, they generate an electrical potential difference that can be measured easily. The magnitude of this nasal PD varies considerably between patients with CF and patients without CF because of differences in how Na^+ and Cl^- ions move. Using a surface electrode to probe various regions of the nasal epithelium, the transepithelial potential in the airway epithelium is measured with respect to the interstitial fluid. Depending on which testing solutions are selected (eg, to block the Na^+ channel or to activate the Cl^- channel), it is possible to determine whether these channels are functional in a patient [55]. Nasal PD measurements also have other uses. Nasal PD can serve as a critical measure for the success of new therapies for CF (outcome measure), including intravenous, oral, or inhaled medications and gene therapy. In addition, nasal PD permits testing of the relationships between genotype and phenotype in terms of specific ion transport defects (Na^+ vs Cl^-) [55]. (Panel C adapted from Collins [53].)

TREATMENT

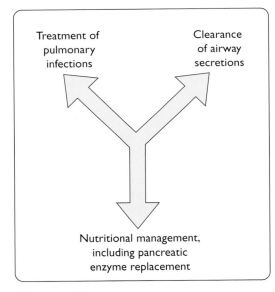

Figure 4-15.
Cornerstones of pulmonary therapy for cystic fibrosis. Treatment of cystic fibrosis is directed toward alleviating symptoms and correcting organ dysfunction. Shown here are the three cornerstones of conventional treatment. Nutritional management is beyond the scope of this chapter; here we focus on airway clearance and treatment of pulmonary infections. We also describe new strategies for managing pulmonary disease, including anti-inflammatory treatments.

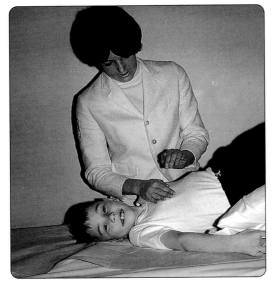

Figure 4-16.
Postural drainage and percussion with vibration. For more than 50 years, this technique has been the primary nonpharmacologic strategy for mobilizing viscous secretions and clearing them from the airways [56]. Postural drainage percussion with vibration is still considered by many the gold standard of therapy, although several

alternative airway clearance techniques (ACTs) exist, including 1) autogenic drainage, which can be performed independently by adolescents and adults; 2) positive expiratory pressure, which involves exhaling against expiratory resistance applied through a mask; and 3) active cycle of breathing technique, an independently performed breathing exercise. These three techniques are less demanding than postural drainage and percussion with vibration and can be performed independently; thus, they are often preferred by patients. Newer ACTs (eg, high-frequency chest percussors and oral oscillators) are less time-consuming and promote independence; however, their effects on patient compliance have not been determined. Although the short-term effect of ACTs on lung function seems limited, lung function appears to deteriorate when they are discontinued. Exercise is considered an important adjunct to ACT, not a replacement. Patients should be encouraged to incorporate ACTs and exercise into their life styles from the time cystic fibrosis is first diagnosed, even when they are asymptomatic. Clinical judgment is the best guide to selecting a regimen that will be most suitable for a particular patient of a given age and circumstance [56].

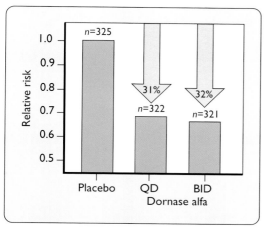

Figure 4-17.

Enzyme therapy effective in clearing airway secretions. Traditional mucolytic therapies, such as *N*-acetylcysteine, confer little benefit in cystic fibrosis (CF) and are rarely used today. However, a cloned enzyme that targets airway DNA is proving efficacious for many patients. Aerosolized recombinant human deoxyribonuclease I (rhDNase, or Pulmozyme ® [Genentech; South San Francisco, CA]) cleaves the DNA residue left by degenerating neutrophils. In doing so, it reduces sputum viscosity and enhances clearance. The enzyme was approved by the US Food and Drug Administration in 1994 for use in CF patients after a clinical trial. The Pulmozyme study enrolled 968 clinically stable patients older than 5 years from 51 CF centers in a randomized, double-blind, placebo-controlled study conducted in conjunction with usual therapy for CF [57]. Patients received 2.5 mg of rhDNase or a placebo once daily (QD) or twice daily (BID) for 24 weeks. Forced expiratory volume in 1 second was improved by approximately 6% in both dosage groups. As shown in the figure, the relative risk of pulmonary exacerbation was significantly reduced by rhDNase. Modest reductions in hospital days and days on parenteral antibiotics were also observed. Similar improvements have been observed in open label studies, including a study conducted in the United Kingdom [58]. Investigators are attempting to identify patient subgroups that will derive maximum benefit from this therapy. Selective β_2-agonists and anticholinergic agents (*eg*, ipratropium bromide) can benefit CF patients who have symptoms of airway hyperresponsiveness due to asthma or other causes. Not all patients benefit from this treatment, however, and the clinical condition of some may even worsen. Thus, patients should be monitored carefully if bronchodilator or anticholinergic therapy is initiated. Because airways inflammation may be an important issue even in the youngest patients with CF, a follow-up study was recently initiated to examine the effects of treatment with dornase alfa of children 6 to 10 years of age with good lung functions (*ie*, FEV_1 95%–96% predicted; FVC 102% predicted) and good nutritional status [60]. In addition, ~20% of the study population had sinusitis, 10% in each of the two cohorts had daily sputum production, and nearly all subjects had pancreatic insufficiency. A total of 474 patients were enrolled into one of the two study cohorts: 235 patients received placebo and 239 patients received dornase alfa. At week 96 of the study, patients receiving dornase alfa demonstrated an initial increase in FEV_1 of 3% that was maintained over the course of the study. FEF 25–75 increased in the dornase alfa group by 8% over the placebo group, and was maintained throughout the study. When researchers looked at pulmonary exacerbations occurring during the study term, the group receiving dornase alfa demonstrated a 34% risk reduction of first exacerbation. These results suggest that early intervention and aggressive therapy in young, relatively healthy patients with CF may provide a substantial reduction in pulmonary exacerbations and a sustained benefit in lung function. (*Adapted from* Fiel [59].)

CLINICAL INDICATIONS FOR INTRAVENOUS ANTIBIOTIC THERAPY IN CYSTIC FIBROSIS

"CF-PANCREAS"
Cough—increased
Fever
Pulmonary function—worsening
Appetite—decreased
Nutritional status—impaired
Complete blood count—leukocytosis with left shift
Radiograph—new infiltrates, overaeration, and mucus plugs
Examination—crackles, wheezes
Activity—decreased
Sputum—thicker, darker, and more abundant

Figure 4-18.

Clinical indications for intravenous antibiotic therapy. Antibiotic therapy for patients with cystic fibrosis has been a cornerstone of treatment for five decades [61]. There is broad consensus regarding the value of intravenous antibiotics for acute pulmonary exacerbations and the indications for its administration. The mnemonic *CF-PANCREAS* covers the signs and symptoms believed to indicate onset of pulmonary exacerbation and the need to initiate treatment. Appropriate antibiotic regimens and special therapeutic considerations for patients with cystic fibrosis are summarized in the figure. The most important aspect of antibiotic therapy for cystic fibrosis is the timely use of appropriate drug combinations. Failure to adhere to these basic principles is the most frequent reason for lack of clinical response. At this time, there is less agreement on the routine use of antibiotics for maintenance than for their use in treating pulmonary exacerbations (*see* Fig. 4-20). The prophylactic use of intravenous antibiotics, a practice that is advocated by Danish physicians, is uncommon in the United States and Canada. (*Adapted from* Schidlow [62].)

A. FIRST-CHOICE ANTIBIOTIC THERAPY IN THE TREATMENT OF PULMONARY BACTERIAL INFECTIONS IN CYSTIC FIBROSIS

Prevalent bacteria	Antibiotic	Dose Child	Adult
Staphylococcus aureus	Cephalothin	25–50 mg/kg every 6 h	1 g every 6 h
	Nafcillin	25–50 mg/kg every 6 h	1 g every 6 h
Haemophilus influenzae and S. aureus	Ticarcillin-clavulanate plus gentamicin	100 mg of ticarcillin/kg and 3.3 mg of clavulanate/kg every 6 h	3 g of ticarcillin and 0.1 g of clavulanate every 6 h
		3 mg every 8 h	3 mg/kg every 8 h
S. aureus and Pseudomonas aeruginosa	Ticarcillin-clavulanate plus tobramycin	100 mg of ticarcillin/kg and 3.3 mg of clavulanate/kg every 8 h	3 g of ticarcillin and 0.1 g of clavulanate every 6 h
		3 mg every 8 h	3 mg/kg every 8 h
P. aeruginosa only	Ticarcillin	100 mg/kg every 6 h	3 g every 6 h
	plus tobramycin	3 mg/kg every 8 h	3 mg/kg every 8 h
P. aeruginosa and Burkholderia cepacia	Ceftazidime	50–75 mg/kg every 8 h	2 g every 8 h
	plus ciprofloxacin	15 mg/kg every 12 h	400 mg every 12 h IV
B. cepacia only	Chloramphenicol	15–20 mg/kg every 6 h	15–20 mg/kg every 6 h
	or trimethoprim-sulfamethoxazole	5 mg of trimethoprim/kg and 25 mg of sulfamethoxazole/kg every 6 h	5 mg of trimethoprim/kg and 25 mg of sulfamethoxazole/kg every 6 h
	or both		

B. ALTERNATIVE ANTIBIOTIC THERAPY IN THE TREATMENT OF PULMONARY BACTERIAL INFECTIONS IN CYSTIC FIBROSIS

Prevalent bacteria	Antibiotic	Dose Child	Adult
Staphylococcus aureus (MRSA)	Vancomycin	15 mg/kg every 6 h	500 mg every 6 h
Haemophilus influenzae and S. aureus	Nafcillin	25–50 mg/kg every 6 h	1 g every 6 h
	plus gentamicin	3 mg/kg every 8 h	3 mg/kg every 8 h
Pseudomonas aeruginosa	Tobramycin	3 mg/kg every 8 h	3 mg/kg every 8 h
	plus ceftazidime,	50 mg/kg every 8 h	2 g every 8 h
	piperacillin,	100 mg/kg every 6 h	3 g every 6 h
	or imipenem	15–25 mg/kg every 6 h	500 mg–1 g every 6 h
	Aztreonam	50 mg/kg every 6 h	2 g every 8 h
	plus amikacin	5–7.5 mg/kg every 8 h	5–7.5 mg/kg every 8 h
P. aeruginosa and Burkholderia cepacia	Ceftazidime	50–75 mg/kg every 8 h	2 g every 8 h
	plus chloramphenicol	15–20 mg/kg every 6 h	15–20 mg/kg every 6 h
	or trimethoprim-sulfamethoxazole	5 mg of trimethoprim/kg IV and 25 mg of sulfamethoxazole/kg every 6 h	5 mg of trimethoprim/kg IV and 25 mg of sulfamethoxazole/kg every 6 h

IV—intravenously; MRSA—mettlicilln-resistant S. aureus.

Figure 4-19.
A and **B**, Bacteria associated with exacerbations of pulmonary infection in patients with cystic fibrosis and appropriate intravenous treatments. Although intravenous aminoglycosides are active against *Pseudomonas aeruginosa*, the large doses that are required increase the risk of nephrotoxic and ototoxic effects. Short-term, high-dose aerosol administration of tobramycin is an efficacious and safe treatment for endobronchial infection with *P. aeruginosa* in patients with clinically stable cystic fibrosis [63]. (*Adapted from* Ramsey [19].)

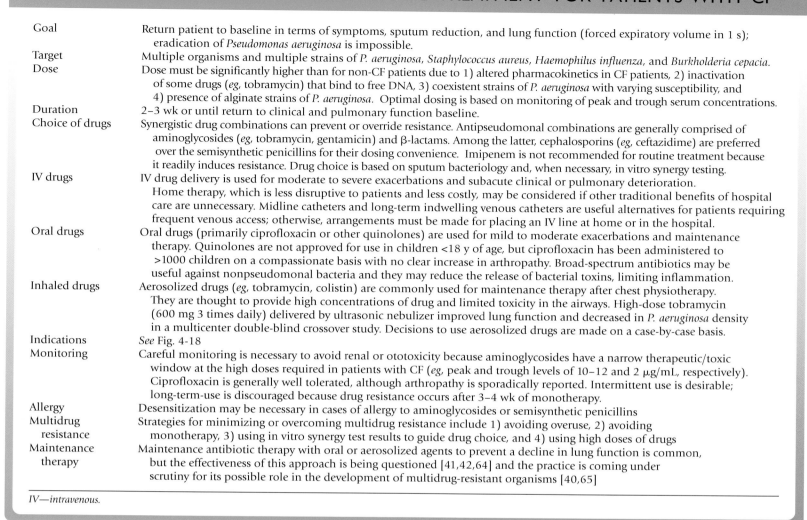

Goal	Return patient to baseline in terms of symptoms, sputum reduction, and lung function (forced expiratory volume in 1 s); eradication of *Pseudomonas aeruginosa* is impossible.
Target	Multiple organisms and multiple strains of *P. aeruginosa, Staphylococcus aureus, Haemophilus influenza,* and *Burkholderia cepacia.*
Dose	Dose must be significantly higher than for non-CF patients due to 1) altered pharmacokinetics in CF patients, 2) inactivation of some drugs (*eg*, tobramycin) that bind to free DNA, 3) coexistent strains of *P. aeruginosa* with varying susceptibility, and 4) presence of alginate strains of *P. aeruginosa.* Optimal dosing is based on monitoring of peak and trough serum concentrations.
Duration	2–3 wk or until return to clinical and pulmonary function baseline.
Choice of drugs	Synergistic drug combinations can prevent or override resistance. Antipseudomonal combinations are generally comprised of aminoglycosides (*eg*, tobramycin, gentamicin) and β-lactams. Among the latter, cephalosporins (*eg*, ceftazidime) are preferred over the semisynthetic penicillins for their dosing convenience. Imipenem is not recommended for routine treatment because it readily induces resistance. Drug choice is based on sputum bacteriology and, when necessary, in vitro synergy testing.
IV drugs	IV drug delivery is used for moderate to severe exacerbations and subacute clinical or pulmonary deterioration. Home therapy, which is less disruptive to patients and less costly, may be considered if other traditional benefits of hospital care are unnecessary. Midline catheters and long-term indwelling venous catheters are useful alternatives for patients requiring frequent venous access; otherwise, arrangements must be made for placing an IV line at home or in the hospital.
Oral drugs	Oral drugs (primarily ciprofloxacin or other quinolones) are used for mild to moderate exacerbations and maintenance therapy. Quinolones are not approved for use in children <18 y of age, but ciprofloxacin has been administered to >1000 children on a compassionate basis with no clear increase in arthropathy. Broad-spectrum antibiotics may be useful against nonpseudomonal bacteria and they may reduce the release of bacterial toxins, limiting inflammation.
Inhaled drugs	Aerosolized drugs (*eg*, tobramycin, colistin) are commonly used for maintenance therapy after chest physiotherapy. They are thought to provide high concentrations of drug and limited toxicity in the airways. High-dose tobramycin (600 mg 3 times daily) delivered by ultrasonic nebulizer improved lung function and decreased in *P. aeruginosa* density in a multicenter double-blind crossover study. Decisions to use aerosolized drugs are made on a case-by-case basis.
Indications	*See* Fig. 4-18
Monitoring	Careful monitoring is necessary to avoid renal or ototoxicity because aminoglycosides have a narrow therapeutic/toxic window at the high doses required in patients with CF (*eg*, peak and trough levels of 10–12 and 2 μg/mL, respectively). Ciprofloxacin is generally well tolerated, although arthropathy is sporadically reported. Intermittent use is desirable; long-term-use is discouraged because drug resistance occurs after 3–4 wk of monotherapy.
Allergy	Desensitization may be necessary in cases of allergy to aminoglycosides or semisynthetic penicillins
Multidrug resistance	Strategies for minimizing or overcoming multidrug resistance include 1) avoiding overuse, 2) avoiding monotherapy, 3) using in vitro synergy test results to guide drug choice, and 4) using high doses of drugs
Maintenance therapy	Maintenance antibiotic therapy with oral or aerosolized agents to prevent a decline in lung function is common, but the effectiveness of this approach is being questioned [41,42,64] and the practice is coming under scrutiny for its possible role in the development of multidrug-resistant organisms [40,65]

IV—intravenous.

Figure 4-20.
Special considerations in antibiotic treatment for patients with cystic fibrosis (CF).

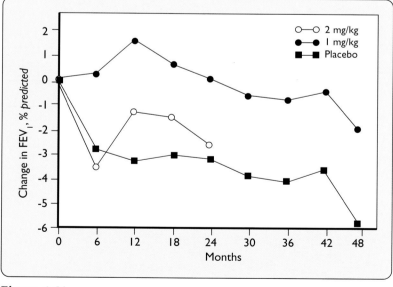

Figure 4-21.
Effects of 4-year anti-inflammatory therapy with prednisone on lung function. Although the initial results of a 4-year double-blind trial of high-dose

(2 mg/kg) alternate-day prednisone in 45 children younger than 12 years of age suggested that treatment was efficacious and without side effects [66], subsequent results were less promising. Growth retardation, glucose intolerance, osteoporosis, and cataracts were reported among 14 of 17 patients observed 6 years after the study [67]. To confirm the efficacy of corticosteroid treatment and to assess adverse effects more thoroughly, a larger study was mounted by the Cystic Fibrosis Foundation Prednisone Trial Group [68]. The results appear in the figure. Investigators enrolled 285 children aged 6 to 14 years with mild to moderate lung disease. The children were randomly assigned to receive high-dose prednisone (2 mg/kg), low-dose prednisone (1 mg/kg), or placebo on alternate days. The high-dose group was terminated early because of growth retardation, glucose abnormalities, and cataract formation [69]. Results were modestly beneficial with respect to forced expiratory volume in 1 second (FEV$_1$), but few other beneficial effects were seen and linear growth retardation was significant after 24 months of therapy. Mean FEV$_1$ (% predicted) declined less relative to baseline among patients receiving low-dose prednisone throughout the entire study; the beneficial effect was seen at 6 months and did not increase later. The mean FEV$_1$ of low-dose prednisone patients was not significantly different from baseline at 48 months. Thus, administration of prednisone in doses of 1 mg/kg every other day may be beneficial in carefully selected patients to curb signs of heightened endobronchial inflammation. (*Adapted from* Eigen *et al.* [68].)

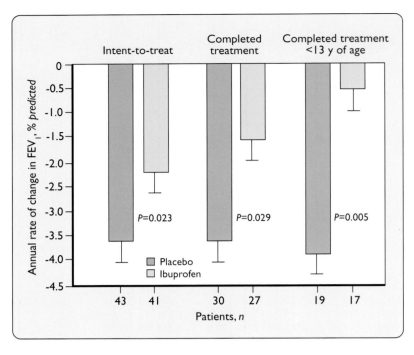

Figure 4-22.

Effects of long-term anti-inflammatory therapy with ibuprofen on the annual rate of change in lung function. Unresolved safety issues with respect to the long-term use of steroids for patients with cystic fibrosis have heightened interest in the use of ibuprofen as a treatment for patients with mild lung disease. Ibuprofen is believed to reduce inflammation by decreasing neutrophil influx and reducing the stimulus for leukotriene B_4, a chemoattractant that is markedly elevated in the airway surface fluid of patients with cystic fibrosis. Because leukotriene B_4 promotes neutrophil adherence, aggregation, migration, degranulation, and superoxide release, inhibition of its production by ibuprofen would inhibit inflammatory damage to the lung. The results of a recent 4-year, randomized, placebo-controlled, double-blind trial of high-dose ibuprofen in 85 cystic fibrosis patients with mild lung disease are shown in the figure [70]. Patients (aged 5 to 39 years) tolerated twice-daily treatment with 20 to 30 mg/kg. The authors concluded that high-dose ibuprofen, taken consistently, significantly slowed the progression of lung disease over the 4-year period without significant toxicity. Compared with placebo, ibuprofen decreased the annual rate of decline of pulmonary measures and Brasfield chest radiographic scores, and preserved the percentage of ideal body weight. For patients meeting the prospective criteria for completing the trial, the annual rate of decline in lung function, measured by the percent predicted forced expiratory volume in 1 second (FEV_1) was 59% lower for the ibuprofen-treated patients. Establishing the appropriate dose by pharmacokinetic studies in each patient is recommended, and monitoring for rare adverse effects is important. Administration of ibuprofen has been recommended, especially for patients aged 5 to 13 years who have mild disease. (*Data from* Konstan *et al.* [70].)

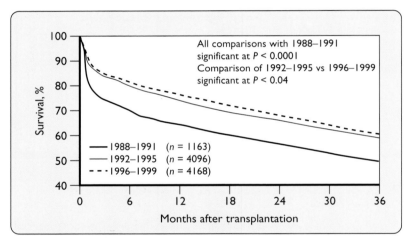

Figure 4-23.

Lung transplantation and improved actuarial survival of patients with cystic fibrosis (CF). Despite treatment advances that have dramatically extended the life expectancy of patients with CF, most patients eventually die of progressive lung disease. Lung transplantation for end-stage CF, first performed in 1985, has altered this scenario for some patients. By 1995,

more than 650 patients had undergone transplantation; bilateral sequential lung transplant is the usual procedure [71]. The long-term implications of this technology for the CF community are unclear. Due to the acute shortage of donor organs, the option of transplantation is available only to a limited number of patients; on average, CF patients wait 1 to 2 years for available organs, and an unacceptably large number of them die while on the waiting list. Consequently, some living donor lobar transplants have also been performed. Although CF presents many additional management challenges once thought to be insurmountable, transplantation has prolonged survival and improved quality of life for hundreds suffering from end-stage disease before surgery. The long-term survival of CF patients does not differ from that of other patients undergoing double-lung transplantation. Despite the clinical challenges posed by their disease, CF patients make good transplantation candidates for a number of reasons, including 1) life-threatening manifestations are usually confined to the respiratory system, 2) patients are relatively young when considered for transplant, and 3) patients have extensive experience in adhering to complex treatment regimens. Data from the International Society of Heart and Lung Transplantation reveal that 1-year actuarial survival is 75% and 3-year survival is 60% for all conditions requiring transplantation [73]. The survival rate for CF patients is similar to that of other patients undergoing transplantation. (*Adapted from* Hosenpud *et al.* [72].)

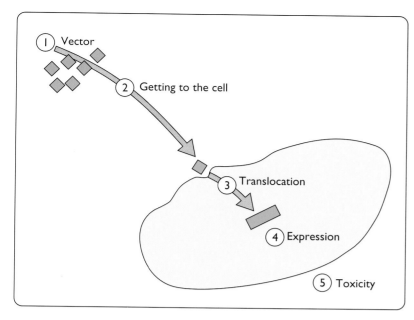

Figure 4-24.

Hurdles to successful gene therapy. Although therapeutic regimens have increased life expectancy and improved the quality of life for thousands of patients, traditional therapies target the signs and symptoms of cystic fibrosis (CF) and a cure for CF remains elusive [73]. An intensive effort to develop gene therapy for CF has been underway since the gene was cloned in 1989. By mid-1995, 10 National Institutes of Health–approved CF gene therapy clinical trials were underway, representing more than half of the total trials approved for all inherited genetic diseases [74]. Most trials have used viral or plasmid vectors, but a new approach uses molecular conjugates designed to draw DNA molecules into cells by receptor-mediated endocytosis [75,76]. Early studies have identified five hurdles to successful gene therapy [77]: 1) Choosing the right vector—vectors must be large enough to incorporate an expression cassette comprising 4.5 KB recombinant human cystic fibrosis transmembrane conductance regulator (CFTR) complementary DNA (cDNA) and a promotor; they should also be stable, nonimmunogenic, and specific for the target cells; ideally, they should also be easily produced and purified. 2) Delivering the vector to the target cell—it is unclear which cells are the most appropriate targets; moreover, viscous CF mucus and humor immunity may serve as barriers. 3) Translocating the genetic information to the nucleus—once the vector has been transferred into the target cell, it must be translocated to the nucleus to express the normal CFTR cDNA. Viral vectors are more efficient than plasmid-liposome systems, but the adenovirus vector is less efficient than anticipated. 4) Expressing the gene—expression of the CFTR protein is thwarted not only by the unexplained loss of the vector genome, but also by late immune mechanisms. 5) Reducing toxicity—toxicity encountered in some human gene therapy trials appears to be related to the vector rather than to the CFTR cDNA. Studies are underway to overcome these hurdles. (*Adapted from* Crystal [77].)

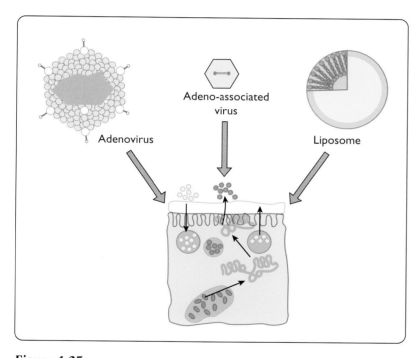

Figure 4-25.

Approaches to gene therapy for cystic fibrosis. Three gene therapy strategies are being investigated. 1) Adenoviruses—replication-deficient recombinant adenoviruses are the best known and most widely studied of the viral vectors [78–86]. In animal models, adenoviruses elicit a cytotoxic T cell–mediated immune response, which is associated with transient lung inflammation after airway administration [80,84,85], and repetitive dosing stimulates production of neutralizing antibodies [87–89]. In clinical trials, efficacy was lower than expected, expression was transient, and molecular evidence of gene transfer did not necessarily predict or correlate with functional correction [90]. Moreover, significant inflammation has been noted in some patients [90–91]. Second- and third-generation vectors that are less easily recognized by the immune system are being developed. Some strategies attempt to disguise the virus by modifying its immunogenic epitopes; another approach is to coat the virus, creating a "stealth" vector [77]. 2) Adeno-associated virus—recombinant adeno-associated virus (AAV) is a small, single-stranded DNA virus, barely large enough to accommodate the expression cassette. Preclinical studies have shown that AAV does not integrate into the genome as readily as expected, making it likely that expression will be transient. Moreover, when integration occurs, it is not site-specific, a problem that raises the specter of mutagenesis from random insertion of AAV genes into the host genome. Recombinant AAV is also difficult to produce [74]. 3) Liposomes—an alternative, nonviral strategy uses plasmid cystic fibrosis transmembrane conductance regulator complementary DNA complexed to a cationic lipid such as DOPE (dioleoylphosphatidylethanolamine). Lipid-mediated gene transfer avoids problems with immunogenicity, and it has successfully transfected genes in animal models [92,93] and in human nasal epithelium [94]. However, it is much less efficient than the viral approach, and gene expression remains low and transient. Investigators are inserting proteins analogous to viruses into their constructs in an effort to improve the yield [77]. Clinical trials for cystic fibrosis using lipid-mediated gene transfer are underway in the United States [74]. Further data are needed regarding the role of the CFTR defect in cystic fibrosis for researchers to determine the level of corrected CFTR expression that is required to effectively treat the disease. While more than 200 trials of gene therapies have been undertaken, no gene therapy has received approval by the US Food and Drug Administration (FDA). (*Adapted from* Wilson [95].)

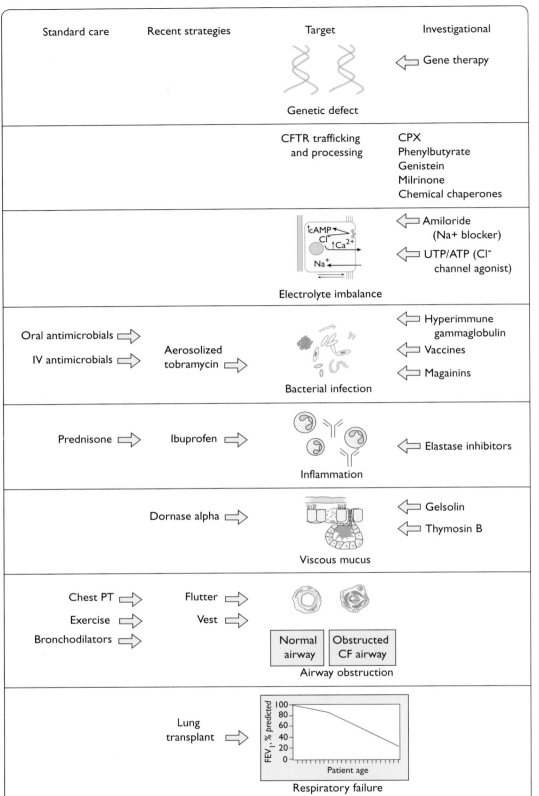

Standard care	Recent strategies	Target	Investigational
		Genetic defect	Gene therapy
		CFTR trafficking and processing	CPX Phenylbutyrate Genistein Milrinone Chemical chaperones
		Electrolyte imbalance	Amiloride (Na+ blocker) UTP/ATP (Cl⁻ channel agonist)
Oral antimicrobials IV antimicrobials	Aerosolized tobramycin	Bacterial infection	Hyperimmune gammaglobulin Vaccines Magainins
Prednisone	Ibuprofen	Inflammation	Elastase inhibitors
	Dornase alpha	Viscous mucus	Gelsolin Thymosin B
Chest PT Exercise Bronchodilators	Flutter Vest	Airway obstruction Normal airway / Obstructed CF airway	
Lung transplant		Respiratory failure	

Figure 4-26.

Current treatments target specific pathophysiologic elements of cystic fibrosis (CF). Although our understanding of the pathogenesis of cystic fibrotic lung disease remains incomplete, a knowledge of the organ-level pathobiology has permitted development of rational and effective management strategies. A broad range of therapies is available to treat the pulmonary symptoms of cystic fibrosis, and several promising treatment strategies are being investigated [27]. IV—intravenous; PT—physiotherapy.

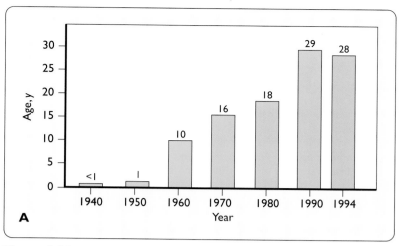

A

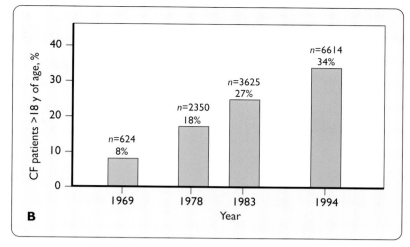

B

Figure 4-27.
Developments in life expectancy of patients with cystic fibrosis (CF) linked to quality of care. **A** and **B**, The median survival age of patients with CF has almost tripled since 1960 (*panel A*), and the number of patients older than 18 years of age has quadrupled since 1969 (*panel B*). The burgeoning number of adult patients comprises a dramatic testimonial to the network of CF clinics that care for pediatric patients throughout North America. Unfortunately, we are less equipped to meet the needs of adults with CF [96]. On reaching adulthood, the care of patients with CF should be transferred to adult programs with personnel with the expertise to meet their special needs. However, many young adults are unable to find age-appropriate caregivers and, therefore, remain under the care of pediatric teams or drift from the health care system altogether.

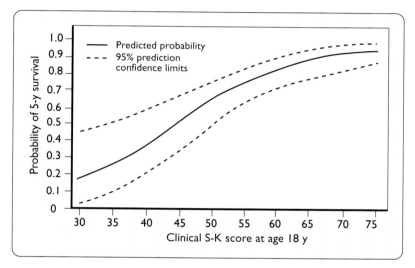

Figure 4-28.
Using clinical scores to predict survival in young adults with cystic fibrosis. Median survival of patients with cystic fibrosis is approximately 29 years. Long-term follow-up of 110 young adults with cystic fibrosis identified factors that predicted 5-year survival. Stepwise logistic regression applied to 11 variables identified Shwachman and Kulczycki (S-K) scores at 18 years of age as the best predictor of survival to age 23 [97]. The S-K scoring system assesses general activity, physical findings, and nutritional status, with 25 points for each and a total of 75 points for normal findings [98]. Median duration of survival for patients with clinical scores of 65 to 75 (12 years) was more than double that of patients with clinical scores of 30 to 49 (5 years). Favorable prognostic factors for long-term survival (*ie*, beyond age 18) include good nutrition, good pulmonary function, high clinical scores, and absence of chronic respiratory colonization with multidrug-resistant organisms [93]. Specialized centers for adult patients with cystic fibrosis make it possible to collect longitudinal historical, physical, and laboratory data that will permit clinicians to respond promptly to subtle changes in any of these indicators; timely intervention is likely to slow disease progression and prolong survival. (*Adapted from* Huang *et al.* [97].)

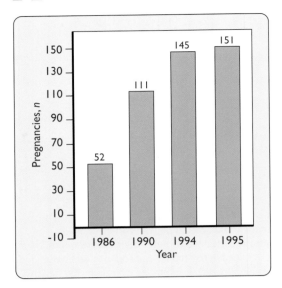

Figure 4-29.

Reproductive issues of men and women with cystic fibrosis (CF). Clinical challenges associated with caring for adult patients with CF are not limited to increasing morbidity and the prospect of death. The number of pregnancies among women with CF has increased 10-fold over the past 30 years [99], and the number nearly tripled in a recent 8-year period. Most women with CF tolerate pregnancy well, despite earlier fears that pregnancy is inherently hazardous for them [100,101]; however, pregnancy may still be contraindicated in most patients with severely compromised pulmonary and pancreatic status. Pregnancy is only one of several issues that were once of little consequence to those who cared for pediatric patients but that are becoming increasingly relevant as the number of adults with CF escalates [102]. Infertility is nearly universal among men with CF as a consequence of congenital bilateral absence of the vas deferens. Options are limited to adoption and artificial insemination by a donor. However, microsurgical epididymal sperm aspiration in combination with in vitro fertilization has been performed successfully [103], and there is no reason to believe that the technology should not be effective among men with CF, provided that sperm count, morphology, and motility are normal.

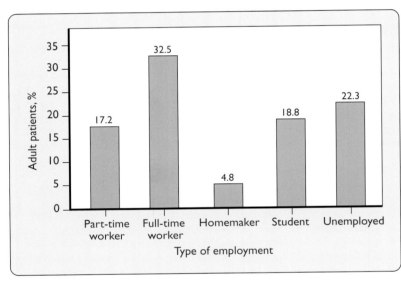

Figure 4-30.

Employment status of adult patients with cystic fibrosis (CF), 1994. Adult patients with CF also present clinicians with complex psychosocial challenges. Approximately 50% of adult CF patients were employed full- or part-time, and almost 20% were students. This demonstrates that many patients pursue their educational and vocational goals successfully in the event of daunting obstacles. The trend toward home-based intravenous therapy, received by 30% of adult patients in 1994 [5], has facilitated these activities. However, the transition to independence is not always easy, nor even possible. Not all patients are able to leave their family homes for college or paid employment, and many of those who become independent face diminished opportunities and a reduced earning capacity because of the constraints of their illness [104–106]. Many patients also face difficulties in obtaining health insurance. Although the resilience of most CF patients is remarkable, the psychosocial costs of increased life expectancy are substantial. Thus, it is important to provide support services appropriate to their age and situation. The situation faced by young adults with CF represents a serious public policy issue. The health care system is not prepared to deal with the growing population of individuals with so-called childhood disorders who have achieved adulthood and are living to a relatively advanced age [96]. The problem is particularly acute for young adults who are not yet integrated into the work force and who lack health insurance. Care for many young adults with CF—and others with chronic diseases—is seriously compromised. Our challenge as caregivers is to develop strategies and mechanisms to ensure that CF patients continue to receive the best possible care as they grow older. (*Adapted from* The New Insights Editorial Board [13].)

REFERENCES

1. Boat TF: Cystic fibrosis. In *Textbook of Respiratory Medicine.* Edited by Murray JF, Nadel JA. Philadelphia: WB Saunders; 1988:1126–1152.

2. FitzSimmons SC: The changing epidemiology of cystic fibrosis. *J Pediatr* 1993, 122:1–9.

3. Welsh MJ, Smith AE: Cystic fibrosis. *Sci Am* 1995, 273:52–59.

4. Taussig LM: Cystic fibrosis: an overview. In *Cystic Fibrosis.* Edited by Taussig LM. New York, NY: Thieme-Stratton Inc; 1984:1–9.

5. Hess JH, Saphir O: Celiac disease: chronic intestinal digestion. *J Pediatr* 1935, 6:1–13.

6. Fanconi G, Uehlinger E, Knaver C: Coeliaksyndrom bei angeborener zystischer pankreas fibromatose und bronchiektasien. *Wien Med Wochenschr* 1936, 86:753–756. (Cited in Rosenfeld MA, Collins FS: Gene therapy for cystic fibrosis. *Chest* 1996, 109:241–252.)

7. Andersen DH: Cystic fibrosis of the pancreas and its relation to celiac disease. *Am J Dis Child* 1938, 56:344–399.

8. Andersen DH, Hodges RG: Celiac syndrome. V. Genetics of cystic fibrosis of the pancreas with a consideration of etiology. *Am J Dis Child* 1946, 72:62–80.

9. di Sant'Agnese PA, Darling RC, Perera GA, Shea E: Abnormal electrolytic composition of sweat in cystic fibrosis of the pancreas: clinical significance and relationship to the disease. *Pediatrics* 1953, 12:549–562.

10. Gibson LE, Cooke RE: A test for concentration of electrolytes in sweat in cystic fibrosis of the pancreas. *Pediatrics* 1959, 23:545–549.

11. Quinton PM: Chloride impermeability in cystic fibrosis. *Nature* 1983, 301:421–422.

12. Knowles MR, Stutts MJ, Spock A, *et al.*: Abnormal ion permeation through cystic fibrosis respiratory epithelium. *Science* 1983, 221:1067–1070.

13. New Insights Editorial Board: A look at the national CF patient registry. *New Insights Into Cystic Fibrosis* 1996, 3:1–6.

14. Kerem BS, Rommens JM, Buchanan JA, *et al.*: Identification of the cystic fibrosis gene: genetic analysis. *Science* 1989, 245:1073–1080.

15. Riordan JR, Rommens JM, Kerem B-S, et al.: Identification of the cystic fibrosis gene: cloning and characterization of complementary DNA. *Science* 1989, 245:1066–1073.

16. Rommens JM, Iannuzzi MC, Kerem B-S, et al.: Identification of the cystic fibrosis gene: chromosome walking and jumping. *Science* 1989, 245:1059–1065.

17. Anderson MP, Gregory RJ, Thompson S, et al.: Demonstration that CFTR is a chloride channel by alteration of its anion selectivity. *Science* 1991, 53:202–205.

18. Stutts MJ, Canessa JC, Olsen M, et al.: CFTR as a cAMP-dependent regulator of sodium channels. *Science* 1995, 269:847–850.

19. Ramsey BW: Management of pulmonary disease in patients with cystic fibrosis. *N Engl J Med* 1996, 335:179–188.

20. Cutting GR: Genotype defect: its effect on cellular function and phenotypic expression. *Sem Respir Crit Care Med* 1994, 15:356–363.

21. Zeitlin PL: Future pharmacological treatments of cystic fibrosis. *Respiration* 2000, 67:351–357.

22. Mickle JE, Cutting GR: Clinical implications of cystic fibrosis transmembrane conductance regulator mutations. In *Clinics in Chest Medicine—Cystic Fibrosis,* Volume 19. Edited by Fiel SB. Philadelphia: WB Saunders; 1999:443–458.

23. Haardt M, Benharouga M, Lechardeur D, et al.: C-terminal truncations destabilize the cystic fibrosis transmembrane conductance regulator without impairing its biogenesis: a novel class of mutation. *J Biol Chem* 1999, 274:21873–21877.

24. Kerem B, Kerem E: The molecular basis for disease variability in cystic fibrosis. *Eur J Hum Genet* 1996, 4:65–73.

25. Wilschanski M, Zielenski J, Markiewicz D, et al.: Correlation of sweat chloride concentration with classes of the cystic fibrosis transmembrane conductance regulator gene mutations. *J Pediatr* 1995, 127:705–710.

26. Welsh MJ, Smith AE: Molecular mechanisms of CFTR chloride channel dysfunction in cystic fibrosis. *Cell* 1993, 73:1251–1254.

27. Mastella G: Relationships between gene mutations and clinical features in cystic fibrosis. *Pediatr Pulmonol* 1995, 11:63–65.

28. Burke W, Aitken ML, Chen S-H, Scott CR: Variable severity of pulmonary disease in adults with identical cystic fibrosis mutations. *Chest* 1992, 102:506–509.

29. The Cystic Fibrosis Genotype-Phenotype Consortium: Correlation between genotype and phenotype in patients with cystic fibrosis. *N Engl J Med* 1993, 329:1308–1313.

30. Marshall BC: Pathophysiology of pulmonary disease in cystic fibrosis. *Sem Res Crit Care Med* 1994, 15:364–374.

31. Birrer P: Consequences of unbalanced protease in the lung: protease involvement in destruction and local defense mechanisms of the lung. *Agents Actions Suppl* 1993, 40:3–12.

32. Smith JJ, Travis SM, Greenberg EP, Welsh MJ: Cystic fibrosis airway epithelia fail to kill bacteria because of abnormal airway surface fluid. *Cell* 1996, 85:229–236.

33. Govan JRW, Nelson JW: Microbiology of cystic fibrosis lung infections: themes and issues. *JR Soc Med* 1993, 86(suppl 20):11–18.

34. Ruef C, Jefferson DM, Schlegel SE, Suter S: Regulation of cytokine secretion by cystic fibrosis airway epithelial cells. *Eur Respir J* 1993, 6:1429–1436.

35. Sibille Y, Marchandise FX: Pulmonary immune cells in health and disease: polymorphonuclear neutrophils. *Eur Respir J* 1993, 6:1429–1443.

36. Warner JO: Immunology of cystic fibrosis. *Br Med Bull* 1992, 48:893–911.

37. Koch C, Høiby N: Pathogenesis of cystic fibrosis. *Lancet,* 1993, 341:1065–1069.

38. McElvaney NG, Doujaiji B, Moan MJ, et al.: Pharmacokinetics of recombinant secretory leukoprotease inhibitor aerosolized to normals and individuals with cystic fibrosis. *Am Rev Respir Dis* 1993, 148:1056–1060.

39. Pier GB, Saunders JM, Ames P, et al.: Opsonophagocytic killing antibody to *Pseudomonas aeruginosa* mucoid exopolysaccharide in older noncolonized patients with cystic fibrosis. *N Engl J Med* 1987, 317:793–798.

40. Prince A, Saiman L: *Pseudomonas aeruginosa* pili bind to asialo GM1 which is increased on the surface of cystic fibrosis epithelial cells. *J Clin Invest* 1993, 92:1875–1880.

41. Stutman HR: Presented at the Ninth Annual North American Cystic Fibrosis Conference, October 11-15, 1995; Dallas, Texas.

42. Beardsmore CS, Thompson JR, Williams A, et al.: Pulmonary function in infants with cystic fibrosis: the effects of antibiotic treatment. *Arch Dis Child* 1994, 71:133–137.

43. Jensen T, Pedersen SS, Hoiby N, et al.: Use of antibiotics in cystic fibrosis: the Danish approach. *Antibiot Chemother* 1989, 42:237–246.

44. Coenye T, Mahenthiralingam E, Henry D, et al.: Classification of Burkholderia cepacia-like biocontrol strains and strains isolated from CF patients as a new member of the B. cepacia complex [abstract]. *Pediatr Pulmonol* 2000, 20:289.

45. Saiman L: Epidemiology and management of infection. In *Highlights.* Bethesda, MD: Cystic Fibrosis Foundation; 1995:26–28.

46. Demko CA, Stern RC, Doerchuk CF: Stenotrophomonas maltophilia in cystic fibrosis. *Pediatr Pulmonol* 1998, 25(5):304–308.

47. Cystic Fibrosis Foundation: Concepts in care: pulmonary complications of cystic fibrosis. *Consensus Conferences* 1991, II:Sect III.

48. Schidlow DV, Taussig LM, Knowles MR: Cystic Fibrosis Foundation Consensus Conference report on pulmonary complications of cystic fibrosis. *Pediatr Pulmonol* 1993, 15:187–198.

49. Boucher RC: Cystic fibrosis. In *Harrison's Principles of Internal Medicine,* edn 13. Edited by Isselbacher KI, Braunwald E, Wilson JD, et al. New York: McGraw-Hill; 1994:1194–1197.

50. Gentile VG, Isaacson G: Patterns of sinusitis in cystic fibrosis. *Laryngoscope* 1996, 106:1005–1009.

51. Sexauer W, Schidlow D, Fiel SB: Unusual manifestations of cystic fibrosis. *Sem Respir Crit Care Med* 1994, 15:375–382.

52. Zrada SE, Isaacson GC: Endoscopic treatment of pediatric ethmoid mucoceles. *Am J Otolaryngol* 1996, 17:197–201.

53. Collins FS: Cystic fibrosis: molecular biology and therapeutic implications. *Science* 1992, 256:774–779.

54. Alton EWFW, Currie D, Logan-Sinclair R, et al.: Nasal potential difference: a clinical diagnostic test for cystic fibrosis. *Eur Respir J* 1990, 3:922–926.

55. Hofmann T, Böhmer O, Bittner P, et al.: Conventional and modified nasal potential difference measurement: clinical use in cystic fibrosis. *Am J Respir Crit Care Med* 1997, 155:1908–1913.

56. Davidson G, McIlwaine M: Airway clearance techniques in cystic fibrosis. *New Insights into Cystic Fibrosis* 1995, 3:6–11.

57. Fuchs HJ, Borowitz DS, Christiansen DH, et al.: The effect of aerosolized recombinant DNase on respiratory exacerbations and pulmonary function in patients with cystic fibrosis. *New Engl J Med* 1994, 331:637–642.

58. Shah PL, Scott SF, Fuchs HJ, et al.: Medium term treatment of stable stage cystic fibrosis with recombinant human Dnase I. *Thorax* 1995, 50:333–338.

59. Fiel SB: Clinical management of pulmonary disease in cystic fibrosis. *Lancet* 1993, 341:1070–1074.

60. Konstan MW, Tiddens HA, Quan JM, et al.: A randomized, placebo-controlled trial of two years' treatment with dornase alfa (Pulmozyme(r)) in cystic fibrosis patients aged 6–10 years with early lung disease [abstract]. *Pediatr Pulmonol* 2000, 20:299.

61. di Sant'Agnese PEA, Andersen DH: Celiac syndrome: IV. Chemotherapy in infections of the respiratory tract associated with cystic fibrosis of the pancreas: observations with penicillin and drugs of the sulfonamide group, with special reference to penicillin aerosol. *Am J Dis Child* 1946, 72:17–61.

62. Schidlow DV: Cystic fibrosis. In *A Practical Guide to Pediatrics.* Edited by Schidlow DV, Smith DSS. Philadelphia: Hanley and Belfus; 1994:75–81.

63. Ramsey BW, Dorkin HL, Eisenberg JD, et al.: Efficacy of aerolised tobramycin in patients with cystic fibrosis. *N Engl J Med* 1993, 328:1740–1746.

64. Sheldon CD, Assoufi BK, Hodson ME: Regular three monthly ciprofloxacin in adult cystic fibrosis patients infected with P. aeruginosa. *Respir Med* 1993, 87:587–593.

65. Accurso FJ: Lung disease in infants with cystic fibrosis. *New Insights Into Cystic Fibrosis* 1996, 4:1–7.

66. Auerbach HS, Williams M, Kirkpatrick JA, Colten HR: Alternate-day prednisone reduces morbidity and improves pulmonary function in cystic fibrosis. *Lancet* 1985, 2:686–688.

67. Donati MA, Haver K, Gerson W, et al.: Long term alternate day prednisone therapy in cystic fibrosis. *Pediatr Pulmonol Suppl* 1990, 5:277

68. Eigen H, Rosenstein BJ, FitzSimmons S, Schidlow DV: A multicenter study of alternate-day prednisone therapy in patients with cystic fibrosis. *J Pediatr* 1995, 126:515–523.

69. Rosenstein BJ, Eigen H: Risks of alternate-day prednisone in patients with cystic fibrosis. *Pediatr* 1991, 87:245–246.

70. Konstan MW, Byard PJ, Hoppel CL, Davis PB: Effect of high-dose ibuprofen in patients with cystic fibrosis. *N Engl J Med* 1995, 332:848–854.

71. Cryz SJ Jr, Wedgwood J, Lang AB, et al.: Immunization of noncolonized cystic fibrosis patients against *Pseudomonas aeruginosa. J Infect Dis* 1994, 169:1159–1162.

72. Hosenpud JD, Bennett LE, Keck BM, et al.: *The Registry of the International Society for Heart and Lung Transplantation Seventeenth Official Report.* 2000, 19(10):909–931.

73. Kotloff RM, Zuckerman JB: Lung transplantation for cystic fibrosis: special considerations. *Chest* 1996, 109:787–798.

74. Rosenfeld MA, Collins FS: Gene therapy for cystic fibrosis. *Chest* 1996, 109:241–252.

75. Curiel DT, Agarwal S, Romer MU, et al.: Gene transfer to respiratory epithelial cells via the receptor-mediated endocytosis pathway. *Am J Respir Cell Mol Biol* 1992, 6:247–252.

76. Gao L, Wagner E, Cotten M, et al.: Direct *in vivo* gene transfer to airway employing adenovirus-polylysine-DNA complexes. *Hum Gene Ther* 1993, 4:17–24.

77. Crystal RG: Gene therapy for cystic fibrosis: lessons learned and hurdles to success. Presented at the Ninth Annual North American Cystic Fibrosis Conference, October 11-15, 1995; Dallas, Texas.

78. Rosenfeld MA, Yoshimura K, Trapnell B, *et al.*: *In vivo* transfer of the human cystic fibrosis transmembrance conductance regulator gene to the airway epithelium. *Cell* 1992, 68:143–155.

79. Rosenfeld MA, Chu CS, Seth P, *et al.*: Gene transfer to freshly isolated human respiratory epithelial cells *in vitro* using a replication-deficient adenovirus containing the human cystic fibrosis transmembrane conductance regulator cDNA. *Hum Gene Ther* 1994, 5:331–342.

80. Englehardt JF, Simon RH, Yang Y, *et al.*: Adenovirus-mediated transfer of the CFTR gene to lung of nonhuman primates: biological efficacy study. *Hum Gene Ther* 1993, 4:759–769.

81. Englehardt JF, Yang Y, Stratford-Perricaudet LD, *et al.*: Direct gene transfer of human CFTR into human bronchial epithelia of xenografts with E1-deleted adenoviruses. *Nature Gen* 1993, 4:27–34.

82. Mastrangeli A, Danel C, Rosenfeld MA, *et al.*: Diversity of airway epithelial cell targets for *in vivo* recombinant adenovirus-mediated gene transfer. *J Clin Invest* 1993, 91:225–234.

83. Rich DP, Couture LA, Cardoza LM, *et al.*: Development and analysis of recombinant adenoviruses for gene therapy of cystic fibrosis. *Hum Gene Ther* 1993, 4:461–476.

84. Yang Y, Nunes FA, Berencsi K, *et al.*: Inactivation of E2a in recombinant adenoviruses improves the prospect for gene therapy for cystic fibrosis. *Nature Genet* 1994, 7:362–369.

85. Zabner J, Petersen DM, Puga AP, *et al.*: Safety and efficacy of repetitive adenovirus-mediated transfer of CFTR cDNA to airway epithelia of primates and cotton rats. *Nat Gen* 1994, 6:75–83.

86. Zabner J, Couture LA, Smith AE, Welsh MJ: Correction of cAMP-stimulated fluid secretion in cystic fibrosis airway epithelia: efficiency of adenovirus-mediated gene transfer *in vivo*. *Hum Gene Ther* 1994, 5:585–593.

87. Wilson JM: Cystic fibrosis: strategies for gene therapy. *Sem Respir Crit Care Med* 1994, 15:439–445.

88. Wilson JM: Gene therapy for cystic fibrosis lung disease with recombinant adenoviruses: host-vector interactions. *Pediatr Pulmonol* 1994, 10:155.

89. Johnson LG: Gene therapy for cystic fibrosis. *Chest* 1995, 107:77S–82S.

90. Knowles MR, Hohneker KW, Zhou Z, *et al.*: A controlled study of adenoviral-vector-mediated gene transfer in the nasal epithelium of patients with cystic fibrosis. *N Engl J Med* 1995, 333:823–831.

91. Crystal RG, McElvaney NG, Rosenfeld MA, *et al.*: Administration of an adenovirus containing the human CFTR cDNA to the respiratory tract of individuals with cystic fibrosis. *Nat Gen* 1994, 8:42–51.

92. Alton EWFW, Middleton PG, Caplen NJ, *et al.*: Non-invasive liposome-mediated gene delivery can correct the ion transport defect in cystic fibrosis mutant mice. *Nat Gen* 1993, 5:135–142.

93. Hyde SC, Gill DR, Higgins CF, *et al.*: Correction of the ion transport defect in cystic fibrosis transgenic mice by gene therapy. *Nature* 1993, 362:250–255.

94. Caplen NJ, Alton RW, Middleton PG, *et al.*: Liposome-mediated CFTR gene transfer to the nasal epithelium of patients with cystic fibrosis. *Nat Med* 1995, 1:39–46.

95. Wilson JM: Prospects for human gene therapy. In *Highlights*. Bethesda, MD: Cystic Fibrosis Foundation; 1995:20–22.

96. Schidlow DV, Fiel SB: Life beyond pediatrics: transition of chronically ill adolescents from pediatric to adult health care systems. *Med Clin North Am* 1990, 74:1113–1120.

97. Huang NN, Schidlow DV, Szatrowski TE, *et al.*: Clinical features, survival rate, and prognostic factors in young adults with cystic fibrosis. *Am J Med* 1987, 82:871–879.

98. Shwachman H, Kulczycki LL: Long-term study of one hundred five patients with cystic fibrosis. *Am J Dis Child* 1958, 96:6–15.

99. Fiel SB, Tullis E: What are the key issues associated with cystic fibrosis in adulthood? In *Highlights*. Bethesda, MD: Cystic Fibrosis Foundation; 1995:17–19.

100. Canny HJ, Corey M, Livingston RA, *et al.*: Pregnancy and cystic fibrosis. *Obstet Gynecol* 1991, 77:850–853.

101. FitzSimmons SC, Winnie G, Fiel S, *et al.*: Effect of pregnancy on women with cystic fibrosis: a one to six year follow-up study. *Am J Respir Crit Care Med* 1995, 151:A742.

102. Kotloff RM: Reproductive issues in patients with cystic fibrosis. *Sem Respir Crit Care Med* 1994, 15:402–413.

103. Hirsh AV, Mills C, Bekir J, *et al.*: Factors influencing the outcome of in-vitro fertilization with epididymal spermatozoa in irreversible obstructive azoospermia. *Hum Reprod* 1994, 9:1710–1716.

104. Aitken ML: Managing cystic fibrosis in adults. *New Insights into Cystic Fibrosis* 1995, 3:7–11.

105. Aspin AJ: Psychological consequences of cystic fibrosis in adults. *Br J Hosp Med* 1991, 45:368–371.

106. Blair C, Cull A, Freeman CP: Psychosocial functioning of young adults with cystic fibrosis and their families. *Thorax* 1994, 49:798–802.

BRONCHIOLITIS OBLITERANS AND OTHER BRONCHIOLAR AIRWAY DISORDERS

5

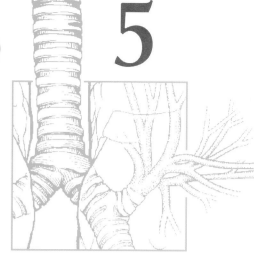
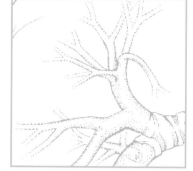
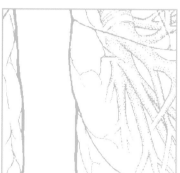

Gary R. Epler &
Thomas V. Colby

Bronchiolar airway disease is an important cause of airflow obstruction. There are several distinct pathologic lesions that correspond to well-defined clinical disorders. Cellular bronchiolitis is the most common disorder and corresponds clinically with a cough that lasts several days or weeks. Diffuse panbronchiolitis has been reported commonly in Japan and is a cause of chronic cough with purulent sputum production and sinusitis. This disorder has been reported in the United States and Europe. The anti-inflammatory action of erythromycin appears to be effective in the management of diffuse panbronchiolitis. The fibrotic restrictive bronchiolitis and obliterative bronchiolitis occurring after fume exposure or infection and associated with connective tissue disease is rare and often has a poor prognosis. Transplantation bronchiolitis obliterans is the major complication and cause of mortality in recipients of bone marrow and lung transplants. In lung transplantation, the lesion represents a form of chronic organ rejection. Risk factors include more frequent and more severe acute rejections and the coexistence of previous organizing pneumonia. The recognition of the distinctive differences among these bronchiolar airway disorders is essential for successful patient care, for a greater understanding of the pathogenesis, and development of new therapeutic advances.

HISTORICAL PERSPECTIVE OF BRONCHIOLAR DISEASE

THE BRONCHIOLAR DISEASES

1901	Bronchiolitis obliterans [1]
1902	Fume-related bronchiolitis obliterans [2]
1904	Postinfectious bronchiolitis obliterans [3,4]
1977	Connective tissue disease-related [5]
1977	Drug-related bronchiolitis obliterans [5]
1982	Bone marrow transplantation bronchiolitis obliterans [6]
1983	Diffuse panbronchiolitis [7]
1984	Heart-lung transplantation bronchiolitis obliterans [8]
1985	Idiopathic BOOP [9]
1987	Respiratory bronchiolitis-interstitial lung disease [10]
1989	Lung transplantation bronchiolitis obliterans [11]
1992	Neuroendocrine cell hyperplasia with airflow obstruction [12]
1995	Microcarcinoid-related bronchiolitis obliterans [13,14]
1996	*Sauropus androgynus*-related bronchiolitis obliterans [15]

BOOP—bronchiolitis obliterans organizing pneumonia.

Figure 5-1.
Major historical milestones of the bronchiolar diseases began when Lange described two patients in 1901 [1]. Then fume and infectious causes were described. Eventually, bronchiolar lesions were described in the connective tissue disorders, after bone marrow transplantation, and after lung transplantation. Obliterative bronchiolitis was then described with neuroendocrine cell hyperplasia and associated with microcarcinoids. Neuroendocrine cell hyperplasia has had a very unusual association with bronchiolitis obliterans from the ingestion of *Sauropus androgynus*, a leafy vegetable used for its alleged effects of body weight reduction and blood pressure control.

Normal Bronchiolar Airway

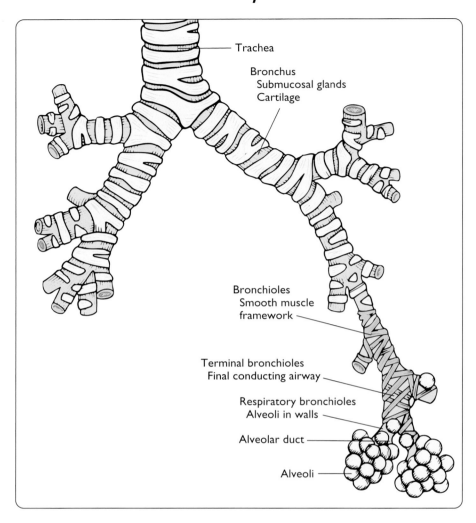

Trachea

Bronchus
Submucosal glands
Cartilage

Bronchioles
Smooth muscle
framework

Terminal bronchioles
Final conducting airway

Respiratory bronchioles
Alveoli in walls

Alveolar duct

Alveoli

Figure 5-2.

Anatomy of the bronchioles. Bronchioles are small airways, up to 1 or 2 mm in diameter, without cartilage or submucosal glands [16]. An estimated 28,000 terminal bronchioles, with diameters of 0.6 mm, comprise the final conducting bronchioles at the 16th generation. The 224,000 respiratory bronchioles are distinguished from the terminal bronchioles by the alveolar sacs in their walls. The respiratory bronchioles terminate at the 13.8 million alveolar ducts and 300 million alveoli.

Normal Alveolar Histology

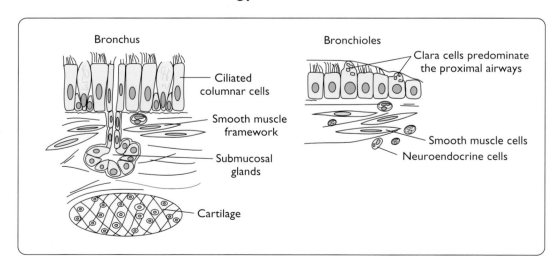

Bronchus

Ciliated
columnar cells

Smooth muscle
framework

Submucosal
glands

Cartilage

Bronchioles

Clara cells predominate
the proximal airways

Smooth muscle cells
Neuroendocrine cells

Figure 5-3.

Normal alveolar histology. Ciliated cells predominate on the surface of the epithelium of the proximal airways, whereas Clara cells comprise the majority of cells in the bronchiolar mucosa [17]. Apically, Clara cells contain membrane-bound secretory granules that probably secrete proteins and may actively secrete surfactant. Neuroendocrine cells reach maximal density in the proximal bronchioles and are rarely found in the terminal bronchioles. These cells occur individually and in clusters, and tend to be concentrated at the bifurcations of the conducting airways. They are a source of biologically active secretory products, including bombesin-like activity (gastrin-releasing peptide), somatostatin, endothelin, serotonin, and calcitonin.

PATHOLOGIC FEATURES OF BRONCHIOLITIS

A. PATHOLOGIC LESIONS OF THE BRONCHIOLES

Cellular bronchiolitis
Follicular bronchiolitis
Mineral dust bronchiolitis
Cigarette smoke respiratory bronchiolitis
Diffuse panbronchiolitis
Constrictive bronchiolitis
Proliferative (intraluminal polyps) bronchiolitis obliterans
Respiratory bronchiolitis-interstitial lung disease
Bronchiolitis obliterans organizing pneumonia

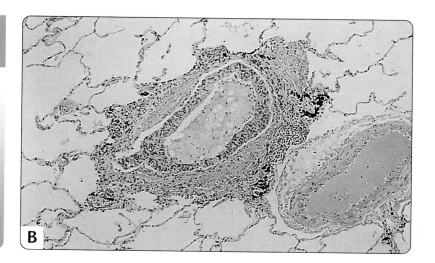

Figure 5-4.

Pathologic lesions of the bronchioles. **A**, The pathologist distinguishes several distinct lesions among the bronchiolar disorders. These are generally airway abnormalities that may involve adjacent alveoli and interstitium. Cellular bronchiolitis is an acute or chronic inflammation of the bronchioles. The inflammation may be submucosal, mural, or peribronchiolar [16]. Follicular bronchiolitis is a descriptive term for a subset of cellular bronchiolitis associated with lymphoid hyperplasia and reactive germinal centers along the small airways and bronchioles [16]. Mineral dust bronchiolitis is the fibrotic thickening of the walls of the terminal and respiratory bronchioles, in some instances with extension into the alveolar ducts [18,19]. This lesion has been described in workers exposed to a variety of inorganic dusts, such as iron oxide, aluminum oxide, asbestos, talc, mica, coal, and silica [19]. Cigarette smoke respiratory bronchiolitis has several features: the bronchioles are thickened as a result of inflammatory edema and cellular infiltrates, the airway wall is distorted because of fibrous tissue scarring in the submucosa and adventitia, and the airway collapses early during expiration due to the destruction of peribronchiolar alveolar attachments and loss of airway-parenchymal interdependence [18]. Airway reactivity may also occur as a result of the inflammatory process. A growing body of evidence suggests that active events triggered by constant cigarette smoking can accentuate airway narrowing and promote a chronic inflammatory process that also

causes the airways to become thick, inflamed, and deformed, and induces emphysematous changes in adjacent tissue. The uncontrolled inflammatory process in the terminal and respiratory bronchioles may lead to destruction of the centrilobular portion of the lung [20]. **B**, Neuroendocrine cell hyperplasia constrictive bronchiolitis is seen in this photomicrograph of lung tissue obtained from a woman with airflow obstruction for several years that became so severe that a lung transplantation was required for her survival. The explanted lung showed diffuse neuroendocrine cell proliferation that involved the bronchioles and was associated with mural fibrosis and mucostasis. The bronchiole shows luminal mucostasis, replacement of mucosal cells with neuroendocrine cells, and fibrotic thickening of the wall associated with focal chronic inflammation. Neuroendocrine cell hyperplasia [12] may occur in patients with peripheral carcinoid tumor; nearly half of these patients may have obliterative bronchiolitis, some with airflow obstruction [13]. In these patients, subepithelial fibrosis varies in severity. In the most severe lesions, the lumen may be replaced with fibrous tissue with few remaining neuroendocrine cells. The investigators who obtained this photomicrograph suggest that neuroendocrine hyperplasia preceded and presumably caused airway fibrosis in this patient. It has also been suggested that airflow blockade in chronic bronchitis may be caused by airway narrowing due to peribronchiolar fibrosis [21]. (*See* Color Plate.)

PATHOLOGIC FEATURES OF CONSTRICTIVE BRONCHIOLITIS

Complete fibrous obliteration of bronchioles

Stenosis due to concentric or eccentric mural fibrosis or granulation of submucosal tissue

Dilation of airways with mucus stasis

Acute or chronic mural inflammation and acute luminal inflammation

Figure 5-5.
Pathologic features of constrictive bronchiolitis. Irreversible scarring and alteration of the bronchioles varies from one airway to the next. The effect of obstruction may appear in distal air spaces. Constrictive bronchiolitis is a late, fibrotic, concentric bronchiolitis that occurs with or without complete obliteration [16]. There is no primary involvement of the distal alveolar ducts and alveoli. The histologic changes associated with constrictive bronchiolitis vary from mild bronchiolar inflammation and scarring to concentric fibrosis with complete obliteration of the bronchioles.

A. GENERAL CHARACTERISTICS OF DIFFUSE PANBRONCHIOLITIS

Largely restricted to Japan

Often associated with HLA antigen Bw54

Chronic sinusitis

Responsive to erythromycin therapy

Pseudomonas infection seen in late stages

Figure 5-6.
Diffuse panbronchiolitis. **A**, Extensive study of diffuse panbronchiolitis continues at a rapid pace. The disorder was initially reported in Japan [7] and has been reported in China, Korea, Europe, the United States, and Latin America [22]. It has been associated with a specific HLA antigen; a major susceptibility gene for diffuse panbronchiolitis has been located on the HLA-B locus on the chromosome 6p21.3 [23]. Erythromycin at 400 to 600 mg for at least 6 months has been an important advance in the treatment of the disorder [24]. **B**, Diffuse panbronchiolitis is seen in this whole mount histologic section, which shows multiple inflammatory nodules that center on small airways. **C**, Diffuse panbronchiolitis is indicated by evidence of peribronchiolar inflammation with interstitial foam cells, as depicted. This is a common and distinctive feature of diffuse panbronchiolitis.

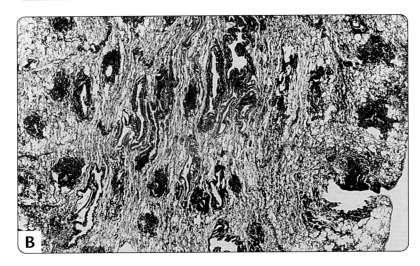

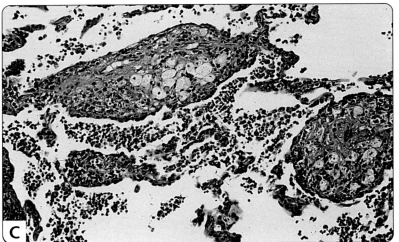

A. BRONCHIOLITIS OBLITERANS ORGANIZING PNEUMONIA

Major pathologic features
  Granulated tissue plugs within lumina of small airways
    extending into alveolar ducts and alveoli

Additional pathologic features
  Fibrinous exudates
  Alveolar accumulation of foamy macrophages
  Inflamed alveolar walls
  Unchanged lung architecture

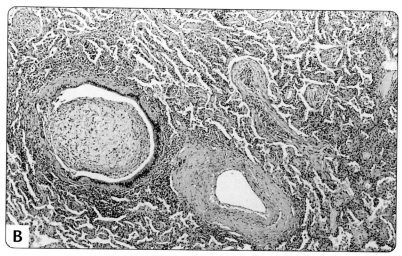

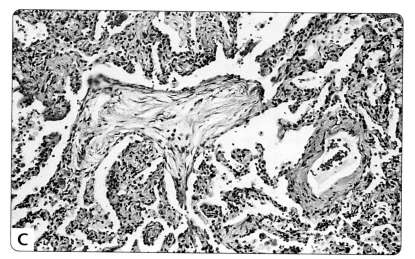

Figure 5-7.

Pathologic features of bronchiolitis obliterans organizing pneumonia (BOOP). **A,** The pathologic features of BOOP include an airway and alveolar component with interstitial involvement in approximately one third of lung biopsy specimens [9,16]. **B,** This photomicrograph of tissue obtained from a patient with bronchiolitis obliterans with intraluminal polyps shows polypoid edematous plugs of granulated tissue within the bronchiolar lumina (*left*) and an organizing pneumonia with airspaces containing similar polypoid tissue in the adjacent lung. The interstitium shows a moderate amount of chronic inflammatory infiltrate. The term *bronchiolitis obliterans with intraluminal polyps* is used because it is more descriptive and more easily understood than *proliferative bronchiolitis obliterans*. It describes a nonspecific reaction to bronchiolar injury that is characterized by an organizing intraluminal exudate and proliferative granulated tissue polyps filling the lumina of terminal and respiratory bronchioles [20]. This reaction usually extends continuously into the alveolar ducts and sometimes into distal alveoli, thus representing an organizing pneumonia [9,14,20]. Conditions associated with this lesion include organizing diffuse alveolar damage (organizing acute respiratory distress syndrome); organizing infections distal to the obstruction; organizing aspiration pneumonia; the organizing phase of toxic fume exposure; connective tissue disorders; hypersensitivity pneumonitis; organizing eosinophilic pneumonia; drug reactions; bone marrow, heart–lung, and lung transplantation; diffuse panbronchiolitis; and BOOP [16]. Respiratory bronchiolitis-interstitial lung disease is seen in smokers and is characterized by mild interstitial infiltrates, fibrosis, and accumulations of macrophages in air spaces surrounding the respiratory bronchioles and alveolar ducts [10]. (*See* Color Plate.) **C,** The most common finding in BOOP is edematous granulated tissue polyps within alveolar ducts, as shown in the figure. (*See* Color Plate.)

CLASSIFICATION OF BRONCHIOLAR DISEASE

CLINICAL CLASSIFICATION OF THE DISEASES OF THE BRONCHIOLES

The airway bronchiolar disorders
    Acute or chronic bronchiolitis
    Cigarette smoke bronchiolitis
    Mineral dust bronchiolitis
    Diffuse panbronchiolitis
    Respiratory bronchiolitis
    Bronchiolitis obliterans, predominately constrictive bronchiolitis
        Idiopathic
        Post-fume exposure
        Rheumatic or connective tissue disorders
        Drug reaction
        After bone marrow and lung transplantation
        Neuroendocrine hyperplasia
        Microcarcinoid tumors
        Sauropus androgynus
    Miscellaneous
        Stevens-Johnson syndrome
        Primary biliary cirrhosis
        IgA nephropathy
        Paraneoplastic pemphigus
The alveloar bronchiolar diseases
    Respiratory bronchiolitis-interstitial lung disease (RB-ILD)
    Bronchiolitis obliterans organizing pneumonia (BOOP)

Figure 5-8.

Clinical classification of bronchiolar disease. The clinician adds information regarding the causes of associated systemic disorders to develop a clinical classification of each bronchiolar disorder. General categories are defined by histologic findings, and specific categories are classified by correlating these findings with the clinical setting. The pathologic lesion associated with bronchiolitis obliterans is virtually always constrictive. Bronchiolitis obliterans with intraluminal polyps is rarely a cause of functionally measurable airflow obstruction. Radiographs of patients with constrictive bronchiolitis usually show airflow obstruction and lobular areas with decreased attenuation and airway dilation; in patients with bronchiolitis obliterans with intraluminal polyps, radiographs show airspace opacification [25,26]. Clinically, scarred constrictive bronchiolitis tends to be associated with fixed airflow obstruction that does not respond to corticosteroid therapy; and proliferative bronchiolitis obliterans is associated with crackles, abnormal diffusing capacity, and an excellent response to corticosteroid therapy. The proliferative (intraluminal polyps) rather than the constrictive bronchiolitic, lesion is the "bronchiolitis obliterans" component of bronchiolitis obliterans organizing pneumonia.

IDIOPATHIC BRONCHIOLITIS OBLITERANS WITH AIRFLOW OBSTRUCTION

Very rare

Associated with progressive dyspnea

Indicated by

Early inspiratory crackles

Chest radiograph: normal or showing small nodular opacities

Poor response to corticosteroid treatment

Figure 5-9.

Idiopathic bronchiolitis obliterans with airflow obstruction. Idiopathic or cryptogenic bronchiolitis obliterans is defined as the disorder that occurs in patients who have no obvious inciting agent or associated systemic disorder, yet who clinically have airflow obstruction and histologically have constrictive bronchiolitis. This disorder continues to be very rare, despite the recent interest in bronchiolar diseases. One report [27] of the chest CT findings in a 68-year-old patient indicated small rounded and branching linear opacities, and thickened, dilated walls of the proximal bronchioles that were connected to peripheral nodules or small ring-like cystic lesions. These findings resembled diffuse panbronchiolitis; however, the linear and nodular opacities in this setting were probably from cellular inflammation. The chest roentgenogram showed micronodular opacities at the bases that had been present in a film 6 years previously. The chest CT findings were unusual, but this report illustrates the typical findings of a patient with idiopathic bronchiolitis obliterans. Dyspnea and a nonproductive cough were present for 1 year. There were fine crackles, a vital capacity of 2.56 L (68% predicted), and FEV_1 of 1.69 L (50% predicted), and an FEV_1/FVC of 66%. The diffusing capacity was 126% predicted. The lung biopsy showed some bronchioles completely replaced by fibrotic scar and others with dilated lumens and mucus stasis. Regarding treatment, 3 months of high-dose prednisone (1 mg/kg) is often needed to determine effectiveness, with tapering doses for 3 months and lower dosages for at least 1 year. Patients who survive the initial episode may stabilize for several years [28] or progress to end-stage airflow disease and cor pulmonale. It is unknown whether progression is a continual fibrosing process or caused by recurrent respiratory infections with incremental loss of function over time. Lung transplantation may be effective for patients who are unresponsive to therapy.

BRONCHIOLITIS OBLITERANS VS BOOP

	Bronchiolitis obliterans	BOOP
Description	Airflow disorder	Interstitial disorder
Chest examination	Early crackles	Late crackles
Chest radiograph	Normal	Patchy infiltrates
Pulmonary function tests	Abnormal FEV_1 and $FEV_1/\%FVC$	Abnormal vital capacity and Dsb
Response to therapy	Poor	Good
Prognosis	Poor	Good

BOOP—bronchiolitis obliterans organizing pneumonia; Dsb—single-breath diffusion capacity; FEV_1—forced expiratory volume in 1 s; $FEV_1/\%FVC$— FEV_1 as a percentage of forced vital capacity.

Figure 5-10.

Comparison of bronchiolitis obliterans with bronchiolitis obliterans organizing pneumonia (BOOP). Bronchiolitis obliterans, the airway disease, is pathologically and clinically distinct from idiopathic BOOP, the interstitial disease [9,29]. Common features include a preceding flu-like illness and dyspnea. Chest findings on auscultation differ, with early inspiratory crackles heard in patients with bronchiolitis obliterans and late inspiratory crackles heard in patients with BOOP. Chest radiographs also differ because they are often normal in patients with bronchiolitis obliterans and show bilateral patchy infiltrates in patients with BOOP. Airflow obstruction is indicated in the former by a reduction in forced expiratory volume in 1 second (FEV_1) and the ratio of FEV_1 to forced vital capacity, and abnormal diffusing capacity is seen in the latter. Response to therapy and prognosis differ markedly: a minimal to moderate response to corticosteroid therapy is expected in patients with bronchiolitis obliterans; no response is expected in patients with disabling disorders. Complete recovery is expected in 65% to 80% of patients with BOOP.

A. TOXIC-FUME BRONCHIOLITIS OBLITERANS

Event	Time	Lesion
Latent period No symptoms or clinical findings	—	Probable early inflammation
Acute respiratory failure Pulmonary edema pattern seen radiographically	4–6 h	Diffuse alveolar damage
Progressive chronic respiratory failure Early inspiratory crackles Normal chest radiograph Severe airflow obstruction	Days to weeks	Constrictive bronchiolitis and bronchiolitis obliterans

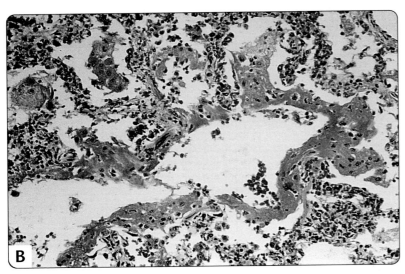 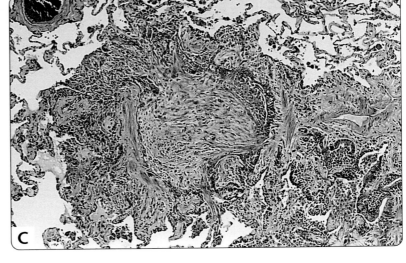

Figure 5-11.

Toxic-fume bronchiolitis obliterans. **A**, Toxic-fume bronchiolitis obliterans has occurred after exposure to nitrogen dioxide and sulfur dioxide. A possible occurrence was described in a 39-year-old truck driver who delivered fly ash. He developed acute respiratory failure requiring hospitalization [30]. His chest radiograph showed bilateral infiltrates. This episode improved rapidly with corticosteroid therapy. After 2 weeks, however, he returned with severe dyspnea. His vital capacity was normal at 5.44 L (102% of predicted), but his forced expiratory volume in 1 second (FEV_1) decreased to 2.13 L (52% of predicted) and the ratio or FEV_1 to forced vital capacity (FEV_1/FVC) had fallen markedly to 39%. It is unknown whether the patient's condition was a result of the direct effect of the fly ash particles or toxic agents, such as nitrogen dioxide (NO_2) or sulfur dioxide (SO_2), adsorbed to the fly ash particles. Smoke inhalation bronchiolitis obliterans was described in a 23-year-old man who was sleeping in his newly constructed house when it caught fire [31]. The synthetic structural materials used to build his house produced gases that contained acrolein,

formaldehyde, acetaldehyde, NO_2, and SO_2 when burned. Smoke inhalation bronchiolitis obliterans has also been described from burning synthetic construction materials in a wood-burning stove [32]. The increased use of potentially toxic chemicals throughout the world has resulted in an increased possibility of exposed workers developing bronchiolar disorders. For example, two workers in a lithium battery factory were accidentally exposed to thionyl-chloride, and one of them developed a prolonged clinical course and findings consistent with bronchiolitis obliterans [33]. This acidic compound is used in the manufacturing process and produces SO_2 and HCl fumes when in contact with water. **B**, Fume (parachlorethylene) inhalation, resulting in acute lung injury, with hyaline membranes lining an alveolar duct. This appearance is typical for most acute fume inhalations. (*See Color Plate.*) **C**, Fume (chlorine) exposure causing a bronchiole to become completely occluded by fibrous tissue. There is some extension of fibrous tissue into the immediately surrounding alveoli, although the lesion is exquisitely bronchiolocentric. (*See Color Plate.*)

PREDISPOSING CONDITIONS TO POSTINFECTIOUS BRONCHIOLITIS OBLITERANS

Viral infection

Mycoplasma infection

Swyer–James or Macleod's syndrome

Figure 5-12.

Conditions associated with postinfectious bronchiolitis obliterans. This condition is rare in adults, although it may occur after a viral or mycoplasmal infection [34]. It is more common in children, especially after infection with respiratory syncytial virus or adenovirus. Swyer–James syndrome is a variant of postinfectious constrictive bronchiolitis that usually develops after a pulmonary infection in infancy or early childhood. It can destroy the alveoli and leads to obliterative bronchiolitis. The computed tomographic scan is a valuable source of information for this diagnosis when evaluated in the presence of decreased lung volume and attenuation values and a marked reduction in vasculature and in the integrity of the main airways [35]. Computed tomographic scans performed at maximal expiration may show air trapping marked by a shift of the mediastinum toward the normal lung.

PREDISPOSING CONDITIONS TO CONNECTIVE TISSUE BRONCHIOLITIS OBLITERANS

Rheumatoid arthritis

Scleroderma

Lupus erythematosus

Ankylosing spondylitis

Sjögren's syndrome

Figure 5-13.

Conditions associated with connective tissue bronchiolitis obliterans. This condition occurs most commonly among women with rheumatoid arthritis, although it has also been reported among patients with other connective tissue disorders, including scleroderma, lupus erythematosus, ankylosing spondylitis, and Sjögren's syndrome. The clinical features are identical to those of idiopathic bronchiolitis obliterans. A histologic pattern of constrictive bronchiolitis or proliferative bronchiolitis obliterans is seen; the latter has a much more favorable course.

DRUG-RELATED BRONCHIOLITIS OBLITERANS

Toxin	Pulmonary lesion	Prognosis
Penicillamine	Constrictive bronchiolitis	Poor
	Proliferative bronchiolitis	Good
Gold	Constrictive bronchiolitis	Poor
	Proliferative bronchiolitis	Good

Figure 5-14.

Drug-related bronchiolitis obliterans. This condition has generally been reported among patients with rheumatoid arthritis receiving gold or penicillamine. The penicillamine-related lesion tends to be constrictive bronchiolitis and has a poor prognosis. Proliferative bronchiolitis obliterans may also occur as a drug-related lesion [16]. Although a cause-and-effect relationship has been difficult to confirm, the possibility of drug-related bronchiolitis obliterans continues to be important clinically. Patients with a connective tissue disorder who are taking these medications and who develop unexplained cough or dyspnea should be evaluated promptly.

A. RISK FACTORS ASSOCIATED WITH BONE MARROW TRANSPLANTATION IN BRONCHIOLITIS OBLITERANS

Allogeneic transplantation

Graft-versus-host disease

Late onset, indicating a poor prognosis

Severe airflow obstruction, indicating a poor prognosis

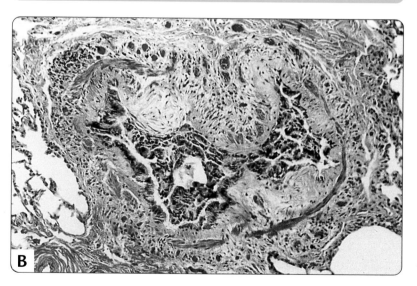

Figure 5-15.

Bone marrow transplantation bronchiolitis obliterans. **A,** Several risk factors have been identified for the development of bronchiolitis obliterans after bone marrow transplantation. The lesion is preceded by findings typical of graft-versus-host disease, including skin rash, mucositis, sicca, and angiitis, usually occurring within 3 months after transplantation. Six months later, the patient develops a cough, then progressive dyspnea. At this late stage, the chest radiograph is normal in 80% of patients; however, the forced expiratory volume in 1 second is severely reduced, and no improvement is seen after bronchodilator inhalation. Response to therapy is poor once severe airflow obstruction has been established. Those with late onset and severe airflow obstruction have the worst prognosis. For these patients, therapy is directed at controlling chronic GVH disease and preventing infection. On the basis of a review of lung biopsy specimens taken from BMT recipients and showing GVH disease, Yousem [36] divided observed morphologic changes into four categories: diffuse alveolar damage, lymphocytic bronchitis/bronchiolitis with interstitial pneumonitis, bronchiolitis obliterans organizing pneumonia, and constrictive bronchiolitis obliterans. The histologic findings for five patients with constrictive bronchiolitis indicated that the airway lumina had been obliterated by dense fibrous scar tissue; the atretic airways could be identified only by their location adjacent to arterioles. All patients had cough and shortness of breath, two died from bronchiolitis obliterans, one was alive with disease by the end of the study, and two had double-lung transplantations. It was noted that this lesion may reflect irreversible pulmonary GVH disease. **B,** This specimen was obtained from a BMT recipient with bronchiolitis obliterans. A bronchiole has been partially compromised by submucosal proliferation of collagen that distorted the lumen. Despite incomplete airway obliteration, this type of lesion may compromise pulmonary function severely. (See Color Plate.)

A. GENERAL CHARACTERISTICS OF LUNG TRANSPLANTATION BRONCHIOLITIS OBLITERANS

Frequency: 10%–50%

Mortality: ≤50%

Acute rejection

May respond to cytolytic immunosuppressive therapy

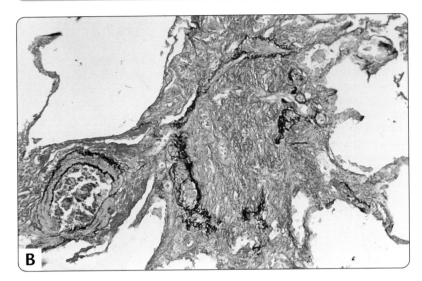

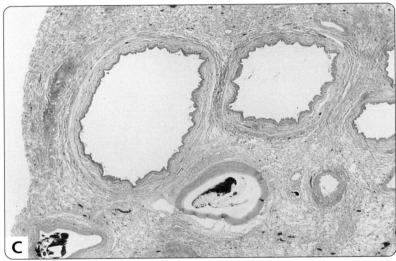

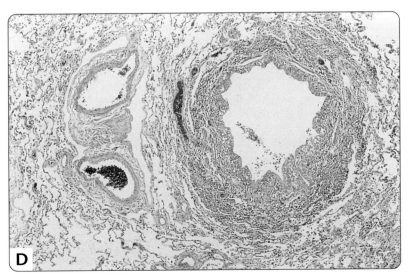

Figure 5-16.

Lung transplantation: bronchiolitis obliterans. **A,** The 1-year survival rate of recipients of lung transplants has improved to 71%. In addition, 46% will survive at least 5 years, yet bronchiolitis obliterans continues to be a serious cause of morbidity and mortality [37]. The cumulative risk of bronchiolitis obliterans may be 60% to 80% from 5 to 10 years after transplantation. The major risk factor appears to be acute rejection; the more frequent and the more severe the rejection, the higher the risk. One study showed that those who had more than three episodes of acute rejection in any 12-month period eventually had a 100% incidence of bronchiolitis obliterans [38]. Factors not correlated with bronchiolitis obliterans include the age or sex of the recipient and donor, the recipient's underlying disease, and whether a single or double transplant was performed. Three patterns of decrement in FEV_1 are characterized by an insidious onset and course. The onset is 12, 15, and 30 months, respectively. All patients in the first group were oxygen dependent after 9 months; none of them survived more than 13 months after diagnosis of bronchiolitis obliterans. Patients in the second and third group had a lower mortality rate. Expiratory chest computerized tomography (CT) films are often helpful for diagnosis of transplant-related bronchiolitis obliterans; however, a study of seven patients indicated that thin-section CT had limited accuracy in diagnosing early bronchiolitis obliterans [4]. Measurements of ventilation distribution can detect obliterative bronchiolitis in recipients of transplants better than conventional pulmonary function testing [41]. Regarding treatment, the bronchiolitis obliterans lesion in these patients may be corticosteroid resistant; cytolitic immunosuppression must be used. Treatment includes cytoloytic drugs such as OKT_3 antithymocyte globulin and antilymphocyte globulin [42]. Other agents include tacrolimus, total lymphoid irradiation, methotrexate, and photochemotherapy. Prevention is a good alternative. The best way to prevent this complication is to eliminate or change clinical events before, during, or after transplantation that will decrease the development of obliterative bronchiolitis [42]. **B,** This specimen was obtained from a patient who underwent lung transplantation and developed bronchiolitis obliterans. A bronchiole has been completely obliterated by fibrous tissue. The original elastica of the bronchiole is highlighted in black by the stain for elastin. **C** and **D,** Patients with lung transplantation bronchiolitis obliterans frequently develop bronchiolectasis (*panel C*) and chronic bronchiolitis (*panel D*), in addition to obliteration of bronchioles.

MISCELLANEOUS DISORDERS ASSOCIATED WITH BRONCHIOLITIS OBLITERANS

Stevens-Johnson syndrome
Primary biliary cirrhosis
IgA nephropathy
Paraneoplastic pemphigus

Figure 5-17.
A, Bronchiolitis obliterans has been associated with aspiration of foreign bodies, esophageal and gastric contents [43,44], and in patients with Stevens-Johnson syndrome and primary biliary cirrhosis [45]. Bronchiolitis obliterans has been reported in a 78-year-old man with IgA nephropathy [46] and is associated with paraneoplastic pemphigus [47]. **B,** This specimen was obtained from a victim of fatal charcoal aspiration [43]. The bronchiole is completely occluded by fibrous tissue, with prominence surrounding the charcoal (the black material). (See Color Plate.)

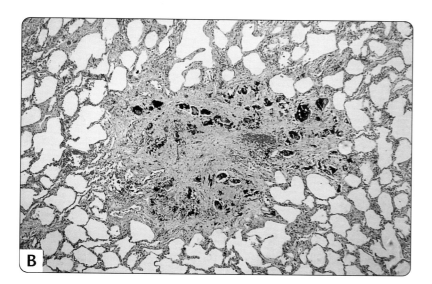

FUTURE CONSIDERATIONS

FUTURE CONSIDERATIONS

Epidemiologic studies of acute and chronic bronchiolitis in the adult
Define the cellular mechanism of diffuse panbronchiolitis
Define the cellular mechanism of bone marrow and lung transplant obliterative bronchiolitis
Develop new therapeutic agents for idiopathic and connective tissue bronchiolitis obliterans
Implement multicenter treatment trials for lung transplant bronchiolitis obliterans

Figure 5-18.
Cellular bronchiolitis associated with cough and wheezing is common as a viral infection in adults; however, epidemiologic studies are needed to determine frequency and clinical characteristics. The cellular mechanisms of diffuse panbronchiolitis and erythromycin treatment are developing gradually, but specific details are needed. Idiopathic, post-fume, and postinfectious bronchiolitis obliterans will continue to be rare. Early treatment with corticosteroid therapy remains the treatment of choice. Connective tissue-related constrictive bronchiolitis obliterans has a poor prognosis, and new forms of treatment are needed. Bronchiolitis obliterans associated with bone marrow and lung transplantation will require intensive investigation to solve the cellular mechanisms for early detection and therapeutic advances. Multicenter immunosuppressive trials are needed to determine their usefulness in the treatment of lung transplant bronchiolitis obliterans. Clinicians must understand the distinction between the bronchiolar disorders. These efforts will result in improved patient care, a greater understanding of the pathogenesis of these disorders, and the development of new therapeutic agents.

REFERENCES

1. Lange W: Ueber eine eigenthumliche erkrankung der kleinen bronchien und bronchilen. *Dtsch Arch Klin Med* 1901, 70:342–364.

2. Fraenkel A: Ueber bronchiolitis fibrosa obliterans, nebst bemerkungen uber lungenhyperamie und indurirende pneumonia. *Dtsch Arch Klin Med* 1902, 73:484–512.

3. Hart C: Anatomische untersuchungen uber die bei masern vorkommenden lungenerkrankungen. *Dtsch Arch Klin Med* 1904, 79:108–128.

4. Jochmann G: Moltrecht, uber seltenere erkrankungsformen der bronchien nach masern und keuchhusten. *Beitrage zur Path Anat zur Allgemeinen Path* 1904, 36:340–352.

5. Geddes DM, Corrin B, Brewerton DA, *et al.*: Progressive airway obliteration in adults and its association with rheumatoid disease. *Q J Med* 1977, 46:427–444.

6. Roca J, Granena A, Rodriguez-Roisin R, *et al.*: Fatal airway disease in an adult with chronic graft-versus-host disease. *Thorax* 1982, 37:77–78.

7. Homma H, Yamanaka A, Shinichi T, *et al.*: Diffuse panbronchiolitis: a disease of the transitional zone of the lung. *Chest* 1983, 83:63–69.

8. Burke CM, Theodore J, Dawkins KD, *et al.*: Post-transplant obliterative bronchiolitis and other late lung sequelae in human heart-lung transplantation. *Chest* 1984, 86:824–829.

9. Epler GR, Colby TV, McLoud TC, *et al.*: Bronchiolitis obliterans organizing pneumonia. *N Engl J Med* 1985, 312:152–158.

10. Myers JF, Veal CF, Shin MS, *et al.*: Respiratory bronchiolitis causing interstitial lung disease: a clinicopathologic study of six cases. *Am Rev Respir Dis* 1987, 135:880–884.

11. McGregor CGA, Dark JH, Hilton CJ, *et al.*: Early results of single lung transplantation in patients with end-stage pulmonary fibrosis. *J Thorac Cardiovasc Surg* 1989, 98:350–354.

12. Aguayo SM, Miller YE, Waldron JA, *et al.*: Idiopathic diffuse hyperplasia of pulmonary neuroendocrine cells and airways disease. *N Engl J Med* 1992, 327:1285–1288.

13. Miller RR, Muller NL: Neuroendocrine cell hyperplasia and obliterative bronchiolitis in patients with peripheral carcinoid tumors. *Am J Surg Pathol* 1995, 19:653–658.

14. Sheerin N, Harrison NK, Sheppard MN, Hansell DM, Yacoub M, Clark TJH: Obliterative bronchiolitis caused by multiple tumorlets and microcarcinoids successfully treated by single lung transplantation. *Thorax* 1995, 50:207–209.

15. Lai RS, Chiang AA, Wu MT, *et al.*: Outbreak of bronchiolitis obliterans associated with consumption of *Sauropus androgynus* in Taiwan. *Lancet* 1996, 348:83–85.

16. Colby TV: Bronchiolitis. *Am J Clin Pathol* 1998, 109:101–109.

17. Thompson AB, Robbins RA, Romberger DJ, *et al.*: Immunological function of the pulmonary epithelium. *Eur Respir J* 1995, 8:127–149.

18. Wright JL, Cagle P, Churg A, *et al.*: Diseases of the small airways. *ARRD* 1992, 146:240–262.

19. Churg A: Mineral dust induced bronchiolitis. In *Diseases of the Bronchioles.* Edited by Epler GR. New York: Raven Press, Ltd.; 1994:139–151.

20. Finkelstein RA, Cosio MG: Disease of the small airways in smokers: smokers' bronchiolitis. In *Diseases of the Bronchioles.* Edited by Epler GR. New York: Raven Press, Ltd.; 1994:115–137.

21. Shelhamer JH, Levine SJ, Wu T, *et al.*: Airway inflammation. *Ann Intern Med* 1995, 123:288–304.

22. Martinez JA, Guimaraes SM, Ferreira RG, Pereira CA: Diffuse panbronchiolitis in Latin America. *Am J Med Sci* 2000, 183–185.

23. Keicho N, Ohashi J, Tamiya G, *et al.*: Fine localization of a major disease-susceptibility locus for diffuse panbronchiolitis. *Am J Hum Genetics* 2000, 66:501–507.

24. Kudoh S, Azuma A, Yamamoto M, Izumi T, Ando M: Improvement of survival in patients with diffuse panbronchiolitis treated with low-dose erythromycin. *Am J Resp Crit Care Med* 1998, 157:1829–1832.

25. Hansell DM, Rubens MB, Padley SP, Wells AU: Obliterative bronchiolitis: individual CT sign of small airways disease and functional correlation. *Radiology* 1997, 203:721–726.

26. Takahasi M, Murata K, Takazakura R, *et al.*: Bronchiolar disease: spectrum and radiological findings. *Eur J Radiol* 2000, 35:15–29.

27. Poletti V, Zompatori M, Boaron M, *et al.*: Cryptogenic constrictive bronchiolitis imitating imaging features of diffuse panbronchiolitis. *Monaldi Arch Chest Dis* 1995, 50:116–117.

28. Kraft M, Mortenson RL, Colby TV, *et al.*: Cryptogenic constrictive bronchiolitis: a clinicopathologic study. *Am Rev Respir Dis* 1993, 148:1093–1101.

29. Epler GR: Bronchiolitis obliterans organizing pneumonia. *Semin Respir Infect* 1995, 10:65–77.

30. Boswell RT, McCunney RJ: Bronchiolitis obliterans from exposure to incinerator fly ash. *J Occup Environ Med* 1995, 37:850–855.

31. Tasaka S, Kanazawa M, Mori M, *et al.*: Long-term course of bronchiectasis and bronchiolitis obliterans as late complications of smoke inhalation. *Respiration* 1995, 62:40–42.

32. Janigan DT, Toomas K, Michael R, McCleave JJ: Bronchiolitis obliterans in a man who used his wood-burning stove to burn synthetic construction materials. *Can Med Assoc* 1997, 156:1171–1173.

33. Konichezky S, Schattner A, Ezri T, *et al.*: Thionyl-chloride–induced lung injury and bronchiolitis obliterans. *Chest* 1993, 104:971–973.

34. Chan E, Kalayanamit T, Lynch DA, *et al.*: Mycoplasma pneumoniae-associated bronchiolitis causing severe restrictive lung disease in adults. *Chest* 1999, 115:1188–1194.

35. Miravitlles M, Alvarez-Castells A, Vidal R, *et al.*: Scintigraphy, angiography and computed tomography in unilateral hyperlucent lung due to obliterative bronchiolitis. *Respiration* 1994 61:324–329.

36. Yousem SA: The histological spectrum of pulmonary graft-versus-host disease in bone marrow transplant recipients. *Hum Pathol* 1995, 26:668–675.

37. Boehler A, Kesten S, Weder W, Speich R: Bronchiolitis obliterans in recipients of single, double, and heart-lung transplantation. *Chest* 1995, 107:973–980.

38. Keller CA, Cagle PT, Brown RW, *et al.*: Bronchiolitis obliterans in recipients of single-, double-, and heart-lung transplantation. *Chest* 1995, 107:973–980.

39. Nathan SD, Ross DJ, Belman MJ, *et al.*: Bronchiolitis obliterans in single-lung transplant recipients. *Chest* 1995, 107:967–972.

40. Lee ES, Gotway MB, Reddy GP, Golden JA, Keith FM, Webb WR: Early bronchiolitis obliterans following lung transplantation: accuracy of expiratory thin-section CT for diagnosis. *Radiology* 2000, 216:472–477.

41. Estenne M, Van Muylem A, Knoop C, Antoine M: Detection of obliterative bronchiolitis after lung transplantation by indexes of ventilation distribution. *Am J Respir Crit Care Med* 2000, 162:1047–1051.

42. Paradis I: Bronchiolitis obliterans: pathogenesis, prevention, and management. *Am J Med Sci* 1998, 315:161–178.

43. Elliot CG, Colby TV, Kelly TM, Hicks HG: Bronchiolitis obliterans after aspiration of activated charcoal. *Chest* 1989, 96:672–674.

44. Rinaldi M, Martinelli L, Volpato G, *et al.*: Gastro-esophageal reflux as cause of obliterative bronchiolitis: a case report. *Transplant Proc* 1995, 27:2006–2007.

45. Chatte G, Streichenberger N, Boillot O, *et al.*: Lymphocytic bronchitis/bronchiolitis in a patient with primary biliary cirrhosis. *Eur Respir J* 1995, 8:176–179.

46. Hernandez JL, Gomez-Roman J, Rodrigo E, *et al.*: Bronchiolitis obliterans and IgA nephropathy. *Am J Respir Crit Care Med* 1997, 156:665–668.

47. Takahashi M, Shimatsu Y, Kazama T, Kimura K, Otsuka T, Hashimoto T: Paraneoplastic pemphigus associated with bronchiolitis obliterans. *Chest* 2000, 117:603–607.

SLEEP

Nancy Collop

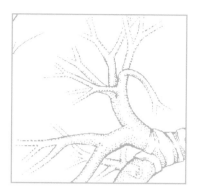
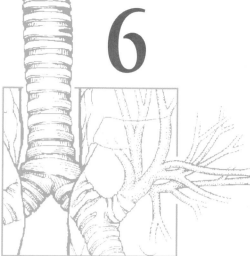
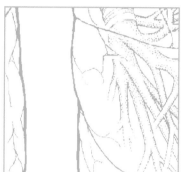

6

People spend approximately one third of their lives asleep. The function of sleep is not completely understood. In 1937, it was discovered that the brain waves changed during sleep. In 1953, the entity of rapid eye movement (REM) sleep was described.

Sleep is a behavioral state in which there is disengagement from the environment. Sleep is not an entirely passive activity because there are areas of the brain that become more active after sleep initiation. Sleep-promoting chemicals have been identified; research on their interactions in the brain continue to expand our knowledge of the mechanisms and role of sleep.

The study of sleep has been enhanced greatly by the development of polysomnography. Amplification of brain waves, the measurement of respiration and cardiac activity, and monitoring of muscle, eye activity, and oxygen saturation give the clinician a plethora of knowledge. The technique of polysomnography is used to assist in the diagnosis of sleep disorders.

The most common sleep disorder is insomnia, which is suffered by one in three Americans each year. The other common sleep disorder is obstructive sleep apnea-hypopnea syndrome, which may afflict up to 5% of the adult population. There is a myriad of other sleep disorders that result in considerable morbidity. Unfortunately, despite the prevalence of sleep complaints, many physicians do not ask their patients about their sleep and potentially miss these disorders.

BRAIN AREAS IMPORTANT TO SLEEP

Anatomic site	Area of sleep involved
Basal forebrain/preoptic area	Sleep initiation
Thalamus	Spindles (stage 2)
Pons, caudal midbrain	Rapid eye movement stage
Raphe nuclei, forebrain	Slow wave sleep
Suprachiasmatic nucleus	Circadian rhythms

Figure 6-1.
Brain areas important to sleep. The areas of the brain that are important to sleep are listed in this table [1].

PHYSIOLOGIC CHANGES OCCURRING WITH SLEEP

Parameter	NREM	REM
Blood pressure	Decreases Stage 1/2, 5% to 9% Stage 3/4, 8% to 14%	Decreases 15% to 20%
Heart rate	Decreases 5% to 8%	Increases to wake levels
Cardiac output	Decreases 7% to 12%	Variable
Body temperature	Decreases with sleep onset	Poikilothermic
Cerebral blood flow	Decreases	Increases
Penile erections	Infrequent	Frequent

Figure 6-2.
Physiologic changes occurring with sleep. There are many normal physiologic changes that occur in humans with sleep onset and some of these effects vary during non-rapid eye movement (NREM) and rapid eye movement (REM) sleep [2].

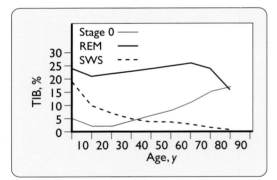

Figure 6-3.
Age-related changes in sleep. This graph depicts some of the changes that occur with aging. Slow wave sleep (SWS) occupies approximately 50% of the sleep time of infants, but with aging it decreases and is often absent in the elderly [3]. Stage random eye movement (REM) sleep, called "active sleep" in newborns, occupies approximately 50% of sleep in infants, then decreases to around 25% of sleep in childhood and stays relatively constant throughout adulthood until tapering off in the elderly. With aging, we also spend more time in bed awake (stage 0); the elderly often spend as much as 20% of the time in bed awake [4]. TIB%—percentage that each stage occurs during the total time in bed; Stage 0—awake.

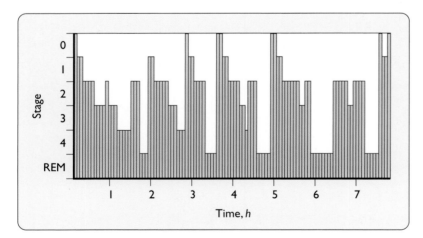

Figure 6-4.
Normal sleep histogram. This figure represents the sleep staging for a young adult with normal sleep. Time across the night is represented on the x-axis in hours. Stage 0 represents wakefulness. Humans cycle through stages 1 to 4 and REM in a characteristic pattern, with stages 3 and 4 (slow wave sleep), predominating the first third of the night. REM sleep occurs after 70 to 100 minutes (average 90 min) and then cycles every 90 minutes thereafter with each progressive REM period lengthening during the night [5–7].

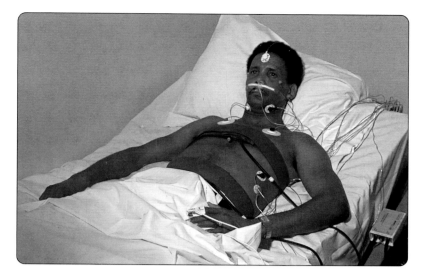

Figure 6-5.
This picture depicts a person ready for polysomnography. He has four electroencephalography leads on his head to measure the brain waves (C3:A2; C4:A1; O2:A1; O1:A2). Only one central lead (C4:A1 or C3:A2) is needed to score sleep according to the criteria set forth by Rechtschaffen and Kales [8]. The occipital leads (O2:A1 and O1:A2) are used to better discern alpha waves. Other leads needed to score sleep mostly help to distinguish REM sleep from wakefulness. The respiratory leads include a nasal-oral thermistor (under the nose) to measure airflow, chest and abdominal belts to measure respiratory effort, and a snore microphone and finger oximetry. Other leads include anterior tibialis electromyography to assess for movement and electrocardiography (lead II).

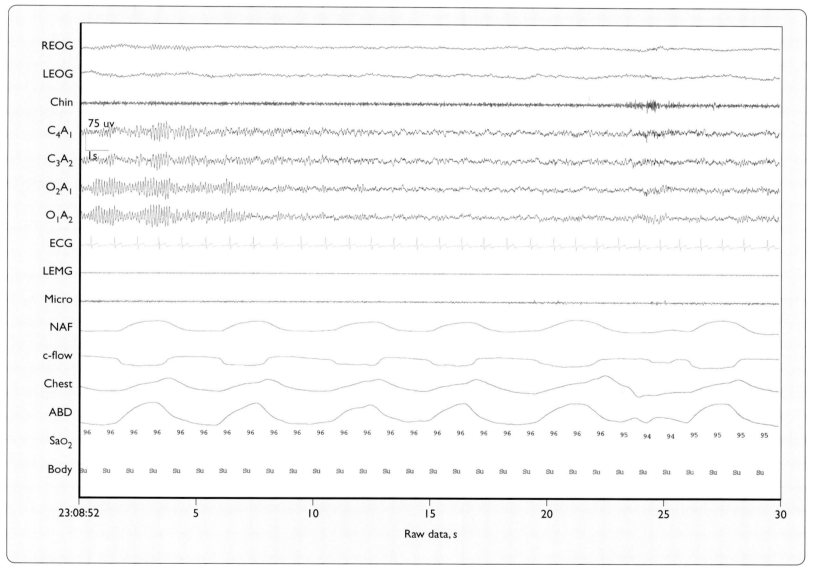

Figure 6-6.
Transition from stage 0 (wakefulness) to stage 1. This is an epoch (30 sec) from an overnight polysomnogram. As can be seen at approximately the 10-second mark, the alpha waves (8–14 cycles/s) disappear and mixed frequency low amplitude waves predominate. This epoch would be scored as stage 1 because more than 15 seconds (50%) of the epoch are stage 1. Stage 1 occupies approximately 2% to 5% of normal sleep. REOG—right electro-oculogram; LEOG—left electro-oculogram; chin—genioglossus electromyogram; C_4A_1, C_3A_2—central electroencephalogram; O_2A_1, O_1A_2—occipital electro-oculogram; Micro—snore microphone; NAF—nasal airflow; c-flow—CPAP flow; Chest—chest respiratory effort; ABD—abdominal respiratory effort; SaO_2—oxygen saturation; Body—body position; Su—supine.

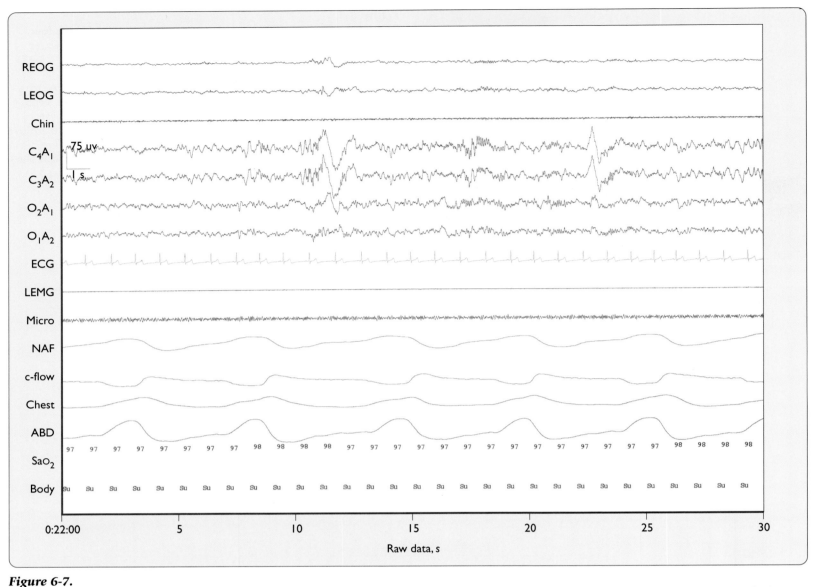

Figure 6-7.

This epoch shows stage 2 sleep, which is characterized by sleep spindles (12–14 cycles/s lasting at least 0.5 s) and K complexes (initial negative [up] deflection followed by a positive [down] deflection lasting 0.5 s). A sleep spindle is seen at 17 seconds and a K complex at 23 seconds. This stage composes most of normal sleep (45%–55%). REOG—right electro-oculogram; LEOG—left electro-oculogram; Chin—genioglossus electromyogram; C_4A_1, C_3A_2—central electroencephalogram; O_2A_1, O_1A_2—occipital electro-oculogram; ECG—electrocardiogram; LEMG—left anterior tibialis electromyogram; Micro—snore microphone; NAF—nasal airflow; c-flow—CPAP flow; Chest—chest respiratory effort; ABD—abdominal respiratory effort; SaO_2—oxygen saturation; Body—body position.

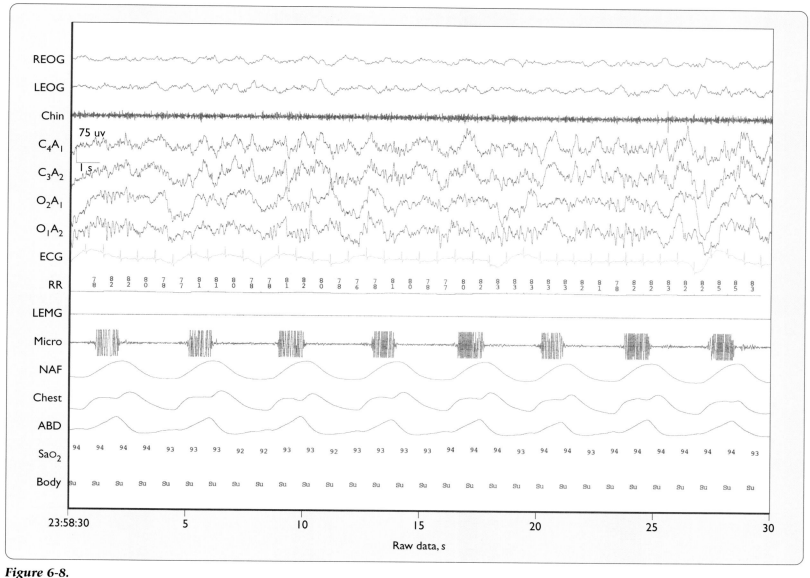

Figure 6-8.

Slow wave sleep. Slow wave sleep is comprised of stages 3 and 4. These stages are characterized by delta waves (0.5–2 cycles/s). An epoch is considered stage 3 if 20% to 50% (6–15 s) of the epoch is dominated by delta waves and stage 4 (if >15 s) is covered with delta waves. The epoch shown demonstrates stage 3. REOG—right electro-oculogram; LEOG—left electro-oculogram; chin—genioglossus electromyogram; C_4A_2, C_3A_2—central electroencephalogram; O_2A_1, O_1A_2—occipital electro-oculogram; ECG—electrocardiogram; RR—the RR interval between QRS complexes on ECG; LEMG—left anterior tibialis electromyogram; Micro—snore microphone; NAF—nasal airflow; Chest—chest respiratory effort; ABD—abdominal respiratory effort; SaO_2—oxygen saturation; Body—body position; Su—supine.

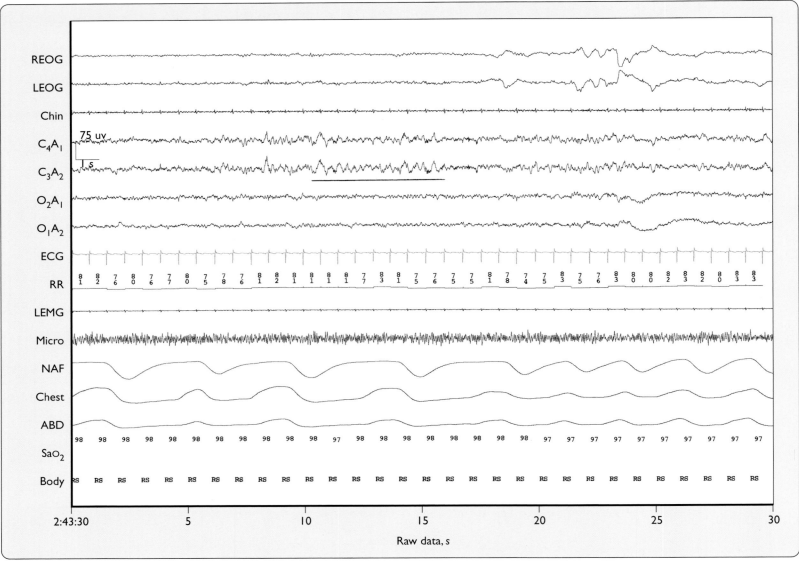

Figure 6-9.
REM sleep. This epoch shows rapid eye movement (REM) stage sleep. It is characterized by loss of muscle tone in the chin electromyogram lead and sharp, rapid eye movements. The EEG will show low voltage waves with the characteristic "sawtooth" or "picket fence" waves (*underlined*) intermittently seen. REOG—right electro-oculogram; LEOG—left electro-oculogram; chin—genioglossus electromyogram; C_4A_1, C_3A_2— central electroencephalogram; O_2A_1, O_1A_2—occipital electro-oculogram; ECG—electrocardiogram; RR—the RR interval between QRS complexes on ECG; LEMG—left anterior tibialis electromyogram; Micro—snore microphone; NAF—nasal airflow; Chest—chest respiratory effort; ABD—abdominal respiratory effort; SaO_2—oxygen saturation; Body—body position.

CLASSIFICATIONS OF INSOMNIA

Types (patients may have more than one)
- Sleep onset: difficulty initiating sleep
- Sleep maintenance: difficulty staying sleep
- Early morning awakening: awakening early and unable to return to sleep

Duration (length of time patient suffers from insomnia)
- Acute: less than 1 month
- Subacute: 1 to 6 months
- Chronic: more than 6 months

Severity (degree of impairment of social or job function)
- Mild: no impairment of function (irritability, fatigue)
- Moderate: some impairment of function
- Severe: major, debilitating impairment of function

Figure 6-10.
Classifications of insomnia. Insomnia is very common, afflicting one third of the population annually. It is more common in women and the elderly. This table lists some common ways in which insomnia is classified [9].

COMMON DISORDERS ASSOCIATED WITH INSOMNIA

Disorder	Description
Adjustment disorder	Most common cause; insomnia related to an anticipated or recent event (death of loved one, anxiety over a test)
Mental disorder	Includes depression, schizophrenia, mania; causes approximately one third of chronic insomnia
Psychophysiologic insomnia [10]	Typically begins in early adulthood; develop learned sleep-preventing behaviors; excessive focus on sleep problem
Restless legs syndrome [11]	Occurs in 10% to 20% of the population; daytime symptom of "creepy-crawly" sensations in legs resulting in irresistible desire to move legs; 80% have periodic limb movements in sleep [12]
Obstructive sleep apnea	5% to 10% of patients with OSA; resolves with treatment
Circadian rhythm disorder	Two general types: advanced sleep phase (fall asleep early and awaken early) and delayed sleep phase (can't fall asleep at scheduled bedtime and can't awaken in the morning) [13]; also includes jet lag
Drug abuse/alcoholism	Includes amphetamines, ephedrine, caffeine, nicotine, some selective serotonin reuptake inhibitors; alcohol induces sleep but alters sleep architecture

Figure 6-11.
Common disorders associated with insomnia [14,15].

TREATMENT FOR INSOMNIA

Category	Example	Action
Medication	Benzodiazepines: triazolam, temazepam, clonazepam	Enhance gamma amino butyric acid (GABA) inhibitory transmission through benzodiazepine receptor
	Benzodiazepine-like: zolpidem, zapelon	$GABA_A$ agonist modulators; very short half-life
	Antidepressants: trazodone, amitryptiline	Best effect in depressive patients with insomnia
	Over-the-counter: melatonin, diphenhydramine (DPH)	Melatonin most efficacious in jet lag, sleep aids with DPH induce drowsiness
Sleep hygiene education	*See* Figure 6-13	Incorporate in all regimens
Stimulus control		Trains patients to associate sleep with the bed and bedroom
Sleep restriction therapy		Inhibit time in bed to time asleep then progressively lengthen sleep time
Biofeedback		Visual/auditory feedback to control a physiologic action

Figure 6-12.
Treatments for insomnia.

SLEEP HYGIENE: RULES FOR A GOOD NIGHT'S SLEEP

1. Go to sleep and awaken at approximately the same time each night and day.
2. Do not exercise or take a hot bath or shower within 1 hour of sleeping.
3. Avoid stimulant drugs or foods after dinner (*eg*, cigarettes, caffeine).
4. Use your bed for only sleeping or sexual activity; do not watch television or engage in other activities in bed.
5. A light snack before bedtime is acceptable, but avoid rich or fatty foods.
6. Keep the bedroom dark, quiet, and at a comfortable temperature during the sleep period.
7. Morning exercise and exposure to sunlight will improve morning wakefulness.
8. Maintain a reasonable weight.
9. Avoid evening naps.
10. Do not drink excessive fluids before bedtime and avoid alcoholic beverages after the evening meal.

Figure 6-13.
Sleep hygiene. This table lists 10 rules for a good night's sleep.

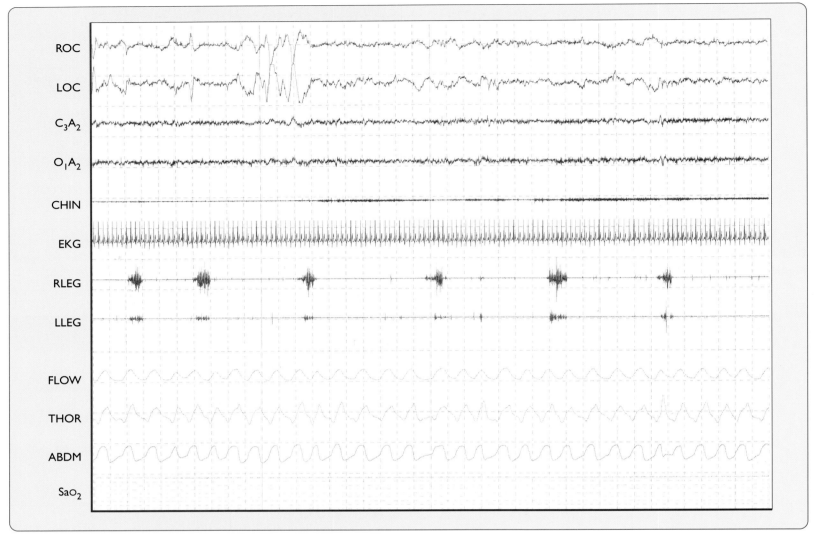

Figure 6-14.
Periodic limb movements (PLM). These are four epochs from a polysomnogram showing periodic limb movements. These are repetitive leg jerks as represented in the leg EMG channel. These typically occur every 20 to 40 seconds and, to be scored as a PLM, require at least four movements. PLM have been associated with restless legs syndrome (RLS), occurring in 80% of those patients; however, only 30% of patients exhibiting PLM have RLS. PLM have also been associated with narcolepsy, sleep apnea, upper airway resistance syndrome, uremia, and CNS disorders. ROC—right electro-oculogram; LOC—left electro-oculogram; C_3A_2—central electroencephalogram; O_1A_2—occipital electro-oculogram; chin—genioglossus electromyogram; EKG—electrocardiogram; RLEG—right anterior tibialis electromyogram; LLEG—left anterior tibialis electromyogram; Micro—snore microphone; FLOW—oronasal airflow; THOR—chest respiratory effort; ABDM—abdominal respiratory effort; SaO_2—oxygen saturation.

CAUSES OF HYPERSOMNIA

Chronic sleep deprivation
Obstructive sleep apnea-hypopnea syndrome
Upper airway resistance syndrome
Narcolepsy
Idiopathic hypersomnia
Kleine-Levin syndrome
Circadian rhythm disorders

Figure 6-15.
Causes of hypersomnia. Most patients at sleep clinics complain of excessive daytime sleepiness [16]. This is associated with poor job and driving performance, difficulty in personal relationships, and poor self-image. Physicians evaluating patients with hypersomnia need to know the differential diagnoses as listed in this table.

Test	Number	Equipment	Length	Normal
MSLT	Four to five nap opportunities	Sleep staging montage, patient lying in bed	20 minutes for sleep onset, up to 35 for REM onset, 2 hours apart	Sleep latency ≥10 minutes; 0 sleep onset REM periods
MWT	Four sleep opportunities	Sleep staging montage, patient sitting in bed	40 minutes, patient encouraged to stay awake, 2 hours apart	Sleep onset ≥20 minutes
ESS	—	Questionnaire	Eight questions with answers of severity ranging from 0 to 3	Score of <10
SSS	—	Questionnaire	Seven sleepiness sentences determined at various times	The higher the number, the sleepier the subject

ESS—Epworth Sleepiness scale; MSLT—multiple sleep latency test; MWT—maintenance of wakefulness test; REM—rapid eye movement; SSS—Stanford Sleepiness scale.

Figure 6-16.

Tests for evaluating excessive daytime sleepiness. MSLT—multiple sleep latency test; MWT—maintenance of wakefulness test; ESS—Epworth Sleepiness scale; SSS—Standford Sleepiness scale.

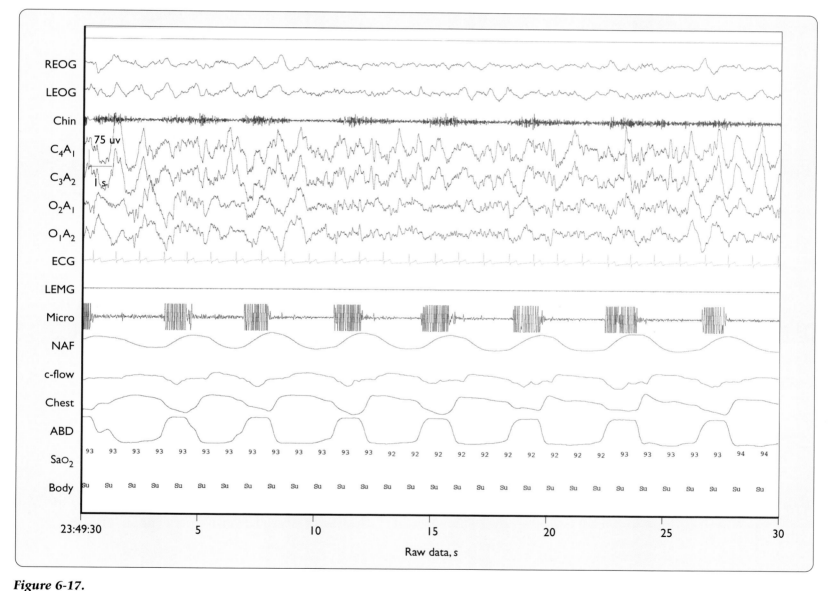

Figure 6-17.

Snoring. This epoch of sleep shows snore signals on the snore microphone channel. It can be seen that these "snores" are occurring during the inspiratory phase (upslope of airflow channel) of inspiration and are not disrupting the patient's sleep. The snores can also be seen with increased amplitude in the chin EMG [17]. REOG—right electro-oculogram; LEOG—left electro-oculogram; chin—genioglossus electromyogram; C_4A_2, C_3A_2—central electroencephalogram; O_2A_1, O_1A_2—occipital electro-oculogram; ECG—electrocardiogram; LEMG—left anterior tibialis electromyogram; Micro—snore microphone; NAF—nasal airflow; c-flow—CPAP flow; Chest—chest respiratory effort; SaO_2—oxygen saturation; Body—body position; Su—supine.

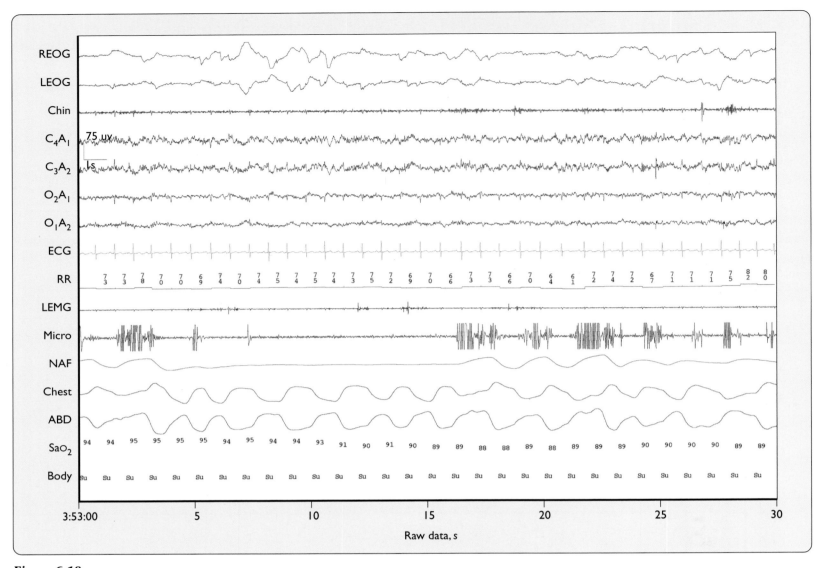

Figure 6-18.

Obstructive apnea [18]. This epoch shows a classic obstructive sleep apnea in which there is loss of airflow for more than 10 seconds, with continued respiratory effort. Oxygen saturation decreases from a high of 95% to a nadir of 88%. REOG—right electro-oculogram; LEOG—left electro-oculogram; Chin—genioglossus electromyogram; C_4A_1, C_3A_2—central electroencephalogram; O_2A_1, O_1A_2—occipital electro-oculogram; ECG—electrocardiogram; RR—the RR interval between QRS complexes on ECG; LEMG—left anterior tibialis electromyogram; Micro—snore microphone; NAF—nasal airflow; Chest—chest respiratory effort; ABD—abdominal respiratory effort; SaO_2—oxygen saturation; Body—body position; Su—supine.

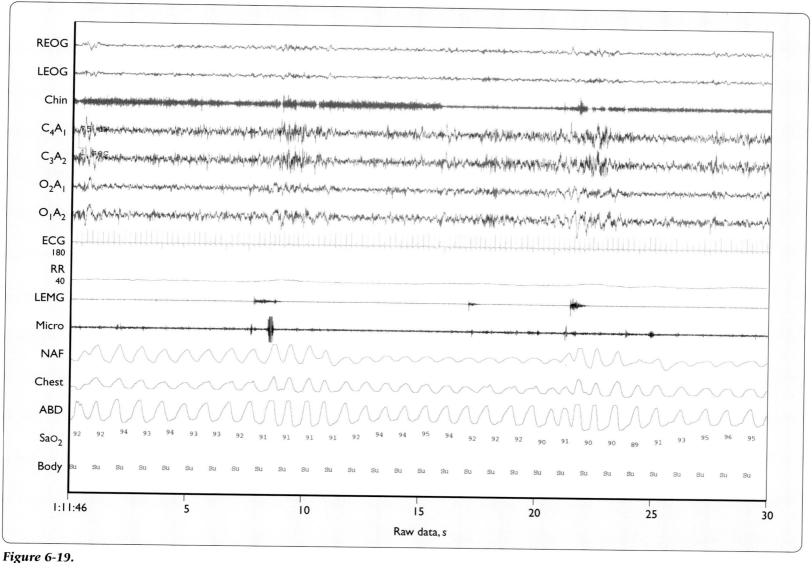

Figure 6-19.

Obstructive hypopnea [19]. This portion of a polysomnogram represents four epochs of sleep (2 min). From approximately 45 seconds to 85 seconds is a hypopnea that is often variably defined. Most sleep laboratories use a definition that requires a reduction in airflow (usually > 50%) lasting at least 10 seconds and ending in an arousal or resulting in a 3% to 4% oxygen desaturation. This example shows a >3% desaturation (95%–89%) after the hypopnea; as the oxygen saturation is recovering, another hypopnea is beginning. REOG—right electro-oculogram; LEOG—left electro-oculogram; Chin—genioglossus electromyogram; C_4A_2, C_3A_2—central electroencephalogram; O_2A_1, O_1A_2—occipital electro-oculogram; ECG—electrocardiogram; LEMG—left anterior tibialis electromyogram; Micro—snore microphone; NAF—nasal airflow; c-flow—CPAP flow; Chest—chest respiratory effort; ABD—abdominal respiratory effort; SaO_2—oxygen saturation; Body—body position; Su—supine.

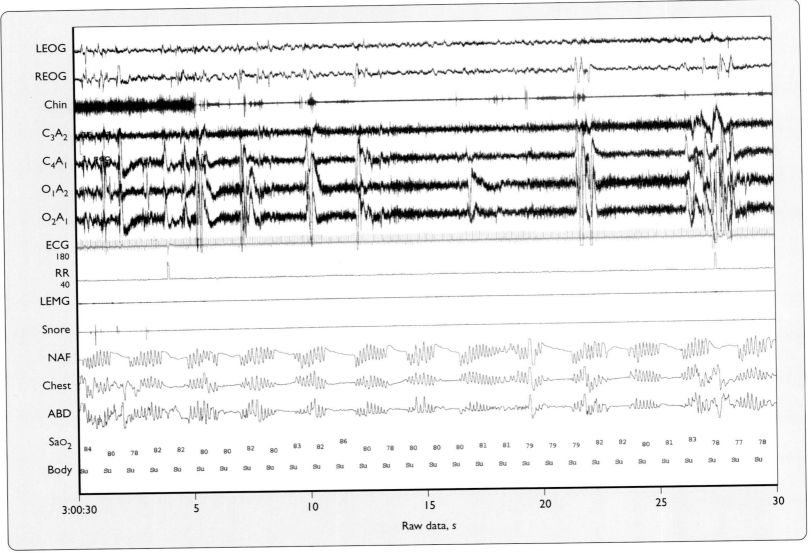

Figure 6-20.

Cheyne-Stokes ventilation (CSR). This figure contains several epochs of a polysomnogram and represents 5 minutes. As can be seen in the flow and effort channels, there is a crescendo followed by a decrescendo pattern resulting eventually in an apnea then repeat of the cycle. This pattern of breathing is seen most commonly in heart failure and central nervous system disorders. Nasal CPAP often eliminates CSR, possibly by altering carbon dioxide levels [20–24]. REOG—right electro-oculogram; LEOG—left electro-oculogram; Chin—genioglossus electromyogram; C_4A_1, C_3A_2—central electroencephalogram; O_2A_1, O_1A_2—occipital electro-oculogram; ECG—electrocardiogram; RR—the RR interval between QRS complexes on ECG; LEMG—left anterior tibialis electromyogram; Micro—snore microphone; NAF—nasal airflow; Chest—chest respiratory effort; ABD—abdominal respiratory effort; SaO_2—oxygen saturation; Body—body position; Su—supine.

REFERENCES

1. Sherin J, Shiroman P, McCarley R, et al.: Activation of ventrolateral preoptic neurons during sleep. *Science* 1996, 271:216–219.

2. Borbeley A: A two-process model of sleep regulation: physiologic basis and outline. *Human Neurobiol* 1982, 1:195–204.

3. Bliwise D: Sleep in normal aging and dementia. *Sleep* 1993, 116:40–81.

4. Maggi S, Langlois J, Minicuci N, et al.: Sleep complaints in community-dwelling older persons: prevalence, associated factors, and reported causes. *J Am Geriatr Soc* 1998, 46:161–168.

5. Shepard J: Gas exchange and hemodynamics during sleep. *Med Clin North Am* 1985, 69:1243–1264.

6. Van de Borne P, Nguyen H, Biston P, et al.: Effects of wake and sleep stages on the 24 h autonomic control of blood pressure and heart rate in recumbent men. *Am J Physiol* 1994, 266:H548–H554.

7. Cardiopulmonary Diagnostics Focus Group: AARC-APT clinical practice guideline. *Respir Care* 1995, 40:1336–1343.

8. Rechtschaffen A, Kales K: A manual of standardized terminology, techniques and scoring system for sleep stages of human subjects. *NIH Publication #204*; 1968.

9. Morin M, Colecchi C, Stone J, et al.: Behavioral and pharmacological therapies for late-life insomnia: a randomized controlled trial. *JAMA* 1999, 281:991–999.

10. Perlis M, Giles D, Mendelson W, et al.: Psychophysiological insomnia: the behavioral model and a neurocognitive perspective. *J Sleep Res* 1997, 6:179–188.

11. Mendelsohn W: Are periodic leg movements associated with a clinical sleep disturbance? *Sleep* 1996, 19(3):219–223.

12. Chesson A, Wise M, Davila D, et al.: Practice parameters for the treatment of Restless Legs Syndrome and Periodic Limb Movement Disorder. *Sleep* 1999, 22(7):961–968.

13. Standards of Practice Committee, American Sleep Disorders Association: The clinical use of the multiple sleep latency test. *Sleep* 1992, 15:268–276.

14. Johns M: Sleepiness in different situations measured by the Epworth Sleepiness Scale. *Sleep* 1994, 17:703–710.

15. Sangal R, Thomas L, Mitler M: Maintenance of Wakefulness Test and Multiple Sleep Latency Test. Measurement of Different Abilities in Patients with Sleep Disorders. *Chest* 1992, 101:898–902.

16. El-Ad B, Korczyn A: Disorders of excessive daytime sleepiness—an update. *J Neurol Sci* 1998, 153:192–202

17. Hoffstein V: Snoring. *Chest* 1996, 109:201–222.

18. American Academy of Sleep Medicine Task Force: Sleep-related breathing disorders in adults: recommendations for syndrome definition and measurement techniques in clinical research. *Sleep* 1999, 22:667–690.

19. Redline S, Sanders M: Hypopnea, a floating metric: implications for prevalence, morbidity estimates, and case findings. *Sleep* 1997, 20(12);1209–1217.

20. White D: Pathophysiology of obstructive sleep apnea. *Thorax* 1995, 50:797–804.

21. Hudgel D: Treatment of obstructive sleep apnea. *Chest* 1996, 109:1346–1358.

22. Javaheri S: A mechanism of central sleep apnea in patients with heart failure. *N Engl J Med* 1999, 341:949–954.

23. Roux F, D'Ambrosio, Mohsenin V: Sleep-related breathing disorders and cardiovascular disease. *Am J Med* 2000, 108:396–402.

24. Trinder J, Merson R, Rosenberg, *et al.*: Pathophysiological interactions of ventilation, arousals, and blood pressure oscillations during Cheyne-Stokes respiration in patients with heart failure. *Am J Respir Crit Care Med* 2000, 162:800–813.

LUNG CANCER

Dessmon Y. H. Tai,
Raed A. Dweik,
Atul C. Mehta, &
Muzaffar Ahmad

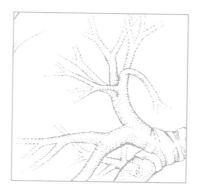

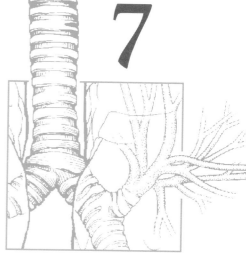

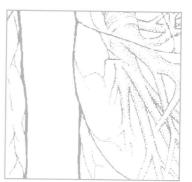

Lung cancer is the leading cause of cancer death in the United States. In the year 2000, lung cancer caused 156,900 deaths and accounted for 28.4% of all cancer deaths and 7% of all deaths. In the same year, 164,100 new cases of bronchogenic carcinoma occurred, accounting for 13.4% of all new cancers [1].

Of greater concern than the overall incidence rate is that the incidence of lung cancer continues to increase in every patient group, except white men. From 1950 to 1988, the overall incidence of new cases increased by 262.8%; this increase was substantially greater among women (511.7%) than men (222.5%). Also of concern is that survival among patients receiving treatment has remained essentially unchanged; during the same time period, the overall 5-year relative survival rate for lung cancer improved minimally, from 6.0% during the period of 1950 to 1954 to 13.4% during the period of 1981 to 1987. Lung cancer accounts for the most years of life lost (2,015,000 years in 1988) due to any cancer [1,2].

Bronchogenic carcinoma has become a worldwide health problem. Successful control of this global epidemic depends on the elimination of tobacco use, avoidance of environmental and occupational exposure to carcinogens, and a better understanding of the biology of lung cancer, which may promote the development of improved prevention and therapeutic strategies [3,4].

This chapter reviews the understanding of lung cancer pathology, its clinical presentation, and diagnostic techniques.

ACQUIRED RISK FACTORS FOR LUNG CANCER

Tobacco smoke
Active
Passive

Environmental factors
Air pollution
Radon progeny: natural decay of uranium

Occupational carcinogens
Proven
Arsenic: copper smelters, glass, and pesticide workers
Asbestos: insulation workers, textile workers, asbestos users
Bischloromethyl ether and chloromethyl methyl ether: textile, paint, chemical, and home insulation workers
Chromium: leather, ceramic, and metal workers; tanners
Diesel exhaust
Ionizing radiation, gamma radiation (x-rays)
Mustard gas: soldiers (warfare), production workers
Nickel and nickel compounds: nickel refinery, smeltery, and electrolysis workers
Radon progeny: uranium miners, fluorspar miners
Soot, tar, mineral oils (polycyclic aromatic hydrocarbons): road workers, roofers, coke oven workers, and iron and steel foundry workers
Vinyl chloride: plastics workers

Suspected
Acrylonitrile
Beryllium
Cadmium and cadmium compounds
Crystalline silica
Electromagnetic fields
Formaldehyde
Man-made mineral fibers (*eg*, rock wool or slag wool)
Wood dust

Dietary influences
Vitamin A deficiency
Vitamin E deficiency
Vitamin C deficiency
Selenium deficiency
High dietary fat/cholesterol intake

Lung diseases
Peripheral pulmonary scar
Pulmonary tuberculosis
Interstitial pulmonary fibrosis
Scleroderma
Pneumoconiosis
Chronic obstructive pulmonary disease

Figure 7-1.

Acquired risk factors for lung cancer. There is a broad range of known and proposed acquired risk factors for lung cancer [2–11]. Chemicals in tobacco smoke are the best known lung carcinogens. Estimates of the proportion of lung cancer attributable to cigarette smoking in developed countries range from 83% to 94% in men and 57% to 80% in women [5]. Radon, an inert gas derived from radium-226 during the natural decay of uranium and found in certain soils and rocks, is the second most frequent cause of lung cancer [3,6]. The incidence of radon-induced lung cancer is increased by smoking [6]. Occupational exposure to carcinogens accounts for about 15% of cases in men and 5% of cases in women. The most common occupational exposure is to asbestos; again, smoking increases the risk of developing the carcinogen-induced lung cancer [2]. Other potential risk factors include a deficiency in vitamins that are thought to protect against lung cancer, and certain chronic lung diseases [10].

MOLECULAR BIOLOGY OF LUNG CANCER

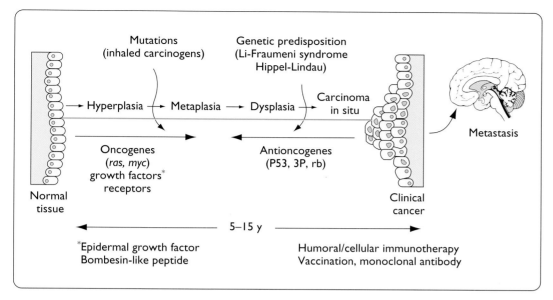

Figure 7-2.
Molecular biology of lung cancer. Cellular proliferation is normally controlled by 1) proto-onco-
genes, which are crucial for normal cellular
functions (including signal transduction and
transcription); 2) tumor suppressor genes, which
regulate transcription; and 3) antioncogenes,
which are recessive growth regulatory genes.
Oncogenes and growth factors, and their receptors, play a central role in tumorigenesis. The loss
of normal antioncogene expression requires
homozygous mutation or deletion; as the number
of mutations increases, the neoplasm progresses
from a hyperplastic lesion to invasive lung cancer.
This may explain the incidence of synchronous
primary lung cancers (estimated to range from
0.26% to 1.33%) and the annual incidence of
2% to 5% for second malignancies after resection
for stage I non–small cell lung cancer [11,12].

MAJOR TYPES OF LUNG CANCER

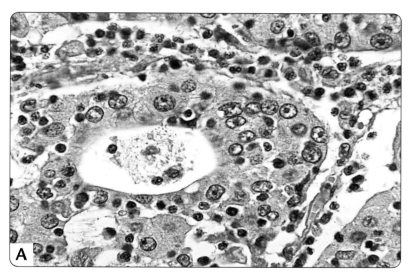

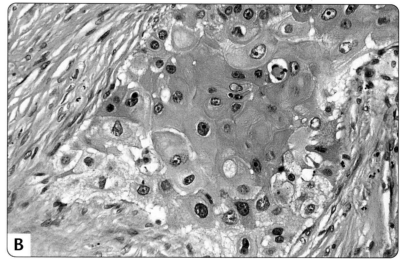

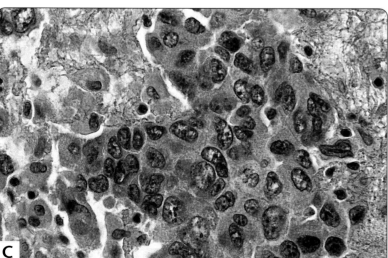

Figure 7-3.
Major types of lung cancer. Ninety percent to 95% of all lung cancers can
be classified under the four major histologic cell types: **A,** Adenocarcinoma
accounts for 33% to 35% of all cases. (*See* Color Plate.) **B,** Squamous
cell carcinoma accounts for 30% to 32% of all cases. (*See* Color Plate.)
C, Large cell carcinoma accounts for 15% to 20% of all cases. (*See*
Color Plate.)

(*Continued on next page*)

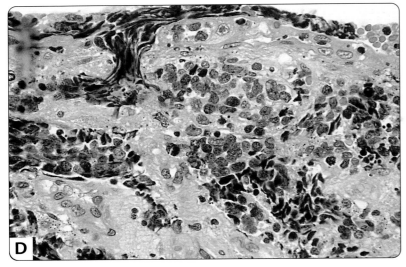 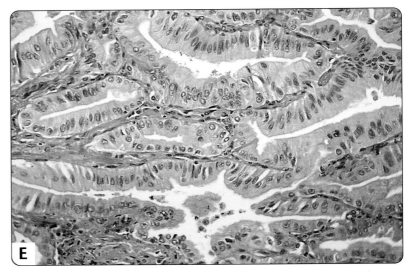

Figure 7-3. (*Continued*)
D, Small cell carcinoma accounts for 20% to 25% of all cases. (*See Color Plate.*) **E,** Bronchioloalveolar cell carcinoma, a subtype of adenocarcinoma, is less common. (*See Color Plate.*)

CLINICAL PRESENTATION OF LUNG CANCER

PRESENTATION OF LUNG CANCER

Local				
Central	**Peripheral**	**Regional**	**Distant**	**Systemic**
Cough	Cough	Horner's syndrome	Bone pain	Weight loss
Hemoptysis	Pain	Pancoast's syndrome	Headache	Anorexia
Pain	Dyspnea	Superior vena cava obstruction	Stroke	Fatigue
Dyspnea		Pleural effusion	Confusion	Fever
Wheezing		Chest pain	Pericardial effusion	
Stridor		Dysphagia	Jaundice	
Pneumonia		Hoarseness (recurrent laryngeal nerve paralysis)	Ascites	
		Elevated hemidiaphragm (phrenic nerve paralysis)	Abdominal pain	
			Hepatomegaly	
			Lymphadenopathy	
			Skin nodules	
			Pulmonary embolism	

Figure 7-4. Clinical presentation of lung cancer. Patients with lung cancer may have local, regional, or metastatic disease [7,9,13,14]. Only 10% to 25% are asymptomatic at the time of diagnosis, when incidental abnormalities are found on chest radiograph [15].

PARANEOPLASTIC SYNDROMES IN LUNG CANCER

System	Syndrome
Endocrine and metabolic	Cushing's syndrome
	SIADH
	Hypercalcemia/PTH-related peptide
	Gynecomastia
	Galactorrhea
	Acromegaly
	Ectopic gonadotropic hormone
	Hyperthyroidism
	Hypercalcitoninemia
	Hypophosphatemia
	Insulin-like activity
	Hyperamylasemia
Neuromuscular	Peripheral neuropathy
	Corticocerebellar degeneration
	Eaton-Lambert syndrome
	Cranial nerve abnormalities
	Necrotizing myelopathy
	Autonomic neuropathy
	Encephalopathy
	Carcinomatous myopathy
Skeletal	Clubbing and pulmonary hypertrophic osteoarthropathy
Dermatologic	Dermatomyositis, polymyositis
	Acanthosis nigricans
	Diffuse hyperpigmentation
	Erythema gyratum repens
	Erythema multiforme
	Pruritus, urticaria
	Tylosis
	Scleroderma
Hematologic	Anemia
	Thrombocytosis
	Nonspecific leukocytosis
	Leukoerythroblastic reaction
	Eosinophilia
	Disseminated intravascular coagulation
	Polycythemia
	Red cell aplasia
	Dysproteinemia
Cardiovascular	Migratory thrombophlebitis
	Nonbacterial verrucous (marantic) endocarditis
	Arterial thrombosis
Renal	Glomerulonephritis
	Proteinuria
	Nephrotic syndrome

PTH—parathyroid hormone; SIADH—syndrome of inappropriate antidiuretic hormone secretion.

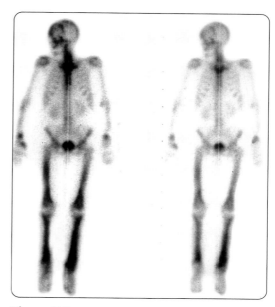

Figure 7-6.
Bone scan showing hypertrophic pulmonary osteoarthropathy. New periosteal bone formation is highlighted in this bone scan of a patient with generalized hypertrophic pulmonary osteoarthropathy, a paraneoplastic disease reported to occur in 2% to 12% of patients with non–small cell lung cancer.

Figure 7-5.
Paraneoplastic syndromes. Paraneoplastic syndromes are reported in 2% to 20% of patients with lung cancer [15–17]. Extrapulmonary nonmetastatic manifestations of these syndromes may precede, coincide with, or follow the diagnosis of lung cancer. Their presence does not necessarily suggest that the lung cancer is unresectable. In some cases, the syndrome resolves immediately after resection of the primary tumor. In incurable cases, treatment of the associated symptoms or biochemical abnormalities— eg, hyperglycemia—may improve the patient's well being.

Types of carcinoma	Frequent location	Initial metastasis	Comments
Squamous cell	Central	Local invasion	Frequent cavitation and obstructive phenomena
			Hypercalcemia
Small cell	Central	Lymphatics	Cavitation rare
			Paraneoplastic syndromes
Adenocarcinoma	Midlung, periphery	Lymphatics	Association with peripheral scars
Large cell	Periphery	Central nervous system, mediastinum	Rapid growth with early metastases
Bronchioloalveolar	Periphery	Lymphatics, local invasion, hematogenous	No correlation with cigarette smoking
			Cavitation rare

Figure 7-7.

Clinical features of specific types of lung cancer. Although the initial presentations of lung cancer are diverse, each type of lung cancer is associated with a specific location, initial pattern of metastasis, and other features [18]. The specific clinical features may be helpful in the differential diagnosis and in selecting an appropriate work-up. (*Adapted from* Kiss [18].)

DIAGNOSIS

Radiography

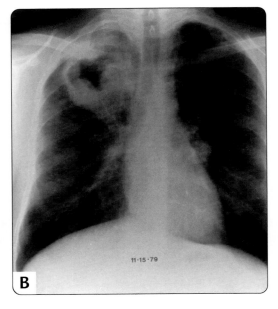

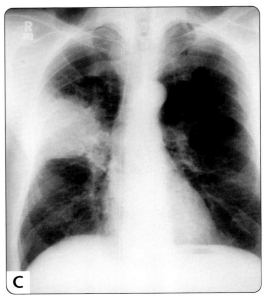

A B C

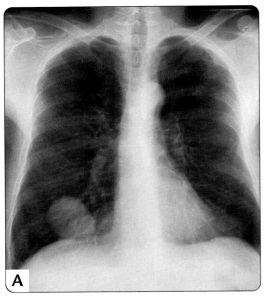

D

Figure 7-8.

Conventional chest radiography. Standard posteroanterior and lateral chest radiographs comprise the primary method of detecting lung cancer. The accuracy of the chest radiograph in the detection of lung cancer is 70% to 88%; in the detection of hilar adenopathy specifically, 61% to 71%; and in the detection of mediastinal adenopathy, 47% to 60% [19]. The detection of abnormalities is helpful in the selection of additional imaging techniques—eg, computed tomographic scans—or interventional procedures for a differential diagnosis and for staging purposes. **A,** Posteroanterior chest radiograph revealing a peripheral lobulated 4-cm mass in the right lower lobe, suggestive of adenocarcinoma. **B,** Posteroanterior chest radiograph showing a right upper lobe lobulated mass with shaggy margins and the classic cavitation, suggestive of squamous cell carcinoma. **C,** Postero-anterior chest radiograph showing a sharply defined peripheral mass more than 4 cm in diameter adjacent to pleura and chest wall, suggestive of large cell carcinoma. **D,** Posteroanterior chest radiograph showing prominent mediastinal adenopathy manifested by lobulated right paratracheal mass and a slight hilar mass, suggestive of small cell carcinoma. Right pleural effusion is also present.

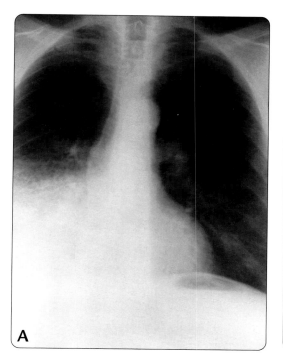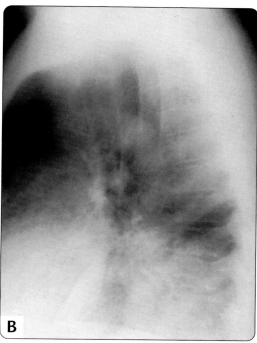

Figure 7-9.
Bronchioloalveolar carcinoma. **A** and **B**, Right lower lobe consolidation with extension to the pleural surface is illustrated on a posteroanterior chest radiograph (*panel A*) and an air bronchogram on lateral chest radiograph (*panel B*).

Bronchoscopy

DIAGNOSTIC YIELD OF VARIOUS BRONCHOSCOPIC TECHNIQUES

Procedure	Histologic type	Average diagnostic yield, % (*range*)	Agreement with definitive diagnosis, % (*range*)
Bronchial washing	Squamous cell	79 (77–81)	93
	Adenocarcinoma	79 (75–83)	50
	Large cell	62 (50–73)	20
	Small cell	65 (64–66)	100
Bronchial brushing	Squamous cell	78 (52–93)	82 (78–87)
	Adenocarcinoma	69 (57–88)	82 (79–85)
	Large cell	62 (20–100)	58 (33–84)
	Small cell	66 (30–95)	80 (72–87)
Forceps biopsy	Squamous cell	75 (63–96)	88 (88–96)
	Adenocarcinoma	55 (50–67)	71 (46–82)
	Large cell	57 (23–80)	31 (20–38)
	Small cell	85 (69–100)	85 (70–100)

Figure 7-10.
Diagnostic yield of various bronchoscopic techniques in lung cancer. The diagnostic yield of the various bronchoscopic techniques in central tumors (squamous cell and small cell carcinoma), which may present as endobronchial masses or submucosal or peribronchial lesions, are acceptable, as demonstrated in the figure [20]. The diagnostic yield in peripheral lesions is better using biplane (40% to 80%) than using conventional single-plane fluoroscopy (10% to 30%). Tumor size also affects diagnostic yield, which is low (28%) in lesions less than 2 cm in diameter but rises to 64% to 80% when the lesion is between 2 and 4 cm in diameter. This may be because tumors larger than 3 cm are supplied by three or more bronchi in 60% of cases, and lesions less than 3 cm are usually supplied by only one bronchus. (*Adapted from* Arroliga and Matthay [20].)

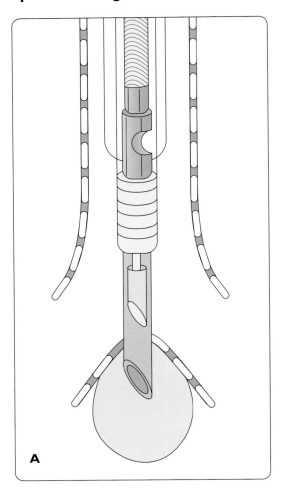

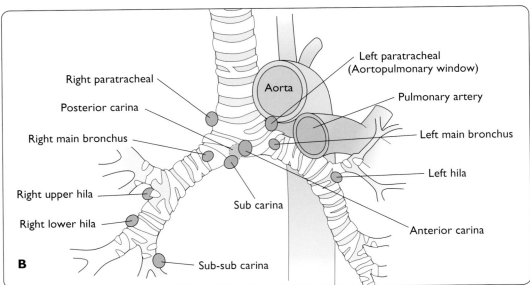

Figure 7-11.
Transbronchial needle aspiration (TBNA). **A** and **B**, TBNA (*panel A*) is particularly useful in evaluating extrabronchial lesions and paratracheal, subcarinal, or hilar lymph nodes (*panel B*). The diagnostic yield of bronchial washing and brushing and forceps biopsy in peripheral lung cancers increases from 48% to 69% with the addition of TBNA. Moreover, it is associated with less bleeding than forceps biopsy [20].

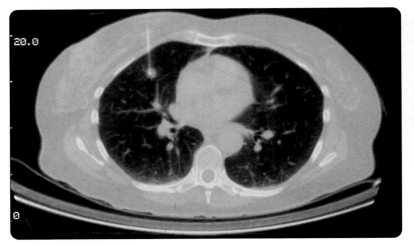

Figure 7-12.
Percutaneous transthoracic needle aspiration (TTNA) using computed tomographic guidance. In peripheral lesions, percutaneous TTNA is reported to have twice the diagnostic yield of bronchoscopy, independent of the size of the lesion [20]. Unfortunately, it is also associated with a higher incidence of adverse events. For example, the incidence of pneumothorax with TTNA is 32% to 36% compared with less than 1% with bronchoscopy. The incidence of bleeding is also greater with TTNA (3.5%) than with bronchoscopy (< 1%).

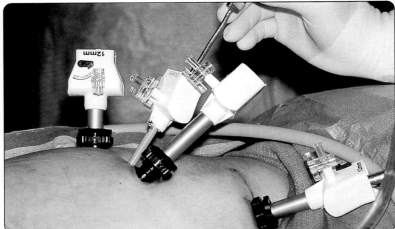

Figure 7-13.
Thoracoscopy. Video-guided thoracoscopic biopsy of pleural and peripheral lung lesions is particularly useful in the diagnosis of pleural metastatic lesion when pleural fluid cytology or "blind" percutaneous needle biopsy yields negative results [15].

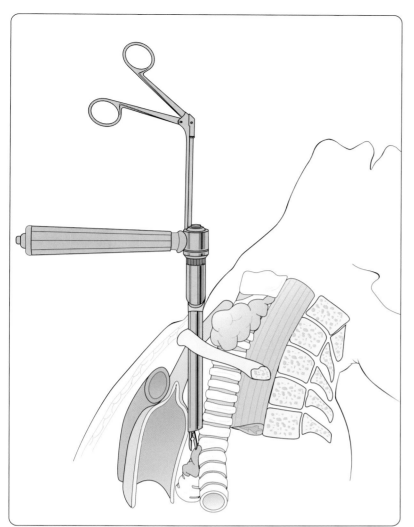

Figure 7-14.
Mediastinoscopy and mediastinotomy. Mediastinoscopy is an invasive, yet safe, procedure that can be used to identify malignant lymph nodes in the superior mediastinum. Mediastinal lymph node metastasis usually denotes unresectability. The introduction of mediastinoscopy has reduced the frequency of staging thoracotomies from 30% to 50% to 5% to 15% [9].

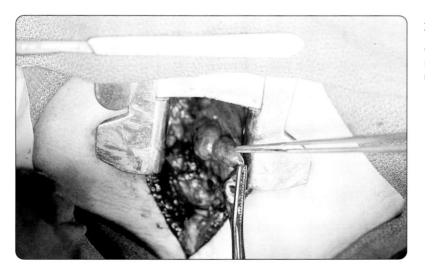

Figure 7-15.
Thoracotomy. Thoracotomy should be considered for establishing a diagnosis in a highly suspicious lesion when the lesion is potentially resectable, the patient is physiologically fit enough for resection, and there is no evidence of distant metastasis [15,17].

SCREENING OF LUNG CANCER

A. INVESTIGATED METHODS (SELECTED) OF LUNG CANCER SCREENING

Method	Design	Findings	Comments
Sputum cytology and CXR			
Mayo Lung Project, 1986	Cytology/CXR every 4 mo; randomized versus usual care	All three found more cases of lung cancer (4%–29% more), increased resectability (up to 44% higher); Mayo found better 5-year survival rates (35% vs 15%)	No disease-specific mortality benefit
Johns Hopkins Lung Project, 1986	Cytology every 4 mo/CXR every year; randomized versus yearly CXR		No disease-specific mortality benefit
Memorial Sloan Kettering Trial, 1984	Cytology every 4 mo/CXR every year; randomized versus yearly CXR		No disease-specific mortality benefit
Low-dose spiral CT			
National Cancer Center Hospital, Japan, 1996	Biannual CT vs biannual CXR; single cohort	15/1369 patients with CA on CT vs four found by CXR; 14/15 stage I	Prevalence data only
Shinshu University, Japan, 1998	Annual CT vs annual CXR; single cohort	19/5483 patients with CA on CT vs eight found by CXR; 16/19 stage I	Prevalence data only
Early Lung Cancer Action Project (ELCAP), 1999	Annual CT vs annual CXR; single cohort	27/1000 patients with CA on CT vs seven found by CXR; 23/27 stage I	Prevalence data only; 23% had noncalcified nodules requiring further imaging
Mayo Trial (ongoing)	Annual CT and sputum cytology	15/1520 patients with CA 9/15 stage I	Prevalence data only, accrual in progress; 51% had noncalcified nodules
Immunocytology			
Lung Cancer Early Detection Working Group (ongoing)	Assay hnRNP A2/B1 in sputum of patients with prior stage I NSCLC resection	Initial data with 15 recurrent cases: 77% sensitive, 67% accurate	Prospective trial underway; goal 1000 subjects
Fluorescence bronchoscopy	No large scale screening trial to date	2.7 times more sensitive than light bronchoscopy by intraepithelial lesions; 6.3 times when invasive CA included in analysis	Practical value questionable; Comparison with video bronchoscopy needed

CA—cancer; CT—computed tomography; CXR—chest radiography; NSCLC—non-small cell lung cancer.

B. SCREENING PITFALLS

Lack of proof of effectiveness

Survival statistics may be misleading in the absence of prospective, randomized controlled data. Mortality may be unchanged because of:

Lead time bias: survival appears longer because of earlier diagnosis, but the ultimate course and outcome of the disease are unchanged (age-adjusted disease-specific mortality unchanged)

Length time bias: less aggressive tumors are detected more often than their true population distribution because they are a longer potential asymptomatic period during which screening may occur. Outcome thereby appears improved in the screened population

Overdiagnosis bias: lesions with no effect on mortality are detected (either very indolent lesions or the patient expires from other causes before appearance of tumor symptoms

Cost

Poor specificity

Figure 7-16.
Lung cancer screening. **A** and **B**, Earlier studies did not demonstrate a mortality benefit, but computed tomography (CT)-based protocols have renewed interest in this area [22–28]. Other potential strategies include tumor marker immunocytology and augmented bronchoscopic surveillance [29,30]. Less than 15% of lung cancer is localized at the time of diagnosis. Treatment of stage I disease is associated with a 5-year survival of 38% to 61%. Advanced lung cancer portends a survival rate of less than 10%. Theoretically, earlier detection and intervention should lead o enhanced resectability and decreased age-adjusted lung cancer mortality [1,31].

STAGING OF LUNG CANCER

INTERNATIONAL TNM STAGING SYSTEM AND STAGE GROUPING FOR LUNG CANCER

TNM definitions

Tumor (T)

T0   No evidence of primary tumor

Tis   Carcinoma in situ

T1   ≤3 cm without evidence of invasion proximal to a lobar bronchus

T2   >3 cm, or tumor of any size involving visceral pleura or main bronchus or associated with atelectasis or obstructive pneumonitis

T3   Any size; extending into the chest wall, diaphragm, mediastinal pleura, or pericardium; or tumor in the main bronchus <2 cm from the carina

T4   Any size invading any of the following: mediastinum, heart, great vessels, trachea, esophagus, vertebral body, carina; or tumor with malignant pleural or pericardial effusion, or with satellite tumor nodules within the ipsilateral primary tumor lobe of the lung

Nodes (N)

N0   No regional nodal involvement

N1   Metastasis to ipsilateral peribronchial or hilar nodes

N2   Metastasis to mediastinal or subcarinal nodes

N3   Metastasis to contralateral hilar or mediastinal nodes; ipsilateral or contralateral supraclavicular or scalene nodes

Distant metastasis (M)

M0   Distant metastasis absent

M1   Distant metastasis present

State groupings

Occult	TX, N0
0	Tis N0
Ia	T1N0M0
Ib	T2N0M0
IIa	T1N1M0
IIb	T2N1M0
	T3N0M0
IIIa	T3N1M0
	T1N2M0
	T3N2M0
IIIb	T1-4N3M0
	T4N0-3M0
IV	Any T, Any N, M1

Figure 7-17.
Staging in non–small cell lung cancer (NSCLC). TNM (tumor, node, metastasis) staging is important in establishing a prognosis in patients with NSCLC. The 5-year postoperative survival rates in patients with pathologic stage I, II, and IIIa NSCLC are 38% to 61%, 24% to 34%, and 13%, respectively [21–23].

STAGING OF SMALL CELL LUNG CANCER

Limited disease (30%–40%)

    Primary tumor confined to one hemithorax

    Ipsilateral hilar lymph nodes

    Ipsilateral and contralateral supraclavicular lymph nodes

    Ipsilateral and contralateral mediastinal lymph nodes

    Ipsilateral pleural effusion, independent of cytology

Extensive disease (60%–70%)

    Metastatic lesions in the contralateral lung

    Distant metastatic involvement (*eg*, brain, bone, liver)

Figure 7-18.
Staging and therapy in small cell lung cancer (SCLC). In patients with SCLC, early metastasis is common, and surgery is curable in about 10% of cases. Staging for SCLC is, therefore, designed to determine if there is limited or extensive disease. The extent of disease affects chemotherapeutic and radiation therapy options and is helpful when estimating survival time. In patients with limited disease, prophylactic cranial irradiation should be considered [21–24].

APPROXIMATE FREQUENCIES OF METASTATIC INVOLVEMENT BY LUNG CANCER

Metastatic site	Frequency All lung cancers, %	Frequency SCLC, %
Central nervous system	20–50	10–30
Cervical lymph nodes	15–60	5 (extrathoracic)
Bone	25	29–35
Adrenal glands	NA	20–40
Liver	1–35	25–28
Heart (including pericardium)	20	NA
Bone marrow	NA	19–50
Pleural effusion	8–15	NA
Pulmonary embolism, infarction	10	NA
Pancoast's syndrome	4–8	NA
Superior vena cava syndrome	4	42.5

NA—data not available; SCLC—small cell lung cancer.

Figure 7-19.
Frequency of metastasis to specific sites. Lung cancer may metastasize to a variety of sites. Because metastatic disease affects treatment options, a careful search for evidence of metastasis should be performed [7,13,16,24,25].

TUMOR MARKERS IN LUNG CANCER

Biomarkers	Adenocarcinoma	Squamous cell	Large cell	Small cell
Carcinoembryonic antigen	++	+	+	+
Tissue polypeptide antigen	+	++	+	-
Squamous cell carcinoma antigen	-	++	-	-
Cytokeratin 19 fragment	+	++	+	-
Ferritin	+	+	+	-
CA 19-9, CA 50, CA 242	+	-	+	-
Neuron-specific enolase	-	-	-	++
Creatine-phosphokinase-BB	-	-	-	+
Chromogranin A	-	-	-	++
Neural cell adhesion molecule	-	-	-	++
Soluble interleukin-2 receptor	-	-	-	+
Bombesin-gastrin/releasing peptide	-	-	-	++
Insulin-like growth factor 1	-	-	-	+
Transferrin	-	-	-	+
Atrial natriuretic peptide	-	-	-	+
Monoclonal antibodies (cluster 5)	-	-	-	++
Lewis Y	-	-	-	+
c-, N-, L-*myc*	-	-	-	++
H-, K-, N-*ras*	++	+	+	-
p53	+	++	+	+

Histotypes of lung cancer

Figure 7-20.
Tumor markers in lung cancer. Molecular genetics and immunohistochemical techniques are being studied for their effectiveness in identifying biomarkers of malignancy. No single specific tumor marker is available for screening asymptomatic patients; however, some are being evaluated for their potential prognostic value when used alone or in combination with other clinical, histopathologic, or biochemical variables [26]. (*Adapted from* Niklinski and Furman [27].)

PROGNOSTIC MARKERS IN STAGE I NON–SMALL CELL LUNG CANCER

Variable	Favorable	Unfavorable
Anatomic and pathologic markers		
Tumor status	T1	T2
Histologic subtype*	Squamous	Large cell
Degree of tumor differentiation	Well differentiated	Poorly differentiated
Lymphatic vessel invasion	Absent	Present
Blood vessel invasion	Absent	Present
Mitotic index	Low	High
Degree of plasma cell infiltration	Present	Absent or minimal
Presence of tumor giant cells	Absent	Present
Adenocarcinoma subtype	Bronchioloalveolar, acinar, papillary	Solid tumor with mucus formation
Molecular genetic markers		
K-*ras* (oncogene) activation	No point mutation	Point mutation at codon 12
ras expression	Absent p21 staining	Strong p21 staining
C-erb B-2 expression	Normal	Increased
p53 (tumor-suppressor gene)	No mutation	Gene mutation present
p53 expression	Normal	Increased
Rb expression	Rb-positive	Rb-negative
bcl-2 expression	bcl-2–positive	bcl-2–negative
Differentiation markers		
Expression of blood group antigen on tumor cell	Conserved	Altered
Expression of H/Le^y/Le^b antigens	Negative staining with MIA-15-5	Positive staining with MIA-15-5
Proliferation markers		
DNA content (flow cytometry)	Diploid	Aneuploid
S-phase fraction (flow cytometry)	Low	High
Mitotic index	<13 mitoses/10 high-powered fields	≥13 mitoses/10 high-powered fields
Proliferation index using Ki-67 nuclear antigen	<3.5	>3.5
Thymidine labeling index	<2.9	>2.9
Nucleolar organizing regions (mean), *n*	<3.8/cell	>3.8/cell
PCNA	<5% of tumor cells stained with PCNA	>5% of tumor cells stained with PCNA
Markers of metastatic propensity		
Intensity of angiogenesis	Low	High
Basement membrane deposition (squamous cell carcinoma)	Extensive	Limited
Soluble interleukin-2 receptor value	Postoperative < preoperative	Postoperative > preoperative
Ability to establish in vitro cell lines	No	Yes

Adenocarcinoma is intermediate in prognostic value.
PCNA—proliferating cell nuclear antigen.

Figure 7-21.

Prognostic factors in stage I non–small cell lung cancer (NSCLC). The three major prognostic factors in NSCLC are stage of the disease, Karnofsky performance status, and weight loss. About 50% of patients with clinical stage I and 30% to 40% with pathologic stage I disease experience recurrence and die after curative resection [28]. Other anatomic, pathologic, and molecular markers reported to be highly predictive of outcome in stage I NSCLC are shown in the figure [28]. (*Adapted from* Strauss *et al.* [28].)

INDICATORS OF A POOR PROGNOSIS IN SMALL CELL LUNG CANCER

	Biochemical		Clinical	Therapeutic
Low	**Elevated**			
Hemoglobin	Leukocytes		Race nonwhite	Slow response rate
Platelets	LDH		Age >60 y	Failure to achieve complete response (?)
Na, Cl	CEA		Male gender	Unable to be resected
Albumin	Gamma-glutamyl transpeptidase		Weight loss	Low-dose density (?)
Uric acid			Extensive disease	No radiotherapy (limited disease) (?)
Bicarbonate			Liver, central nervous system, marrow sites/increasing number of sites	

CEA—carcinoembryonic antigen; LDH—lactate dehydrogenase.

Figure 7-22.
Prognostic markers in small cell lung cancer. Although the 5-year survival rate among patients with limited disease is only 10% to 20%, use of prognostic factors may help in selecting patients for more specific, intensive treatment to prolong survival and achieve a cure. (*Adapted from* Skarin [29].)

CONTRAINDICATIONS FOR PNEUMONECTOMY OR LOBECTOMY

Predicted postoperative FEV_1 <40%, or 0.8 L

$Paco_2$ >45 mm Hg

Pao_2 <50 mm Hg

Pulmonary hypertension (mean pulmonary artery pressure >30 mm Hg)

Cor pulmonale

Maximum oxygen consumption <10 mL/kg/min

Intractable congestive cardiac failure

Intractable ventricular arrhythmia

Recent myocardial infarction (<3 mo)

FEV_1—forced expiratory volume in 1 s.

Figure 7-23.
Treatment of non–small cell lung cancer (NSCLC). Surgery is the primary curative therapy for stage I and II NSCLC and is being used increasingly as a component of multimodality in locally advanced disease (stage IIIa and IIIb) [30]. Contraindications for surgery are listed in the figure. Approximately two thirds of patients with surgically resected pathologic stage I disease will be cured. The 5-year survival for pathologic stage II is 25% to 50%; for stage IIIa, it is 15% to 34%. Regarding recurrences, local recurrences are more likely to be squamous cell carcinoma and distal metastases are more likely to be adenocarcinoma.

MANAGEMENT OF PATIENTS WITH LUNG CANCER

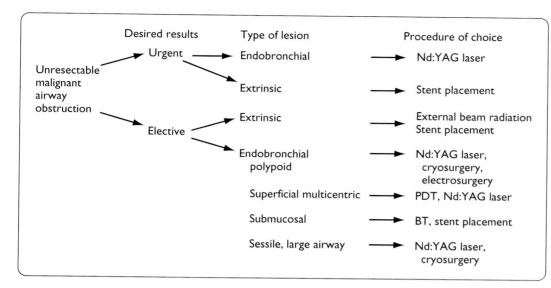

Figure 7-24.
Algorithm for the palliative management of airway obstruction caused by malignancy. Approximately 40% of lung cancer deaths occur as a result of locoregional disease, from either airway or vascular involvement. Airway obstruction may result from exophytic or submucosal lesions, or extrinsic compression. Palliative management of airway obstruction can be extremely helpful in properly selected patients [31]. BT—brachytherapy; Nd:YAG—neodymium:yttrium-aluminum-garnet; PDT—photodynamic therapy.

REFERENCES

1. Landis SH, Murray T, Bolden S, Wingo PA: Cancer statistics, 1998. *CA Cancer J Clin* 1998, 48:6–29.

2. Beckett WS: Epidemiology and etiology of lung cancer. *Clin Chest Med* 1993, 14:1–15.

3. Davila DG, Williams DE: The etiology of lung cancer. *Mayo Clin Proc* 1993, 68:170–182.

4. Roth JA: Molecular events in lung cancer. *Lung Cancer* 1995, 12(suppl 2):S3–S15.

5. Kabat GC: Recent developments in the epidemiology of lung cancer. *Semin Surg Oncol* 1993, 9:73–79.

6. Samet JM: The epidemiology of lung cancer. *Chest* 1993, 103:20S–29S.

7. Iannuzzi MC, Toews GB: Neoplasms of the lung. In *Internal Medicine*. Edited by Stein JH. St Louis: Mosby; 1994:1733–1741.

8. Ernster VL, Mustacchi P, Osann KE: Epidemiology of lung cancer. In *Textbook of Respiratory Medicine*, vol 2, edn 2. Edited by Murray JF, Nadel JA. Philadelphia: WB Saunders; 1994:1504–1527.

9. Carr DT, Holoye PY, Hong WK: Bronchogenic carcinoma. In *Textbook of Respiratory Medicine*, vol 2, edn 2. Edited by Murray JF, Nadel JA. Philadelphia: WB Saunders; 1994:1528-1596.

10. Pastorino U: Lung cancer chemoprevention. *Cancer Treat Res* 1995, 72:43–74.

11. Bhatia R, Lopipero P, Smith AH: Diesel exhaust exposure and lung cancer. *Epidemiology* 1998, 9:84–91.

12. Gazdar AF: The molecular and cellular basis of human lung cancer. *Anticancer Res* 1994, 13:261–268.

13. Ferguson MK: Synchronous primary lung cancers. *Chest* 1993, 103:398S–400S.

14. Hinson JA, Perry MC: Small cell lung cancer. *CA Cancer J Clin* 1993, 43:216–225.

15. Karsell PR, McDougall JC: Diagnostic tests for lung cancer. *Mayo Clin Proc* 1993, 68:288–296.

16. Stauffer JL: Pulmonary diseases: neoplastic and related diseases. In *Current Medical Diagnosis & Treatment*, edn 33. Edited by Tierney LM Jr, McPhee SJ, Papadakis MA. Norwalk: Appleton & Lange; 1994:241–247.

17. Matthay RA, Carter DC: Lung neoplasms. In *Chest Medicine: Essentials of Pulmonary and Critical Care Medicine*, edn 2. Edited by George RB, Light RW, Matthay MA, Matthay RA. Baltimore: Williams & Wilkins; 1990:353–379.

18. Patel AM, Davila DG, Peters SG: Paraneoplastic syndromes associated with lung cancer. *Mayo Clin Proc* 1993, 68:278–287.

19. Kiss GT: Pulmonary diseases: carcinoma of the lung. In *Practical Guide to the Care of the Medical Patient*, edn 2. Edited by Ferri F. St Louis: Mosby Year Book; 1991:519–524.

20. Swensen SJ, Brown LR: Conventional radiography of hilum and mediastinum in bronchogenic carcinoma. *Radiol Clin North Am* 1990, 28:521–538.

21. Arroliga AC, Matthay RA: The role of bronchoscopy in lung cancer. *Clin Chest Med* 1993, 14:87–98.

22. Fontana RS, Sanderson DR, Woolner LB, Taylor WF, Miller WE, Muhm JR: Lung cancer screening: the Mayo Program. *J Occup Med* 1986, 28:746–750.

23. Tockman M: Survival and mortality from lung cancer in a screened population: the Johns Hopkins study. *Chest* 1986, 89:325S–326S.

24. Melamed MR, Flehinger BJ, Zaman MB, Heelan RT, Perchick WA, Martini N: Screening for early lung cancer: results of the Memorial Sloan-Kettering study in New York. *Chest* 1984, 86:44–53.

25. Kaneko M, Eguchi K, Ohmatsu H, Kakinuma R, Naruke T, Suemasu K, Moriyama N: Peripheral lung cancer: screening with detection with low-dose spiral CT versus radiography. *Radiology* 1996, 201:798–802.

26. Sone S, Takashima S, Li F, et al.: Mass screening for lung cancer and mobile spiral computed tomography scanner. *Lancet* 1998, 351:1242–1245.

27. Henschke CI, McCauley DI, Yankelevitz DF, et al.: Early lung cancer action project: overall design and findings from baseline screening. *Lancet* 1999, 354:99–105.

28. Patz EF, Goodman PC, Bepler G: Screening for lung cancer. *N Engl J Med* 2000, 343:1627–1633.

29. Tockman MS, Mulshine JL, Piantadosi S, et al.: Prospective detection of preclinical lung cancer: results from two studies of heterogeneous nuclear ribonucleoprotein A2/B1 overexpression. *Clin Cancer Res* 1997, 3:2237–2246.

30. Lam S, Kennedy T, Unger M, et al.: Localization of bronchial intraepithelial lesions by fluorescence bronchoscopy. *Chest* 1998, 113:696–702.

31. Stitik FP: The new staging of lung cancer. *Radiol Clin North Am* 1994, 32:635–647.

32. Mountain CF: Revision in the international system for staging lung cancer. *Chest* 1997, 111:1710–1717.

33. Patel AM, Dunn WF, Trastek VF: Staging systems of lung cancer. *Mayo Clin Proc* 1993, 68:475–482.

34. Johnson BE: Management of small-cell lung cancer. *Clin Chest Med* 1993, 14:173–187.

35. Patel AM, Peters SG: Clinical manifestations of lung cancer. *Mayo Clin Proc* 1993, 68:273–277.

36. Ferrigno D, Buccheri G: Clinical applications of serum markers for lung cancer. *Respir Med* 1995, 89:587–597.

37. Niklinski J, Furman M: Clinical tumour markers in lung cancer. *Eur J Cancer Prev* 1995, 4:129–138.

38. Strauss GM, Kwiatkowski DJ, Harpole DH, et al.: Molecular and pathologic markers in stage I non-small-cell carcinoma of the lung. *J Clin Oncol* 1995, 13:1265–1279.

39. Skarin AT: Analysis of long-term survivors with small-cell lung cancer. *Chest* 1993, 103:440S–444S.

40. Ruckdeschel JC: Therapeutic options for treatment of small cell and non-small cell lung cancer. *Curr Opin Oncol* 1993, 5:323–334.

41. Dweik RA, Mehta AC: Bronchoscopic management of malignant airway disease. *Clin Pulm Med* 1996, 3:43–51.

PULMONARY NEOPLASMS OTHER THAN LUNG CANCER

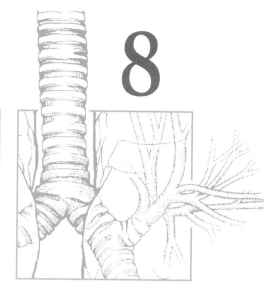

8

Raed A. Dweik, Carol Farver, & Peter B. O'Donovan

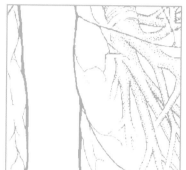

Pulmonary neoplasms other than the four major primary bronchogenic carcinomas include typical and atypical carcinoids, hamartomas, mucous gland tumors, papillomas, juvenile laryngotracheal papillomatosis, mesenchymal tumors, sclerosing hemangiomas, intravascular bronchioloalveolar tumors (epithelioid hemangioendotheliomas), teratomas, blastomas, and inflammatory pseudotumors. Although many of these tumors are rare, they need to be considered in the differential diagnosis when a patient presents with a lung nodule or a mass. This chapter reviews the clinical presentation and the radiographic and histologic features of these tumors.

CARCINOID TUMORS

Typical Carcinoid Tumors

DISTINGUISHING FEATURES OF TYPICAL AND ATYPICAL CARCINOID TUMORS

Feature	Typical carcinoid tumor	Atypical carcinoid tumor
Histologic pattern	Neuroendocrine	Neuroendocrine
Mitoses	Absent or rare	Increased (up to 10/10 high-power fields)
Necrosis	Rarely seen	Characteristic, usually central
Nuclear anaplasia	Usually absent	Characteristic
Regional lymph node metastasis at presentation	5%–10%	40%–48%
Distant metastasis at presentation	Rare	20%
Disease-free survival at 5 y	>95%	40%

Figure 8-1.

Clinical and histologic differences between typical and atypical carcinoids. Carcinoid tumors of the lung are low-grade malignancies and constitute less than 4% of lung primary neoplasms [1,2]. Carcinoids are neuroendocrine tumors and are divided into typical carcinoids and the more aggressive atypical carcinoid tumors [3]. (*Adapted from* Arroliga *et al.* [4].)

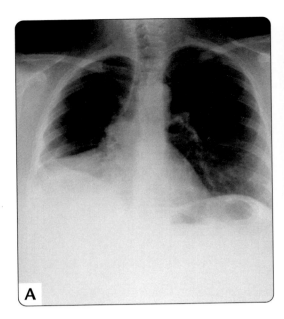

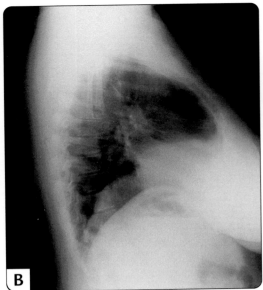

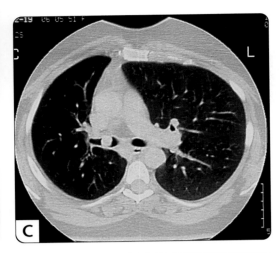

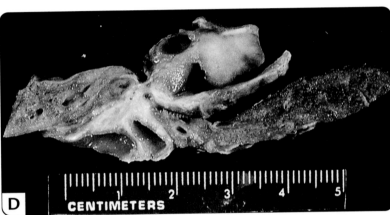

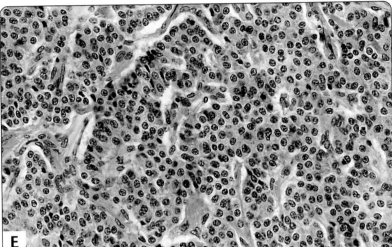

Figure 8-2.

Typical carcinoid tumors. **A** and **B,** Posteroanterior (*panel A*) and lateral (*panel B*) chest radiographs of a patient with carcinoid tumor of the bronchus intermedius. The tumor resulted in right middle lobe collapse. **C,** Computed tomographic scan of the same patient, demonstrating a well-circumscribed lesion in the bronchus intermedius. Notice the loss of volume of the right lung. In approximately 80% of the cases, typical carcinoids are located in the central airways and the chest radiograph shows segmental or lobar atelectasis, with or without postobstructive pneumonia [5–7]. Lesions in the periphery, however, are usually well demarcated, round, and radiopaque, with sharp and often notched margins [6]. Hilar adenopathy is uncommon in either presentation and, if present, is probably due to inflammation [6]. Cavitation is uncommon, although it may occur in atypical carcinoid. Other uncommon radiologic features of typical carcinoids include calcification and satellite nodules [5,6]. Because of their central location, the most common symptoms of typical carcinoid tumors include cough, hemoptysis, dyspnea, and wheezing. Up to 50% of patients are asymptomatic [7,8]. Pulmonary carcinoid tumors can occur in almost any location in the lungs from the trachea to the lung periphery [8]. Typical carcinoids are four times more likely than atypical carcinoids (see Fig. 8-3) to be central in location [7]. **D,** Gross specimen of a carcinoid tumor, obtained from a different patient. Notice the well-encapsulated, yellow, homogenous, endobronchial mass protruding into the lumen of the airway. (*See Color Plate.*) **E,** Microscopic specimen of a typical carcinoid tumor. The tumor is composed of nests of cells with slightly spindled nuclei, finely stippled chromatin, and a "salt-and-pepper" pattern. The cells have moderate amounts of pink cytoplasm that lack distinct borders. The cell nests are highlighted by intervening congested vessels. The degree of nuclear pleomorphism is mild to moderate, and mitotic figures are rare. The histologic pattern in central tumors may be different from that in peripheral tumors [9]. Although both usually have medium-sized, uniform epithelial cells with limited nuclear pleomorphism and limited mitoses, the pattern of cell growth in peripheral lesions may be less organized, more crowded, and without orientation. A spindle pattern is also more common in peripheral carcinoid tumors [9,10]. (*See Color Plate.*)

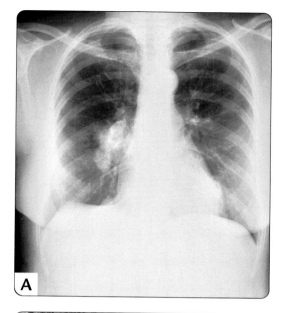

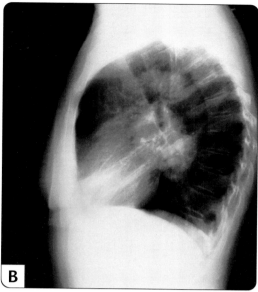

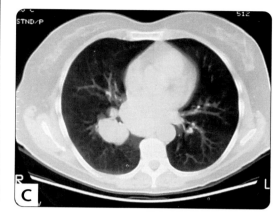

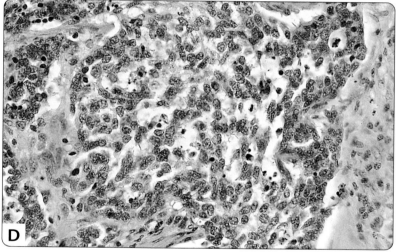

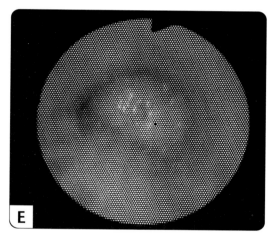

Figure 8-3.

Atypical carcinoid tumors. **A** and **B,** Posteroanterior (*panel A*) and lateral (*panel B*) chest radiographs of a patient with an atypical carcinoid presenting as a right middle lobe infiltrative mass. The chest radiograph of patients with atypical carcinoid usually shows a round or ovoid mass, 1.5 to 10 cm in diameter. The mass may be lobulated or spiculated, or it may have smooth borders. Atypical carcinoids are more common peripherally than typical carcinoids [11]. **C,** On computed tomographic scans of the chest, atypical carcinoids are significantly larger than typical carcinoids, and lymph node involvement may be seen in as many as 40% of cases [11]. Endobronchial growth and obstruction are less common than in typical carcinoid [11]. **D,** Microscopic studies demonstrate that, unlike typical carcinoids, atypical carcinoid tumors are necrotic and have an increased number of mitotic

figures [3,4,9,10]. These tumors show patterns of discrete nests of cells separated by a fibrovascular stroma. Architectural features are more varied in atypical carcinoids. The cells have a fine granular eosinophilic cytoplasm and their borders tend to be indistinct. The nuclei are predominantly ovoid and hyperchromatic. They are also anaplastic and have larger and more numerous nucleoli than the nuclei of typical carcinoids [3,4,9–11]. (*See* Color Plate.) **E,** On bronchoscopic examination, typical and atypical carcinoid lesions are described as having a polypoid, shiny, glistening, vascular appearance [6]. Contrary to the earlier belief that bronchoscopic biopsy may put patients at risk of significant bleeding, several recent reports show that significant hemorrhage is not a major problem [2,6,12]. (Panel E *courtesy of* A.C. Mehta, MD.)

Hamartoma

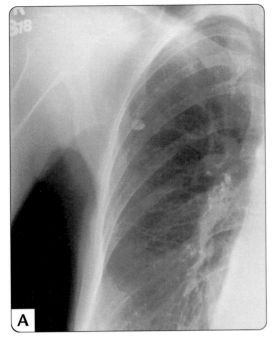

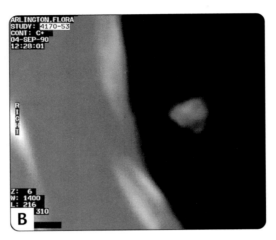

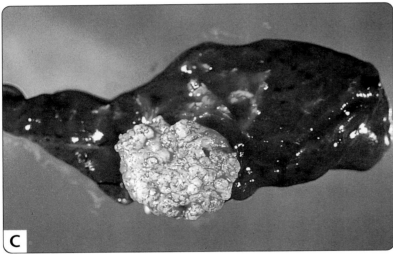

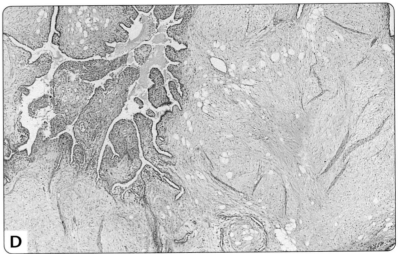

Figure 8-4.

Hamartomas. Hamartoma is the most common benign pulmonary tumor. It accounts for 6% to 8% of solitary pulmonary nodules (SPNs). Most patients with hamartomas are asymptomatic. The most common presentation is an SPN that is usually detected incidentally on a chest radiograph. Approximately 10% of hamartomas grow endobronchially and may present with cough, dyspnea, wheezing, or hemoptysis [13–15]. **A,** Posteroanterior chest radiograph of a patient with a hamartoma presenting incidentally as a right upper lobe solitary nodule. The chest radiograph in patients with hamartoma is rarely diagnostic. It usually shows a round, homogenous, occasionally lobulated peripheral opacity. Calcification is seen in 10% of cases, but the classically described "popcorn" calcification is rare. Although most hamartomas are 2 to 3 cm in size, their size may range from 1 to 8.5 cm, and tumors involving a whole lobe have been reported [13,14]. **B,** Computed tomographic scan of a patient with a solitary nodule

suggestive of a hamartoma. A computed tomographic scan of the chest may be helpful in determining whether an SPN is a hamartoma. Nodules less than 2.5 cm in diameter and containing fat or having a typical benign calcification pattern—as demonstrated in this scan—suggest the diagnosis of hamartoma [15]. **C,** Gross specimen showing a hamartoma as a well-circumscribed, smooth mass that "shells out" of the surrounding lung. On gross examination, hamartomas are usually gray-pink, well circumscribed, uniform, and rubber-hard but not encapsulated [16]. (See Color Plate.) **D,** Microscopic specimen, with benign lobules of cartilage entrapping adjacent air spaces. Other mesenchymal elements, including fat and smooth muscle, can be seen. Histologically, a hamartoma may contain cartilage, fat, or both. It may also contain entrapped epithelium that is not an intrinsic part of the tumor. Chronic inflammation and fibrosis may also be evident in lung tissue adjacent to the lesion [16]. (See Color Plate.)

Mucous Gland Tumors

TUMORS ARISING FROM THE TRACHEOBRONCHIAL MUCOUS GLANDS AND THEIR DUCTS

Adenoid cystic carcinomas (cylindromas)
Mucoepidermoid carcinomas
Mixed (pleomorphic) adenomas
Cystadenomas
Oxyphilic bronchial gland adenomas

Figure 8-5.
Mucous gland tumors. These rare tumors arise from the exocrine cells of the mucous glands and their ducts in the trachea and bronchi. Patients with mucous gland tumors usually present with symptoms of bronchial obstruction. Histologically, these tumors have features similar to those of salivary gland tumors.

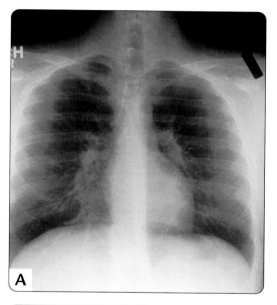

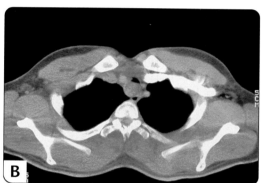

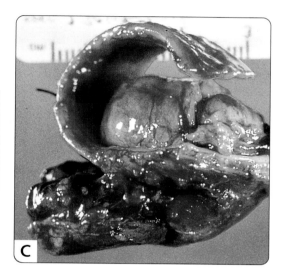

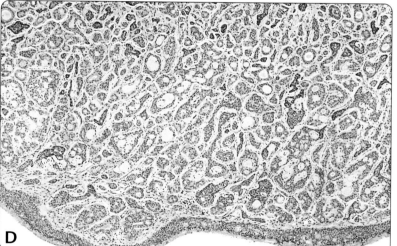

Figure 8-6.
Adenoid cystic carcinoma. **A,** Posteroanterior chest radiograph of a patient who had dry cough and dyspnea on exertion, which progressed in the past 3 months to dyspnea at rest. On physical examination, he was found to have stridor. The large mass in the trachea turned out to be an adenoid cystic carcinoma. The etiology of adenoid cystic carcinoma is unknown, and smoking does not seem to be a predisposing factor. Almost 80% of these tumors arise from the trachea and mainstem bronchi and the rest from lobar bronchi. About 10% may arise in the periphery [17]. **B,** Computed tomographic scan of the chest of the same patient, showing a mass obstructing the trachea. **C,** Gross specimen, obtained from another patient, demonstrating a firm, polypoid, tan-pink mass infiltrating the bronchial wall. Adenoid cystic carcinomas grow slowly and are locally invasive. Symptoms are usually caused by bronchial obstruction and include dyspnea, wheezing, cough, recurrent pneumonia, and hemoptysis [17]. (*See* Color Plate.) **D,** The histologic features of adenoid cystic carcinomas are similar to those of salivary gland tumors [18]. Malignant glands infiltrate the underlying bronchial epithelium. These glands have a microcystic, cribriform, and trabecular pattern. The cystic spaces contain acidic mucin. A thickened basement membrane surrounds the glands. Surgical resection by lobectomy or pneumonectomy is the treatment of choice. Recurrence is common and multiple procedures may be needed [18]. Adenoid cystic carcinomas show poor response to radiotherapy or chemotherapy, but prolonged survival (up to 20 years) is common due to the slow growth of the tumor [18]. (*See* Color Plate.)

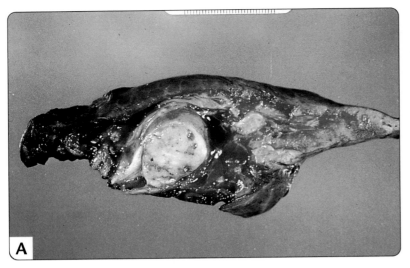 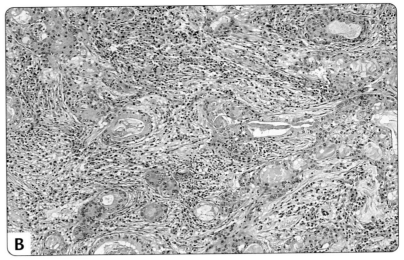

Figure 8-7.

Mucoepidermoid carcinoma. **A,** Gross pathology of a low-grade mucoepidermoid carcinoma appearing as a spherical, tan-white mass occluding the bronchus. Based on microscopic histopathology and clinical behavior, mucoepidermoid tumors can be divided into low- and high-grade tumors. Low-grade tumors are grossly well-circumscribed, exophytic, endobronchial lesions. (*See Color Plate.*) **B,** Microscopic specimen showing a low-grade tumor that contains a mixture of solid and cystic components. The glandular component predominates and cellular atypia is absent [19,20]. Notice the malignant glands with abundant mucinous cystic spaces filled with weakly acidic mucous substance invading the bronchial epithelium. More solid areas of transitional cells or nonkeratinizing squamous cells are seen adjacent to these cystic areas. Some cells appear to be between glandular and squamous. Mitoses are rare or absent. High-grade tumors are larger than low-grade tumors. They also have a predominantly solid component and marked atypia and mitotic activity [20]. Clinically, patients with the more aggressive high-grade tumors have a worse prognosis. (*See Color Plate.*)

Papilloma

CLASSIFICATION OF BENIGN PAPILLOMAS OF THE TRACHEOBRONCHIAL TREE

Tumor	Cell type	Clinical presentation

Multiple papillomas
   Juvenile
   Adult
	Squamous	Young children; larynx

Solitary papilloma	Squamous	Adults; lobar and segmental bronchi
Solitary papilloma	Columnar or cuboidal with or without squamous metaplasia	Adults; may undergo malignant transformation
Inflammatory polyps	Columnar	Patients with chronic respiratory infections

Figure 8-8.

Papillomas. Squamous papillomas of the upper and lower respiratory tract are exophytic tumors derived from the surface epithelium and bronchial mucous glands [21]. A classification schema for these tumors appears in the figure [22]. The most common type of papilloma is juvenile papillomatosis, which occurs primarily in children and most commonly in the larynx [22,23]. Extension to the trachea, proximal bronchi, or both occurs in 5% of cases, and the lung parenchyma is involved in less than 1% of cases [23]. The symptoms are those of an obstructive airway lesion, *ie*, wheezing, dyspnea, cough, and hemoptysis [23,24]. (*Adapted from* Maxwell *et al.* [22].)

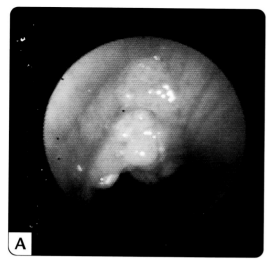

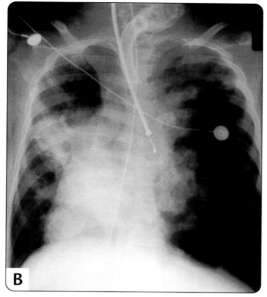

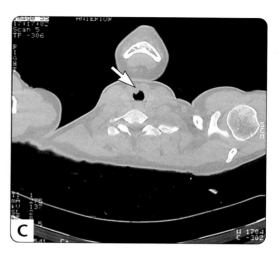

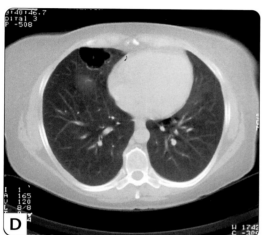

Figure 8-9.

Juvenile papillomatosis. **A,** Bronchoscopy of a patient with juvenile papillomatosis, demonstrating typical pink, polypoid, exophytic lesions with a "bunch-of-grapes" appearance [23]. Juvenile papillomas are benign tumors caused by the human papilloma virus, especially types 6 and 11 [23,25]. Malignant transformation can occur, especially in adults, in parenchymal lesions, and after radiation therapy [26]. (*See Color Plate.*) **B,** Radiograph of a patient with pulmonary parenchymal extension of tracheobronchial papillomas. These parenchymal lesions occur in less than 1% of cases, and tend to undergo a transformation into squamous cell carcinoma [23,26]. **C** and **D,** Computed tomographic scans of a patient with a tracheal lesion (*arrow; panel C*) and cavitary parenchymal involvement (*panel D*). Histologically, these papillomas consist of a core of fibrous connective tissue covered by squamous epithelium [21–23]. There is no curative therapy for these tumors, and they tend to recur. Standard management consists of laser excision of the lesions [23]. Other palliative approaches include the use of lymphoblastoid interferon-α [23,27] and photodynamic therapy [23,28,29]. Acyclovir and leukocyte interferon have not been useful [23,30]. (Panel A *courtesy of* A.C. Mehta, MD.)

MESENCHYMAL TUMORS OF THE LUNG

MESENCHYMAL PULMONARY NEOPLASMS

Benign	Malignant*
Leiomyoma*	Fibrosarcoma
Fibroma	Leiomyosarcoma
Bronchial lipoma	Malignant fibrous histiocytoma
Cavernous hemangioma	Liposarcoma
Endobronchial schwannoma	Extraosseous osteosarcoma
Granular cell tumor	Chondrosarcoma
Neurofibroma	Rhabdomyosarcoma
	Hemangiopericytoma
	Carcinosarcoma

Need to exclude metastasis from extrapulmonary sites.

Figure 8-10.

Mesenchymal tumors of the lung. Patients with benign mesenchymal tumors of the lung usually present with bronchial obstruction and atelectasis or with a solitary pulmonary nodule on a chest radiograph. Leiomyomas are the most common soft-tissue tumors of the lung and resemble uterine leiomyomas histologically. Although primary pulmonary leiomyomas and leiomyosarcomas have been reported [31], most smooth muscle tumors of the lung are well-differentiated metastases from extrathoracic (usually uterine) leiomyosarcomas. Several other mesenchymal tumors can be found in the lung and are listed here [31].

OTHER PULMONARY NEOPLASMS

Tumor	Age, y (range)	Male-to-female ratio	Clinical presentation	Cells of origin	Diagnosis/therapy	Prognosis	Notes
Sclerosing hemangioma [32,33]	30s (15–69)	1:4	60%–80% asymptomatic nodule; hemoptysis, cough, chest pain	Pulmonary epithelial cells	Surgical resection	Excellent	4 histologic patterns: solid, hemorrhagic, papillary, sclerotic
Intravascular bronchoalveolar tumor—epithelioid hemangioendothelioma [34–36]	30s (12–61)	1:4	45% asymptomatic; pleuritic pain, cough, progressive dyspnea, weight loss, clubbing	Endothelial	Surgical resection	Poor; >60% die of disease within 1–15 y of diagnosis	Multiple resections may be necessary
Teratoma [37,38]	Young adults (10–30)	1:1	Mainly asymptomatic; chest pain, hemoptysis, cough	Multiple: endodermal, mesodermal, ectodermal	Surgical resection	Benign (mature), malignant (immature)	Metastatic germ cell tumors need to be excluded
Blastoma [39–42]	40s (10–60)	2.6:1	Mainly asymptomatic nodule; hemoptysis, chest pain, cough, dyspnea, fever	Epithelial, mesenchymal, (histology resembles fetal lung)	Surgical resection	Poor (similar to adenocarcinoma); 2 of 3 recur	May herald other dysplastic and neoplastic diseases in patient and family
Primary melanoma [43,44]	Adults (29–80)	1:1	Cough, sputum, hemoptysis, dyspnea, weight loss	Epithelial	Surgical resection	11-y survival reported	Exclude metastasis
Inflammatory pseudotumor—plasma cell granuloma [45–47]	Children*, young adults, adults (11–64)	1:1	Cough, chest pain, hemoptysis (if endobronchial)	Plasma cells	Surgical resection	Recurs in 10%–20% of cases if incompletely excised	May represent pulmonary reaction to previous (infectious?) insult

*Most common pulmonary neoplasm in children.

Figure 8-11.
Clinical and pathologic characteristics of additional pulmonary neoplasms.

REFERENCES

1. Bertelsen S, Aasted A, Lund C, et al.: Bronchial carcinoid tumors: a clinicopathologic study of 82 cases. *Scand J Thorac Cardiovasc Surg* 1985, 19:105–111.

2. Hurt R, Bates M: Carcinoid tumors of the bronchus: a 33 year experience. *Thorax* 1984, 39:617–623.

3. Paladugu RR, Benfield JR, Pak HY, et al.: Bronchopulmonary Kulchitzky cell carcinomas: a new classification scheme for typical and atypical carcinoma. *Cancer* 1985, 55:1303–1311.

4. Arroliga AC, Carter D, Matthay RA: Other primary neoplasms of the lung. In *Pulmonary and Critical Care Medicine.* Edited by Bone RC, et al. St. Louis: Mosby Yearbook; 1993:1–16.

5. Davila DG, Dunn WF, Tazelaar HD, et al.: Bronchial carcinoid tumors. *Mayo Clinic Proc* 1993, 68:795–803.

6. Nessi R, Basso Ricci P, Vasso Ricci S, et al.: Bronchial carcinoid tumors: radiologic observations in 49 cases. *J Thorac Imaging* 1991, 6:47–53.

7. Warren WH, Faber LP, Could VE: Neuroendocrine neoplasm of the lung: a clinicopathologic update. *J Thorac Cardiovasc Surg* 1989, 98:321–332.

8. Wilkens EW, Grillo HC, Moncure AC, et al.: Changing times in surgical management of bronchopulmonary carcinoid tumor. *Ann Thorac Surg* 1984, 38:339–342.

9. Froudarakis M, Fournel P, Burgard G, et al.: Bronchial carcinoids: a review of 22 cases. *Oncology* 1996, 53:153–158.

10. DeCaro LF, Paladugu R, Benfield JR, et al.: Typical and atypical carcinoids within the pulmonary APUD tumor spectrum. *J Thorac Cardiovasc Surg* 1983, 86:528–536.

11. Foster BB, Mueller NL, Miller RR, et al.: Neuroendocrine carcinomas of the lung: clinical, radiologic, and pathologic correlation. *Radiology* 1989, 170:441–445.

12. Rozenman J, Pausner R, Lieberman Y, et al.: Bronchial adenoma. *Chest* 1987, 92:145–147.

13. Gjevre JG, Meyers JL, Prakash UBS: Pulmonary hamartomas. *Mayo Clin Proc* 1996, 71:14–20.

14. Van den Bosh JMM, Wagenaar SS, Corrin B, et al.: Mesenchymoma of the lung (so called hamartoma): a review of 154 parenchymal and endobronchial cases. *Thorax* 1987, 42:790–793.

15. Caskey CJ, Templeton PA, Zerhouni EA: Current evaluation of the solitary pulmonary nodule. *Radiol Clin North Am* 1990, 28:511–520.

16. Perez-Atayde AR, Seiler MW: Pulmonary hamartoma: an ultrastructural study. *Cancer* 1984, 53:485–492.

17. Li W, Ellerbrolk NA, Libshitz HI: Primary malignant tumors of the trachea: a radiological and clinical study. *Cancer* 1990, 66:894–899.

18. Spencer H: Bronchial mucous gland tumor. *Virchows Arch [A]* 1979, 383:101–115.

19. Klacsman PG, Olson JL, Eggleston JC: Mucoepidermoid carcinomas of the bronchus: an electron microscopic study of the low grade and the high grade variants. *Cancer* 1979, 43:1720–1733.

20. Yousem SA, Hochholzer L: Malignant fibrous histiocytoma of the lung. *Cancer* 1987, 60:2532–2541.

21. Spencer H, Dail DH, Arneaud J: Non-invasive bronchial epithelial papillary tumors. *Cancer* 1980, 45:1486–1497.

22. Maxwell RJ, Gibbons JR, O'Hara MD: Solitary squamous papilloma of the bronchus. *Thorax* 1985, 40:68–71.

23. Dweik RA, Patel SR, Mehta AC: Tracheal papillomatosis. *J Bronchology* 1994, 1:226–227.

24. Kramer SS, Wehaunt WD, Stocker JT, Kashima H: Pulmonary manifestations of juvenile laryngotracheal papillomatosis. *AJR Am J Roentgenol* 1985, 144:687–694.

25. Quiney RE, Wells M, Lewis FA, et al.: Laryngeal papillomatosis: correlation between severity of the disease and presence of HPV6 and 11 detected by in situ DNA hybridization. *J Clin Pathol* 1989, 42:694–698.

26. Lie ES, Engh V, Boysen M, et al.: Squamous cell carcinoma of the respiratory tract following laryngeal papillomatosis. *Acta Otolaryngol (Stockh)* 1994, 114:209–212.

27. Leventhal BG, Kashima HK, Mounts P, et al.: Long-term response of recurrent respiratory papillomatosis to treatment with lymphatoid interferon α-n1. *N Engl J Med* 1991, 325:613–617.

28. Dweik RA, Mehta AC: Bronchoscopic management of malignant airway disease. *Clin Pulm Med* 1996, 3:43–51.

29. Kavuru MS, Mehta AC, Eliachar I: Effect of photodynamic therapy and external beam radiation therapy on juvenile laryngotracheal papillomatosis. *Am Rev Resp Dis* 1990, 141:509–510.

30. Morrison GAJ, Evans JNG: Juvenile respiratory papillomatosis: acyclovir reassessed. *Int J Paediatr Otorhinolaryngol* 1993, 26:193–197.

31. Tench WD, Dail D, Gmelich JT, et al.: Benign metastasizing leiomyomas: a review of 21 cases [abstract]. *Lab Invest* 1978, 38: 367–368.

32. Katzenstein AA, Gmelich JT, Carrinton CB: Sclerosing hemangioma of the lung: a clinicopathologic study of 51 cases. *Am J Surg Pathol* 1980, 4:343–356.

33. Yousem SA, Wick MR, Singh G, et al.: So-called sclerosing hemangiomas of the lung: an immunohistochemical analysis with comparison with fetal lung in its pseudoglandular stage. *Am J Clin Pathol* 1990, 93:167–175.

34. Van Kasteren ME, Van der Wurff AA, Palmen FM, et al.: Epithelioid haemangioendothelioma of the lung: clinical and pathological pitfalls. *European Resp J* 1995, 8:1616–1619.

35. Weiss SW, Ishak KG, Dail DH, et al.: Epithelioid hemangioendothelioma and related lesions. *Semin Diag Pathol* 1986, 3:259–287.

36. Miettinen M, Collan Y, Halttunen P, et al.: Intravascular bronchoalveolar tumor. *Cancer* 1987, 60:2471–2475.

37. Ashley DJB: Origin of teratomas. *Cancer* 1973, 32:390–394.

38. Collier FC, Dowling EA, Plott D, et al.: Teratoma of the lung. *Arch Pathol* 1959, 68:138–142.

39. Yousem SA, Hochholzer L: Primary pulmonary hemangiopericytoma. *Cancer* 1987, 59:549–555.

40. Priest JR, Watterson J, Strong L, et al.: Pleuropulmonary blastoma: a marker for familial disease. *J Pediatr* 1996, 128:220–224.

41. Koss MN, Hochholzer L, O'Leary T: Pulmonary blastomas. *Cancer* 1991, 67:2368–2381.

42. Novotny JE, Huiras CM: Resection and adjuvant chemotherapy of pulmonary blastoma: a case report. *Cancer* 1995, 76:1537–1539.

43. Bagwell SP, Flynn SD, Cox PM, et al.: Primary malignant melanoma of the lung. *Am Rev Respir Dis* 1989, 139:1543–1547.

44. Jennings TA, Axiotis CA, Kress Y, et al.: Primary malignant melanoma of the lower respiratory tract. *Am J Clin Pathol* 1990, 94:649–655.

45. Dweik RA, Goldfarb J, Alexander F, Stillwell PC: Actinomycosis and plasma cell granuloma, coincidence or coexistence: patient report and review of the literature. *Clin Pediatr* 1997, 36:229–233.

46. Biselli R, Ferlini C, Fattorossi A, et al.: Inflammatory myofibroblastic tumor (inflammatory pseudotumor). *Cancer* 1996, 77:778–784.

47. Hancock BJ, Di Lorenzo M, Youssef S, et al.: Childhood primary pulmonary neoplasms. *J Pediatr Surg* 1993, 28:1133–1136.

SOLITARY PULMONARY NODULE

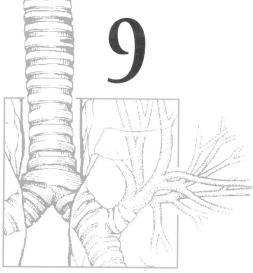
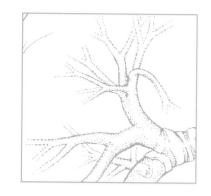
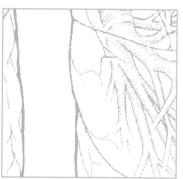

9

Pyng Lee,
Omar A. Minai,
Atul C. Mehta, &
Muzaffar Ahmad

The finding of a solitary pulmonary nodule (SPN) on a chest radiograph is a common problem in pulmonary medicine. SPNs are seen in approximately one in 500 chest radiographs and are caused by a variety of conditions ranging from infectious granulomas to lung cancer [1]. An estimated 130,000 new benign or malignant SPNs are discovered each year in the United States, of which 20% to 40% are malignant [2]. Because asymptomatic bronchogenic carcinomas commonly present as SPNs [3] and surgical resection results in a 5-year survival of 40% to 80% [4], it is important to identify them promptly to ensure optimal treatment. Similarly, it is important to avoid the morbidity and mortality associated with thoracotomy in patients with benign disease. Thus, the work-up for SPN focuses on distinguishing benign from malignant nodules. This chapter describes how clinicians can distinguish the two in a practical manner.

DEFINITION

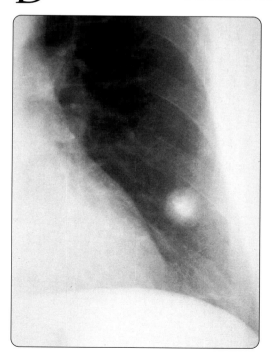

Figure 9-1.
Chest radiograph of a solitary pulmonary nodule (SPN). SPN is defined as a single spherical lesion ≤3 cm in diameter, surrounded by aerated lung and not associated with mediastinal adenopathy, atelectasis, pneumonitis, or satellite lesions [1,5]. Lesions >3 cm in diameter are referred to as masses; 80% to 90% of these masses are malignant [6].

DIFFERENTIAL DIAGNOSIS

DIFFERENTIAL DIAGNOSIS OF SOLITARY PULMONARY NODULES

Malignant

Bronchogenic carcinoma
  Adenocarcinoma
  Squamous cell carcinoma
  Large cell carcinoma
  Small cell carcinoma
Bronchial carcinoid
Metastases
  Breast
  Renal
  Colon
  Head and neck
  Sarcoma
  Germ cell
  Thyroid
  Others

Benign

Infectious granulomas
  Tuberculosis
  Coccidiomycosis
  Histoplasmosis
Noninfectious granulomas
  Sarcoid
  Wegener's granulomatosis
Nongranulomatous infections
  Echinococcal cyst
  Ascariasis
  Pneumocystis carinii
Benign tumors
  Hamartoma
  Lipoma
  Fibroma
Congenital
  Arteriovenous malformations
  Bronchogenic cyst
Miscellaneous
  Rheumatoid nodule
  Amyloid
  Pulmonary infarction

Figure 9-2.
Common causes of solitary pulmonary nodules. Infectious granulomas, bronchogenic carcinoma, and metastatic disease are the most common causes of solitary pulmonary nodules.

DISTRIBUTION OF MALIGNANT AND BENIGN LESIONS IN SELECT STUDIES

Study	Cases, *n*	Malignant, %	Benign, %	Bronchogenic, %	Granuloma, %
Steele [10]	887	36	64	32	53
Walske [11]	217	36	64	34	54
Nandi *et al.* [12]	239	67	33	65	25
Toomes *et al.* [7]	955	49	51	38	24
Stoller *et al.* [2]	67	69	31	58	15
Libby *et al.* [13]	40	52	48	45	21
Rubins *et al.* [14]	370	79	21	71	11
Total	2775	50 (*n* = 1383)	50 (*n* = 1392)	43 (*n* = 1202)	34 (*n* = 934)

Figure 9-3.
Causes of solitary pulmonary nodules (SPN). Benign processes are the most common causes of SPNs, although their incidence has decreased over time. In the largest series, slightly more than 50% of the surgically resected nodules were benign and 80% were caused by infectious granulomas, with tuberculosis and fungal infections as the most common causes [7]. While most of the malignant nodules are bronchogenic carcinomas, metastases and bronchial carcinoids account for 10% to 30% and 1%, respectively [8]. Adenocarcinoma and large cell carcinoma are the most common histologic subtypes. (*Adapted from* Mehta *et al.* [9].)

DIAGNOSIS

STAGING AND SURVIVAL IN LUNG CANCER

Stage	Patients, *n*	Survival at 1 y, %	Survival at 5 y, %
Clinical TNM*			
cIA	687	91	61
cIB	1189	72	38
cIIA	29	79	34
cIIB	357	59	24
cIIIA	511	50	13
cIIIB	1030	34	5
cIV	1427	19	1
Pathologic TNM†			
pIA	511	94	67
pIB	549	87	57
pIIA	76	89	55
pIIB	375	73	39
pIIIA	399	64	23

*Staging based on all diagnostic and evaluative information obtained before the institution of treatment or decision for no treatment.
†Staging based on pathologic examination of resected specimens.
TNM—tumor, node, metastasis.

Figure 9-4.
Cumulative proportion of patients with bronchogenic carcinoma surviving 5 years, by clinical stage of disease. Bronchogenic carcinomas presenting as solitary pulmonary nodules that are resected early usually correspond to TNM (tumor, node, metastasis) stage I; patients with these lesions have a median 5-year survival of approximately 50% to 60% [15]. While it may be possible for the clinician to distinguish between benign and malignant nodules based on clinical and radiographic features and with modern imaging techniques, such as spiral computed tomography and positron emission tomography, most nodules cannot be differentiated by these tests alone. Tissue specimens are required for a final diagnosis. (*Adapted from* Mountain [15].)

History

IMPORTANT FEATURES TO BE INVESTIGATED IN PATIENTS WITH SOLITARY PULMONARY NODULES

Age
Area of residence
History of smoking
History of chest trauma
History of intra- or extrathoracic malignancy

Figure 9-5.
Factors suggesting the nature of solitary pulmonary nodules (SPN). A detailed medical history can help the clinician identify patients who are more likely to have malignant SPNs. Among the many risk factors studied, age, smoking, and history of malignancy have been shown to be the most useful. A benign process is the causative factor in most SPNs found in patients younger than 35 years of age and in two thirds of patients younger than 50 years [16]. Smoking [17] and prior cancer increase the likelihood of malignancy. It has been reported that more than 80% of SPNs found in patients with previous extrathoracic cancer are malignant at thoracotomy [18]. Area of residence and travel to areas with high prevalence rates for tuberculosis, coccidiodomycosis, or histoplasmosis are important considerations because they may suggest that the nodule is benign.

Imaging Studies

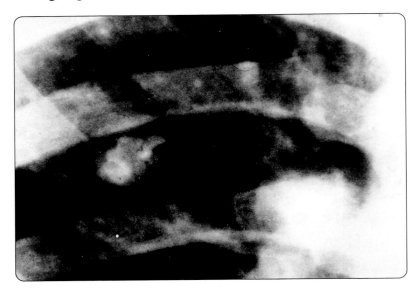

Figure 9-6.
Chest radiograph of harmartoma presenting as a solitary pulmonary nodule (SPN). An SPN can be detected on chest radiograph when it is 8 to 10 mm in diameter [19]. It is usually seen in frontal and lateral views. If it is visualized in only one view, an extrapulmonary cause should be ruled out. Approximately 20% of patients with extrathoracic malignancy have multiple lesions at thoracotomy even when they appear as an SPN on chest radiograph [18]. Growth rate, calcification, nodule size, and appearance of nodule edges are helpful characteristics in differentiating malignant from benign SPNs on chest radiograph. Other features such as cavitation and satellite lesions are less reliable. Previous chest radiographs are invaluable for determining the growth rate and doubling time (dT) of the nodule and should be obtained for comparison even if they are reportedly negative. Growth rate (dT) is the time necessary for the nodule to double in volume; approximately 30 doublings are required to produce a lesion that is 1 cm in diameter. A dT of 16 to 450 days is consistent with a malignant process [20]. A dT of more than 500 days strongly suggests that the nodule is benign; no growth for more than 2 years is considered one of the features of benignity.

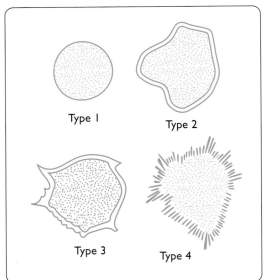

Type 1   Type 2

Type 3   Type 4

Figure 9-7.
Classification of nodular margins. Nodule margins are divided into four categories, with types 3 and 4 suggesting malignancy and types 1 and 2 suggesting benignity [21]. Nodule margins are better appreciated with computed tomography (*see* Fig. 9-9) than plain film. (*Adapted from* Siegelman *et al.* [21].)

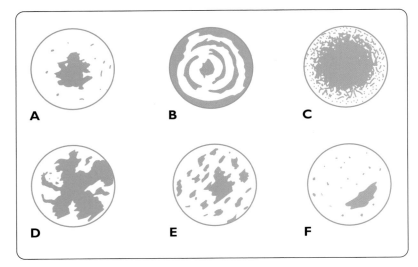

A   B   C

D   E   F

Figure 9-8.
Calcification patterns in solitary pulmonary nodules. Calcification often suggests a benign process [5]. Patterns of calcification that may be present in a solitary pulmonary nodule include central (*A*), laminated (*B*), diffuse (*C*), popcorn (*D*), stippled (*E*), and eccentric (*F*). A solitary pulmonary nodule with a stippled or eccentric pattern of calcification must be considered indeterminate and requires further work-up [22]. Central, laminated, or diffuse calcification patterns suggest a benignity. The presence of popcorn calcification is characteristic of hamartoma, but this is rare, occurring in approximately 5% to 10% of cases. Computed tomography is also more sensitive than the plain film for the detection of calcification (*see* Fig. 9-9). (*Adapted from* Siegelman *et al.* [21].)

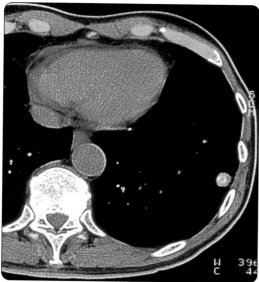

Figure 9-9.

Computed tomographic (CT) scan of a patient with solitary pulmonary nodule (SPN). CT scans provide better representation of nodule margins and calcification pattern than plain film radi-

ographs. CT scans also provide better definition of other characteristics such as fat and vascular connections. For example, the diagnostic feature of hamartoma on CT consists of focal high attenuation due to calcium and low attenuation due to fat. The degree of enhancement seen on a CT scan after injection of nonionic contrast dye can be helpful in distinguishing malignant nodules from benign nodules because the blood supply of malignant lesions is qualitatively and quantitatively different from that of benign lesions [23]. Using an attenuation of 20 Hounsfield Units (HU) as the threshold for a positive test result, the sensitivity and specificity for malignancy are 95% to 100% and 70% to 93%, respectively [24]. False-negative results with this technique could be further minimized by the use of SPN-to-aorta enhancement ratio [24]; this ratio may be complementary to the 20 HU threshold value for the identification of malignant nodules. Other advantages of CT scan include staging of the tumor, detection of multiple lesions, and guiding transthoracic needle aspiration and bronchoscopic biopsies. In recent years, there has been renewed interest in lung cancer screening using low dose CT scan [25–27]. Based on the results of the Early Lung Cancer Action Program (ELCAP), which showed that low dose CT, when compared with chest radiograph, detected noncalcified nodules three times more commonly (23% vs 7%), malignancy four times more commonly (2.7% vs 0.7%), and stage I malignancies six times more commonly (2.3% vs 0.4%). Moreover, the sizes of the malignancies detected on low dose CT were smaller than those detected on chest radiograph, even within stage I; 96% of these CT-detected lung cancers were resectable. Similarly, studies conducted in Japan also showed that low dose CT markedly enhanced the detection of malignancies by 10 times with an average nodule size of 12 mm versus 30 mm in diameter by chest radiograph; 82% of these lung cancers were stage I [26,27]. High resolution CT is more sensitive than CT in delineating tumor-bronchus relationships. An air bronchogram leading to an SPN increases the likelihood of malignancy [28,29]. However, helical CT is useful in detecting nodules smaller than 5 mm in diameter [30] and in evaluating areas of the lung that are difficult to examine because of respiratory motion (eg, the lung bases adjacent to the diaphragm). CT densitometry based on a phantom reference is not part of the SPN work-up because of the high false-negative rate.

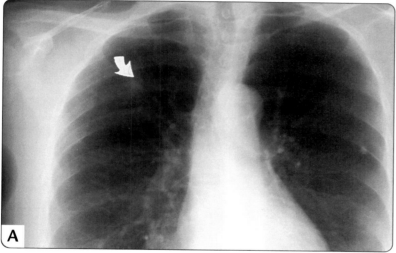
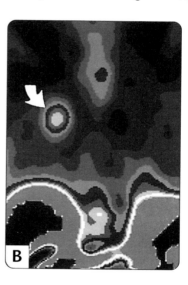

Figure 9-10.

A, Chest radiograph demonstrating a solitary pulmonary nodule (*arrow*). **B**, Positron emission tomographic (PET) scan of the same lesion is shown with greater uptake of F-18 fluorodeoxyglucose (FDG) than surrounding normal tissue (*arrow*). In one study, PET-FDG classified 27 of 30 nodules less than 3 cm in diameter correctly with a specificity of 80% and a sensitivity of 95% [31]. PET-FDG was shown to be superior to the traditional Bayesian approach in classifying lesions as benign or malignant [32]. A decision-analysis model used to assess its cost-effectiveness demonstrated that a CT-plus-PET strategy decreased surgical procedures by 15% and a total estimated cost savings of $91 to $2200 per patient [33]. Another potential benefit of PET-FDG is the detection of occult metastases and improved staging. False-negative results can occur in scar adenocarcinoma, carcinoids, bronchioloalveolar carcinoma, and tumors smaller than 10 mm in diameter [31,34,35]. False-positive results can occur in hyperglycemia, caseating granulomas with active inflammation, and Histoplasma organisms [36]. (*See Color Plate.*)

Biopsy Procedures

SUCCESS RATE OF FLEXIBLE BRONCHOSCOPY

Study	Patients, n	Overall, %	Transbronchial biopsy, %	Cytology brush, %	Cytology wash, %	Size of lesion	
						<2 cm, %	>2 cm, %
Stringfield et al. [37]	27	48	28	31	24	33	50
Cortese and McDougall [38]	48	60	46	40	43	0	66
Radke et al. [39]	97	56	52	33	—	29	64
Fletcher and Levin [40]*	101	36	27	16	4	13	46
Wallace and Deutsch [41]*	133	20	20	12	9	5	34
Shiner et al. [42]*	71	68	65	37	10	—	68
Chechani [43]	49	73	57	52	35	54	75

Some patients did not have all the procedures (brushings, washings, transbronchial biopsies) done.

Figure 9-11.

Flexible bronchoscopy. In most cases, a solitary pulmonary nodule cannot be classified as benign or malignant on the basis of clinical and radiographic characteristics alone. Other options available for making a tissue diagnosis include flexible bronchoscopy, percutaneous needle aspiration, video-assisted thoracotomy, and open thoracotomy. The success rate of flexible bronchoscopy in diagnosing solitary pulmonary nodule is summarized in the figure. Although brush biopsy and bronchial washing (lavage) play important complementary roles, bronchoscopic lung biopsy is the most sensitive sampling method, with an overall success rate of 36% to 68% [9]. Nodule size and location affect the diagnostic yield with flexible bronchoscopy. For lesions less than 2 cm in diameter, the diagnostic yield is 21%; for lesions larger than 2 cm, it is 57%. If the CT reveals a bronchus leading to the lesion, the yield is 60% [44]. For nodules located in the middle third of the chest, the yield is much higher than for nodules located in the outer third [9]. (*Adapted from* Mehta et al. [9].)

DIAGNOSTIC YIELD OF BRONCHOALVEOLAR LAVAGE

Study	Patients, n	Bronchoalveolar lavage yield
Shiner et al. [42]	71	9/38 (24%)
Pirozynski [45]	145	52/145 (40%)
		94/145 (65%)*
de Garcia et al. [46]	35	10/35 (28%)
Total	251	71/218 (33%)

Includes patients in whom malignant cells were present but correct cell type could not be identified.

Figure 9-12.

Diagnostic yield of bronchoalveolar lavage in patients with solitary pulmonary nodules. Bronchoalveolar lavage complements the bronchoscopic brush biopsy. However, with a diagnostic yield of only 28% to 65%, it is a less reliable diagnostic method than bronchoscopic lung biopsy (see Fig. 9-11). (*Adapted from* Mehta et al. [9].)

INDICATIONS FOR A HIGHER DIAGNOSTIC YIELD WITH FLEXIBLE BRONCHOSCOPY

Solitary pulmonary nodule >2 cm

Positive "bronchus sign" on high-resolution computed tomography

Strong clinical suspicion of malignancy

Location in the middle or inner third on chest radiography

Percutaneous needle aspiration is contraindicated

Figure 9-13.

Factors that increase the diagnostic yield of flexible bronchoscopy. In addition to nodule size and location, the diagnostic yield with flexible bronchoscopy is increased by a positive "bronchus sign" on computed tomography. (*Adapted from* Mehta et al. [9].)

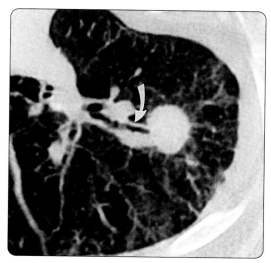

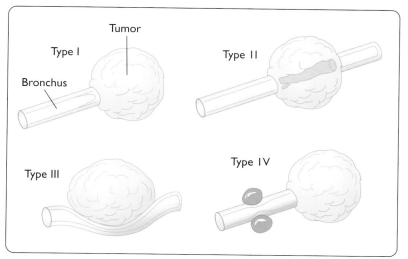

Figure 9-14.
"Bronchus sign" on computed tomography. The term *bronchus sign* was used to describe the computed tomographic finding of a bronchus (*arrow*) leading directly to or contained within a nodule or mass. The presence of a bronchus sign indicates a higher diagnostic yield (60%) with flexible bronchoscopy than if the sign is absent (14%) [47].

Figure 9-15.
Classification of nodule bronchus relationships. Based on its anatomic relationship with the bronchus, the solitary pulmonary nodule (SPN) is classified as one of four types: *type 1*, in which the bronchial lumen is patent up to the tumor; *type 2*, in which the bronchus is contained in the tumor mass; *type 3*, in which the tumor compresses and narrows the bronchus, but the bronchial mucosa is intact; or *type 4*, in which the proximal bronchial tree is narrowed by peribronchial or submucosal spread of the tumor or by enlarged lymph nodes [48]. When high-resolution computed tomography indicates that the SPN is a type-1 or type-2 lesion, conventional sampling methods (transbronchial biopsy with brushing and washing) will be adequate to obtain a tissue diagnosis. However, if the SPN is a type-3 or type-4 lesion, transbronchial needle aspiration may be the diagnostic procedure of choice. Complications of flexible bronchoscopy methods include pneumothorax (1%–3.8%) [49] and significant bleeding (<2%) [50]. (*Adapted from* Tsuboi *et al.* [48].)

INDICATIONS FOR PERCUTANEOUS NEEDLE ASPIRATION*

Small nodules <2 cm

Peripheral location of the solitary pulmonary nodule (outer third of the lung)

Negative flexible bronchoscopy in an indeterminate lesion accessible to percutaneous needle aspiration

---

* *These patients should have no contraindication to percutaneous needle aspiration, such as inability to hold breath, severe pulmonary hypertension, or bleeding diathesis.*

Figure 9-16.
Percutaneous needle aspiration (PCNA). PCNA is preferred for tissue diagnosis of small (<2 cm) and peripheral nodules (outer third of the lung), for which the diagnostic yield of flexible bronchoscopy is very low. The choice of fluoroscopy, ultrasound, or computed tomography (CT) guidance for PCNA is based on lesion characteristics (size and location) and the experience of the radiologist. CT is better for the biopsy of nodules adjacent to vascular struc-

tures or nerves and nodules that are not seen on fluoroscopy. Fluoroscopy allows real-time monitoring of the needle course and is often easier in patients who are less cooperative with breath-holding. Transthoracic ultrasonography can be used only to guide biopsy of peripheral lung lesions and not direct biopsy of most lung nodules because air in the lung parenchyma blocks ultrasound beams [51]. Magnetic resonance imaging (MRI) may play a bigger role in the future with the development of open configuration magnets that allow more rapid evaluation of needle position [52]. The diagnostic yield of PCNA varies between studies, ranging from 43% to 97% [53,54]. PCNA is successful in obtaining a diagnosis in 65% of nodules larger than 1 cm in diameter and in more than 80% of nodules larger than 2 cm. PCNA can be used to identify 95% of malignant nodules [55] and, therefore, has a significant negative predictive value. However, it yields a specific diagnosis in 70% of benign nodules [53]; thus, a nonspecific diagnosis of so-called benign nodules on PCNA does not rule out malignancy [56] and a repeat PCNA or removal of SPN is advisable if clinical suspicion for malignancy is high. Some new technical advances such as the addition of core biopsy to routine fine-needle aspiration (FNA) may enhance the accuracy of benign diagnoses. In a study of 50 patients, the accuracy of benign diagnoses increased from 31% with FNA alone to 69% with core biopsy. The addition of core samples did not increase the accuracy of malignant diagnoses [57]. The utility of on site cytologic examination could also increase the success rate of PCNA and minimize complication risks and discomfort to patients [58]. Complications of the procedure include pneumothorax (30%) and bleeding.

INDICATIONS FOR VIDEO-ASSISTED THORACOSCOPIC SURGERY

Indeterminate nodule that is peripheral (outer one third of lung) and inaccessible to flexible bronchoscopy or computed tomography–guided needle aspiration (small lesion, located under ribs or scapula or near area of emphysema or bullous disease)

Wedge resection of indeterminate or malignant solitary pulmonary nodule in a patient with limited pulmonary reserve who cannot tolerate thoracotomy and wedge resection

Figure 9-17.
Indications for video-assisted thoracoscopic surgery (VATS). VATS may be a less invasive option than open thoracotomy when an indeterminate nodule cannot be classified as benign by flexible bronchoscopy or percutaneous needle aspiration. Open lung resection, lobectomy, or pneumonectomy, if required, can be performed during the same procedure if the solitary pulmonary nodule is malignant [59]. (*Adapted from* Fein *et al.* [60].)

Figure 9-18.
Indications for open thoracotomy. Open thoracotomy is the procedure of choice for malignant solitary pulmonary nodules. The mortality rate varies from 1.4% for segmentectomy to 6.2% for pneumonectomy [61]. (*Adapted from* Fein *et al.* [60].)

MANAGEMENT

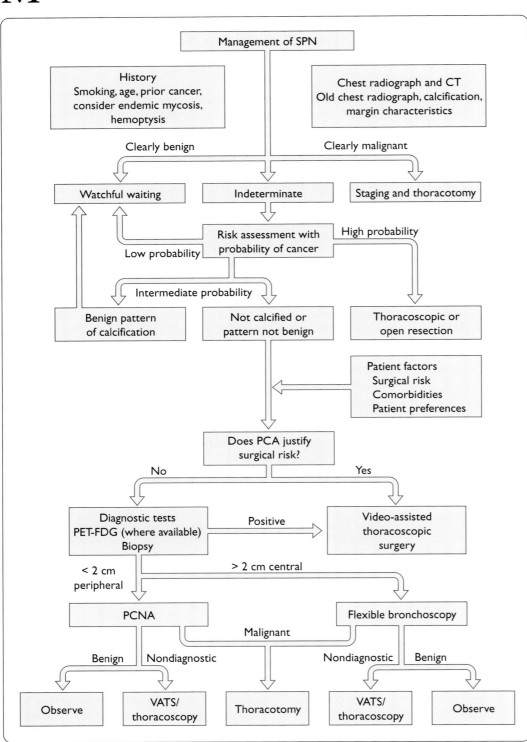

Figure 9-19.
Algorithm for management of the solitary pulmonary nodule (SPN). Based on a detailed history, physical examination, and the results of noninvasive studies such as chest radiographs and CT scans, an SPN can be categorized as benign, indeterminate, or malignant. "Watchful waiting," an active process that involves close monitoring and serial chest radiographs, may be used for patients with SPNs that are probably benign (eg, a nodule in a patient younger than 35 years of age who has no additional risk factors or a nodule that becomes smaller or remains stable for a 2-year period). For malignant SPNs, thoracotomy and resection of the nodule is advocated. For indeterminate nodules, variables such as nodule characteristics, patient's age, history of smoking, and prior malignancy must be considered. Based on the literature and cost-effectiveness analyses, the approach to patients with indeterminate nodules favors PET scanning because it allows more precise risk stratification. This is important particularly in older patients with concurrent medical illnesses in whom the surgical risk is high and avoiding unnecessary surgery is essential. If the PET scan is negative, serial chest radiograph or CT scan follow-up is justified. Similarly, a positive PET scan justifies the risk associated with surgery because malignancy is likely. As for patients without comorbidities who have a relatively high risk for cancer, early thoracotomy is an option. However, in clinical situations in which potential differences between choice strategies are small, patient preference may play an important role in the decision making.

REFERENCES

1. Good CA, Wilson TW: The solitary circumscribed pulmonary nodule: study of 705 cases encountered roentgenographically in a period of three and one-half years. *JAMA* 1958, 66:210–215.

2. Stoller JK, Ahmad M, Rice TW: Solitary pulmonary nodule. *Cleve Clin J Med* 1988, 55:68–74.

3. Stitik FP, Tockman MS: Radiographic screening in early detection of lung cancer. *Radiol Clin North Am* 1978, 16:347–366.

4. Shields TW: Surgical therapy for carcinoma of the lung. *Clin Chest Med* 1993, 14:121–147.

5. Lilington GA: Management of solitary pulmonary nodules. *Dis Mon* 1991, 37:271–318.

6. Zerhouni EA, Stilik FP, Siegelman SS, Naidich DP: CT of the pulmonary nodule: a national cooperative study. *Radiology* 1986, 160:319–327.

7. Toomes HG, Delphendahl A, Manke HG, Vogt-Moykopf I: The coin lesion of the lungs: a review of 955 resected coin lesions. *Cancer* 1983, 51:534–537.

8. Davila DG, Dunn WF, Tazelaar HD, Pairolero PC: Bronchial carcinoid tumors. *Mayo Clin Proc* 1993, 68:795–803.

9. Mehta AC, Kathawalla SA, Chan CC, Arroliga AC: Role of bronchoscopy in the evaluation of SPN. *J Bronchol* 1995, 4:315–322.

10. Steele JD: The solitary pulmonary nodule: report of a co-operative study of resected asymptomatic solitary pulmonary nodules in males. *J Thorac Cardiovasc Surg* 1963, 46:21–39.

11. Walske BR: The solitary pulmonary nodule: a review of 217 cases. *Dis Chest* 1966, 49:302–304.

12. Nandi PL, Tang SC, Mok CK, et al.: Pulmonary coin lesions: a review of 239 cases. *Aust NZ J Surg* 1981, 51:56–58.

13. Libby DM, Henschke CI, Yankelevitz DF: The solitary pulmonary nodule: update 1995. *Am J Med* 1995, 99:491–496.

14. Rubins JB, Rubins HB: Temporal trends in the prevalence of malignancy in resected solitary pulmonary lesions. *Chest* 1996, 109:100–103.

15. Mountain CF: Revisions in the international system for staging lung cancer. *Chest* 1997, 111:1710–1717.

16. Cummings SR, Lillington GA, Richard RJ: Estimating the probability of malignancy in solitary pulmonary nodules. *Am Rev Respir Dis* 1986, 134:449–452.

17. US Surgeon General: The health consequences of smoking: cancer. Washington DC: US Department of Health and Human Services; 1982: publication no. 82-50179.

18. Neifield JP, Michaelis LL, Doppman JL: Suspected pulmonary metastases: correlation of chest x-ray, whole lung tomogram and operative findings. *Cancer* 1977, 39:383–387.

19. Goldmeier E: Limits of visibility of bronchogenic carcinoma. *Am Rev Respir Dis* 1965, 91:232–239.

20. Steele JD, Buell P: Asymptomatic solitary pulmonary nodule: host survival, tumor size and growth rate. *J Thorac Cardiovasc Surg* 1973, 65:140–151.

21. Siegelman SS, Khouri NF, Leo FP, et al.: Solitary pulmonary nodule: CT assessment. *Radiology* 1986, 160:307–312.

22. Swensen SJ, Jett JR, Payne S, et al.: An integrated approach to the evaluation of the solitary pulmonary nodule. *Mayo Clin Proc* 1990, 65:173–186.

23. Swenson SJ, Brown LR, Colby TV; et al.: Pulmonary nodules: CT evaluation of enhancement with iodinated contrast material. *Radiology* 1995, 194:393–398.

24. Zhang M, Kono M: Solitary pulmonary nodules: evaluation of blood flow patterns with dynamic CT. *Radiology* 1997, 205:471–478.

25. Henschke CI, Miettinene OS, Yankelevitz DF, et al.: Early Lung Cancer Action Project: overall design and findings from baseline screening. *Lancet* 1999, 354:99–105.

26. Kaneko M: Computed tomography screening for lung carcinoma in Japan. *Cancer* 2000, 89:2485–2488.

27. Sone S, Takashima S, Li F, et al.: Mass screening for lung cancer with mobile spiral computed tomography scanner. *Lancet* 1998, 351:1242–1245.

28. Naidich DP, Harkin TJ: Airway and lung: correlation of CT with fiberoptic bronchoscopy. *Radiology* 1995, 197:1–12.

29. Kuniyama K, Tateishi R, Higashiyama M, et al.: Prevalence of air-bronchograms in small peripheral carcinomas of the lung on thin-section CT: comparison with benign tumors. *AJR Am J Roentengol* 1991, 156:921–924.

30. Remy-Jardin M, Remy J, Girand F, Marquette CH: Pulmonary nodule detection with thick-section spiral CT versus conventional CT. *Radiology* 1992, 182:809–816.

31. Dewan NA, Gupta NC, Redepenning LS, et al.: Diagnostic efficacy of PET-FDG imaging in solitary pulmonary nodules. *Chest* 1993, 104:997–1002.

32. Dewan NA, Shehan CJ, Reeb SD, et al.: Likelihood of malignancy in a solitary pulmonary nodule: comparison of Bayesian analysis and result of FDG-PET scan. *Chest* 1997, 112:416–422.

33. Gambhir SS, Shepherd JE, Shah BD, et al.: Analytical decision model for the cost-effective management of solitary pulmonary nodules. *J Clin Oncol* 1998, 16:2113–2125.

34. Higashi K, Ueda Y, Seki H, et al.: Fluorine-18-FDG PET imaging is negative in bronchioloalveolar lung carcinoma. *J Nucl Med* 1998, 39:1016–1020.

35. Erasmus JJ, McAdams HP, Patz EF, et al.: Evaluation of primary pulmonary carcinoid tumors using FDG-PET. *AJR* 1998, 170:1369–1373.

36. Gupta NC, Frank AR, Dewan NA, et al.: Solitary pulmonary nodules: detection of malignancy with PET with 2-[F-18]-fluoro-2-deoxy-D-glucose. *Radiology* 1992, 184:441–444.

37. Stringfield JT, Markowitz DJ, Bentz RR, et al.: The effect of tumor size and location on diagnosis by fiberoptic bronchoscopy. *Chest* 1977, 72:474–476.

38. Cortese DA, McDougall JC: Biopsy and brushing of peripheral lung cancer with fluoroscopic guidance. *Chest* 1979, 75:141–145.

39. Radke JR, Conway WA, Eyler WR, Kvale PA: Diagnostic accuracy in peripheral lung lesions: factors predicting success with flexible fiberoptic bronchoscopy. *Chest* 1979, 76:176–179.

40. Fletcher EC, Levin DC: Flexible fiberoptic bronchoscopy and fluoroscopically guided transbronchial biopsy in the management of solitary pulmonary nodules. *West J Med* 1982, 136:477–483.

41. Wallace JM, Deutsch AL: Flexible fiberoptic bronchoscopy and percutaneous needle lung aspiration for evaluating the solitary pulmonary nodule. *Chest* 1982, 81:665–671.

42. Shiner RJ, Rosenman J, Katz I, et al.: Bronchoscopic evaluation of peripheral lung tumors. *Thorax* 1988, 43:887–889.

43. Chechani V: Bronchoscopic diagnosis of solitary pulmonary nodules and lung masses in the absence of endobronchial abnormality. *Chest* 1996, 109:620–625.

44. Naidich DP, Sussman R, Kutcher WL, et al.: Solitary pulmonary nodule: CT-bronchoscopic correlation. *Chest* 1988, 93:595–598.

45. Pirozynski M: Bronchoalveolar lavage in the diagnosis of peripheral primary lung cancer. *Chest* 1992, 102:372–374.

46. de Garcia J, Bravo C, Miravitilles M, et al.: Diagnostic value of bronchoalveolar lavage in peripheral lung cancer. *Am Rev Respir Dis* 1993, 147:649–652.

47. Gaeta M, Pandolfo I, Volta S, et al.: Bronchus sign on CT in peripheral carcinoma of the lung: value in predicting results of transbronchial biopsy. *AJR Am J Roentengol* 1991, 157:1181–1185.

48. Tsuboi E, Ikeda S, Tajima M; et al.: Transbronchial biopsy smear for the diagnosis of peripheral pulmonary carcinoma. *Cancer* 1967, 20:687–698.

49. Blasco LH, Sanchez Hernandez IM, Villena G, et al.: Safety of the transbronchial biopsy in outpatients. *Chest* 1991, 99:562–565.

50. Cordasco EM Jr, Mehta AC, Ahmad M: Bronchoscopically induced bleeding: a summary of nine years Cleveland Clinic experience and review of the literature. *Chest* 1991, 100:1141–1147.

51. Targhetta R, Bourgeois JM, Marty-Double C, et al.: Peripheral pulmonary lesions: ultrasonic features and ultrasonically guided fine needle aspiration biopsy. *J Ultrasound Med* 1993, 12:369–374.

52. Steiner P, Erhart P, Heske N, et al.: Active biplanar MR tracking for biopsies in humans. *AJR Am J Roentgenol* 1997, 169:735–738.

53. Levine MS, Weiss JM, Harrell JH, et al.: Transthoracic needle aspiration biopsy following negative fiberoptic bronchoscopy in solitary pulmonary nodules. *Chest* 1988, 93:1152–1155.

54. Khouri NF, Stitik FP, Erozan YS, et al.: Transbronchial needle aspiration biopsy of benign and malignant lung lesions. *AJR Am J Roentgenol* 1985, 144:281–288.

55. Westcott JL: Percutaneous transthoracic needle biopsy. *Radiology* 1988, 169:593–601.

56. Calhoun P, Feldman PS, Armstrong P: The clinical outcome of needle aspiration of the lung when cancer is not diagnosed. *Am Thorac Surg* 1986, 41:592–596.

57. Boiselle PM, Shepard JA, Mark EJ, et al.: Routine addition of an automated biopsy device to fine-needle aspiration of the lung: a prospective assessment. *AJR Am J Roentgenol* 1997, 169:661–666.

58. Satambrogio L, Nosotti M, Bellaviti N, et al: CT-guided fine-needle aspiration cytology of solitary pulmonary nodules: a prospective, randomized study of immediate cytologic evaluation. *Chest* 1997, 112:423–425.

59. Ginsberg RT: Thoracoscopy: a cautionary note. *Ann Thorac Surg* 1993, 56:801–803.

60. Fein AM, Feinsilver SH, Ares CA: The solitary pulmonary nodule: a systemic approach. In *Fishman's Pulmonary Diseases and Disorders*, edn 3. Edited by Fishman AP. New York: McGraw Hill; 1998:1727–1737.

61. Ginsberg RJ, Hill LD, Eagan RT, et al.: Modern thirty-day operative mortality for surgical resection in lung cancer. *J Thorac Cardiovasc Surg* 1983, 86:654–658.

PLEURAL AND CHEST WALL TUMORS

10

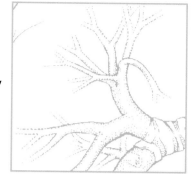
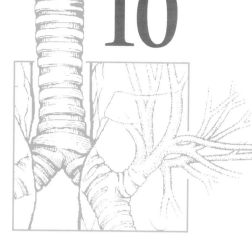
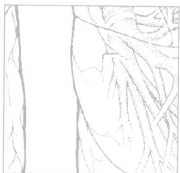

Saeed U. Khan, Mani S. Kavuru,
Carol Farver, Moulay Meziane,
& Thomas W. Rice

Compared with neoplasms of the lung parenchyma, pleural and chest wall tumors are uncommon. Furthermore, primary pleural and chest wall tumors need to be distinguished from the more common metastatic disease as well as benign and reactive processes that may affect the pleural space. This chapter considers various aspects of pleural and chest wall tumors, the emphasis being on pathology and diagnostic radiology. Tumors metastatic to the pleural space are not considered here.

The most common primary pleural tumor is malignant mesothelioma. The diagnosis is usually based on a spectrum of clinical findings, typical computed tomographic (CT) findings, and consistent pathologic findings on electron microscopy and immunohistochemical stains. None of these findings are pathognomonic, however, and the differential diagnosis usually involves mesothelioma versus adenocarcinoma. Typical radiographic findings suggesting malignant mesothelioma include a unilateral pleural effusion, with an ipsilateral shift of the mediastinum toward the pleural effusion and bilateral pleural plaques and/or thickening or, lobulation on a CT scan. A CT scan is essential for the initial diagnosis and staging of mesothelioma, according to the newly proposed TNM (tumor, node, metastasis) classification system [1]. Magnetic resonance imaging does not appear to offer an advantage over the CT scan in the management of patients with mesothelioma [2]. A diagnosis is usually established by thoracoscopy. Pleural fluid cytology and closed pleural biopsy are usually inadequate to firmly establish a diagnosis and, with the widespread use of thoracoscopy, open surgical biopsy is infrequently performed for diagnosis [3]. Much has been published about the pathology of mesothelioma, but no monoclonal antibody specific for mesothelioma has been found to differentiate it from adenocarcinoma. A recent study suggests that the best means of differentiating between these tumors involves the use of a panel of antibodies, carcinoembryonic antigen, B72.3, and Leu-M1.

Overall, the prognosis for patients with malignant mesothelioma remains grim. Symptomatic therapy remains the best approach for most patients managed outside of clinical trials. Surgical procedures (pleurectomy with decortication or the radical extrapleural pneumonectomy) rarely offer a cure. Combination chemotherapy, with or without radiotherapy, does not appear more efficacious than single-agent therapy and does not prolong survival.

Primary chest wall tumors usually arise from soft tissue, bone, or cartilage. These tumors may present as painless chest wall masses or as painful, ulcerating lesions. Their evaluation should include a CT scan of the chest and a bone scan to evaluate the extent of the mass as well as assess its metastasis. The need for a preoperative histologic diagnosis and whether needle biopsy or an incisional biopsy is preferred remains controversial. The strongest argument in favor of a preoperative diagnosis is it can be used to identify patients with Ewing's sarcoma, plasmacytoma, or embryonal rhabdomyosarcoma, whose primary therapy consists of combination chemotherapy.

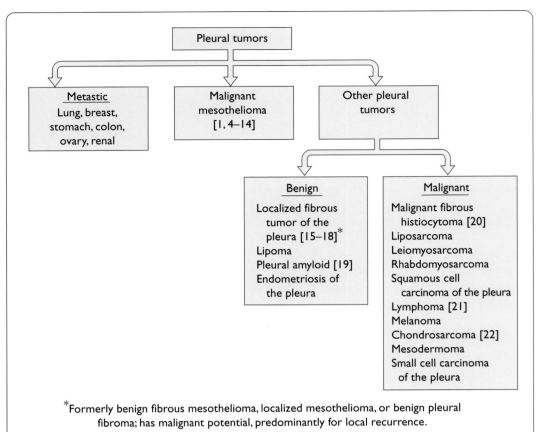

Figure 10-1.
Overview of the differential diagnosis for pleural tumors. Malignant mesothelioma is the most common primary pleural tumor.

CLINICAL FEATURES OF MALIGNANT MESOTHELIOMA

Age	40–70 y
Male-to-female ratio	5:1
Risk factors	Asbestos exposure, *eg*, shipyard workers, miners
	Spouse of asbestos worker
	Irradiation
	Beryllium exposure
Latency period after asbestos exposure	30–45 y
Type of asbestos fiber	Crocidolite ≥ amosite > tremolite > chrysotile
Incidence	Nonasbestos exposure—1:1,000,000
	Asbestos exposure—0.2–2:100
History of asbestos exposure	13%–76%
Smoking history	36%–71%
Symptoms to diagnosis	
<6 mo	70%
>6 mo	28%
Survival without treatment (after diagnosis)	6.8–15 mo

Figure 10-2.
Epidemiologic and clinical features of malignant mesothelioma [9–11].

INTERNATIONAL STAGING SYSTEM FOR MALIGNANT MESOTHELIOMA

T—Primary tumor

T1a	Tumor limited to ipsilateral parietal pleura
T1b	Ipsilateral parietal and visceral pleura
T2	Ipsilateral pleura plus involvement of diaphragm and/or extension of visceral tumor into underlying lung parenchyma
T3	Ipsilateral pleura plus involvement of mediastinal fat, endothoracic fascia, soft tissues of chest wall, and/or pericardium
T4	Locally advanced, unresectable tumor with extension to chest wall, peritoneum, contralateral pleura, mediastinal organs, spine, and myocardium

N—Lymph nodes

NX	Regional lymph nodes cannot be assessed
N0	No regional lymph node metastases
N1	Metastases in the ipsilateral bronchopulmonary or hilar lymph nodes
N2	Metastases in the subcarinal or the ipsilateral mediastinal lymph nodes, including the ipsilateral internal mammary nodes
N3	Metastases in the contralateral mediastinal, contralateral internal mammary, or ipsilateral or contralateral supraclavicular lymph nodes

M—Metastases

MX	Presence of distant metastases cannot be assessed
M0	No distant metastasis
M1	Distant metastasis present

Stage	Description
Stage I	
Ia	T1aN0M0
Ib	T1bN0M0
Stage II	T2N0M0
Stage III	Any T3M0
	Any N1M0
	Any N2M0
Stage IV	Any T4
	Any N3
	Any M1

Figure 10-3.
International staging system for malignant mesothelioma. (*Adapted from* International Mesothelioma Interest Group [1].)

TREATMENT OPTIONS FOR MALIGNANT MESOTHELIOMA

Debulking surgery
    Extrapleural pneumonectomy
    Pleurectomy
Radiation [12]
    External beam irradiation
    Implantation of radioactive isotopes
Chemotherapy [9]
    Doxorubicin, cyclophosphamide, *cis*-platinum

Figure 10-4.
Treatment options for malignant mesothelioma. The surgical options for patients with malignant mesothelioma include the radical extrapleural pneumonectomy, which involves removal of the parietal and mediastinal pleura, lung, and ipsilateral half of the diaphragm. Surgery is rarely curative. Combination chemotherapy–with or without radiation therapy–does not appear to have any advantage over single-agent therapy.

PROGNOSIS FOR MALIGNANT MESOTHELIOMA

	Therapeutic options	
	EPP	Pleurectomy
Mortality, %	6–31	1.5–11
Median survival, *mo*	9.3–13.3	9–21
1-y survival, *mo*	28–70	30–80
2-y survival, *mo*	10–48	8.9–32
5-y survival, *mo*	3.5–28.5	—

EPP—extrapleural pneumonectomy.

Figure 10-5.
Prognosis for patients with malignant mesothelioma treated with surgery. Extrapleural pneumonectomy does not offer added advantage over pleurectomy and carries a higher mortality rate [12,13].

CHEST WALL TUMORS

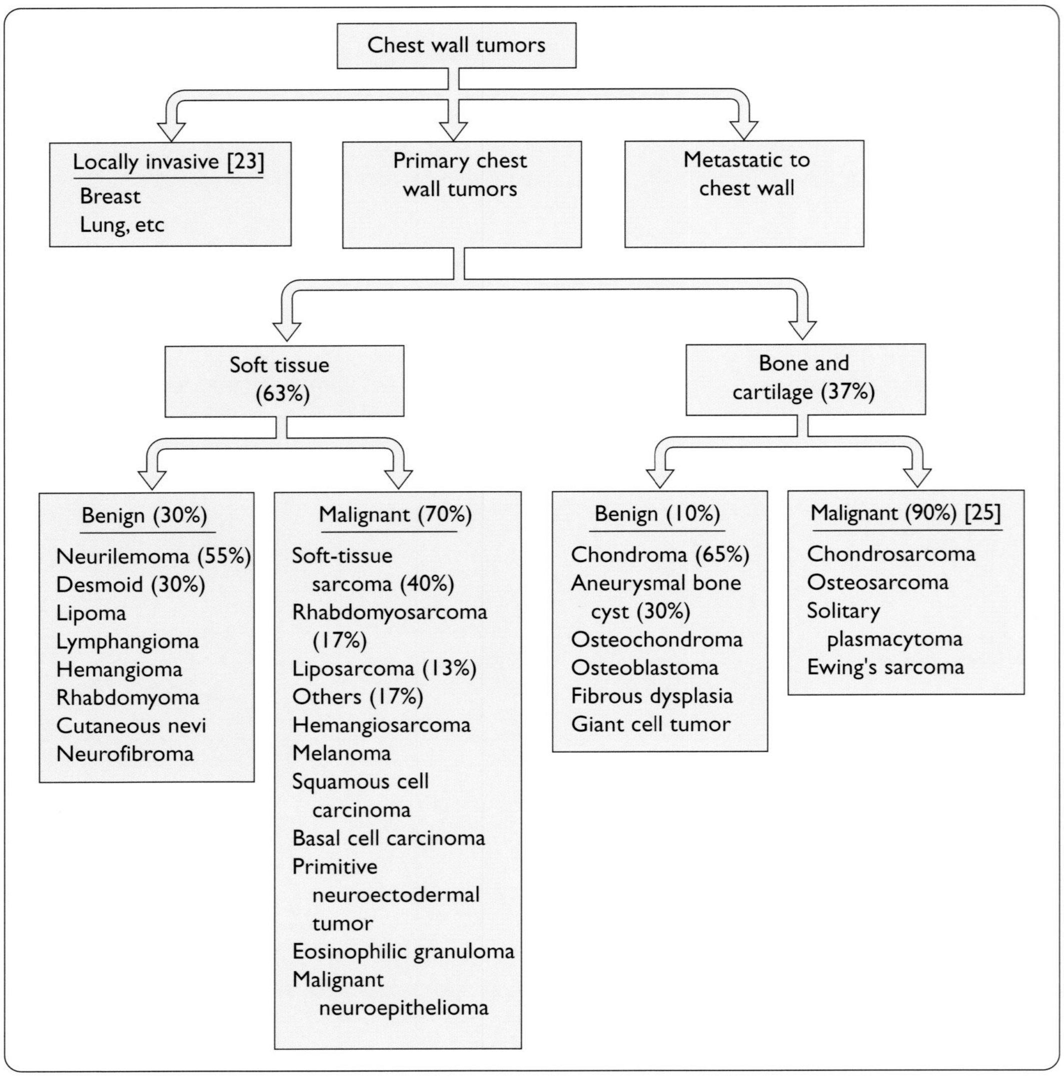

Chest wall tumors
Locally invasive [23]
Breast
Lung, etc
Primary chest wall tumors
Metastatic to chest wall
Soft tissue (63%)
Bone and cartilage (37%)
Benign (30%)
Neurilemoma (55%)
Desmoid (30%)
Lipoma
Lymphangioma
Hemangioma
Rhabdomyoma
Cutaneous nevi
Neurofibroma
Malignant (70%)
Soft-tissue sarcoma (40%)
Rhabdomyosarcoma (17%)
Liposarcoma (13%)
Others (17%)
Hemangiosarcoma
Melanoma
Squamous cell carcinoma
Basal cell carcinoma
Primitive neuroectodermal tumor
Eosinophilic granuloma
Malignant neuroepithelioma
Benign (10%)
Chondroma (65%)
Aneurysmal bone cyst (30%)
Osteochondroma
Osteoblastoma
Fibrous dysplasia
Giant cell tumor
Malignant (90%) [25]
Chondrosarcoma
Osteosarcoma
Solitary plasmacytoma
Ewing's sarcoma

Figure 10-6.
Overview of the differential diagnosis for chest wall tumors [23–30]. These tumors usually arise from soft tissue or bone and cartilage.

CLINICAL FEATURES OF COMMON MALIGNANT CHEST WALL TUMORS

	Soft-tissue sarcoma	Chondrosarcoma	Ewing's sarcoma	Osteosarcoma	Plasmacytoma
Incidence in chest wall, %	6	15	15	3	20
Male-to-female ratio	2:1	1.3:1	1.6:1	1.5:1	2.4:1
Age, *y* (*mean*)	<1–86 (38)	5–86 (49)	2–39 (16)	11–78 (42)	35–75 (59)
Site	—	Rib 43%	Rib 55%	Rib 34%	Rib 62%
		Scapula 36%	Scapula 34%	Scapula 32%	Scapula 4%
		Sternum 16%	Sternum 3%	Sternum 26%	Sternum 12%
		Clavicle 5%	Clavicle 8%	Clavicle 8%	Clavicle 21%
Symptoms					
Mass only, %	73	43	3	16	21
Mass and pain, %	13	37	8	68	17
Pain only, %	1	12	6	10	54
Others, %	2	7	2	5	8
Incidence, %	35	18	75	68	40–60
Site of metastasis	Lung, pleura, brain, liver, spleen	Lung, liver, bone	Lung, bone, brain, lymph nodes	Lung, bone, colon	

Figure 10-7.
Clinical features of common malignant chest wall tumors [23–30]. Overall, these tumors are relatively uncommon. Most patients are symptomatic with a mass involving the soft tissues or rib and scapula.

	Soft-tissue sarcoma	Chondrosarcoma	Ewing's sarcoma	Osteosarcoma	Plasmacytoma
Treatment	Complete resection	Complete resection	Combination chemotherapy followed by radiotherapy; limited role for resection	Resection followed by postoperative chemotherapy protocol	Chemotherapy plus radiotherapy/resection for local control
Local recurrence rate after resection, %	27	39	—	10	—
5-y survival, %	49–90	27–64	48	15	38
Indicators of poor prognosis	Metastasis High-grade histology Pain	Metastasis Age >50 y Local recurrence	Metastasis	Metastasis Sternal tumor Incomplete resection	Multiple myeloma

Figure 10-8.

Treatment and prognosis for chest wall tumors [23–30]. Treatment depends on the histology of the primary malignant tumor. Resection is the primary therapy in all cases except those involving Ewing's sarcoma and plasmacytoma.

PATHOLOGY OF PLEURAL TUMORS

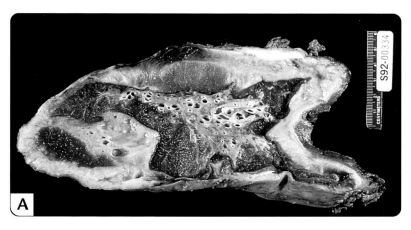

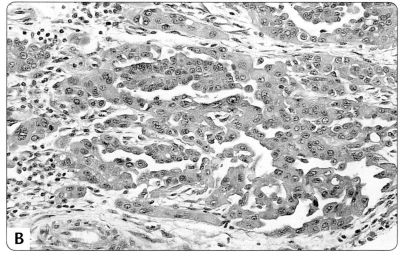

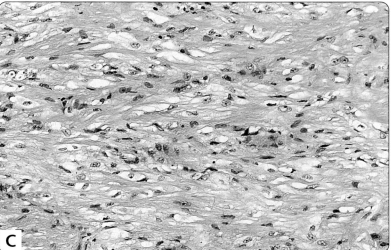

Figure 10-9.

Malignant mesothelioma. **A,** Gross specimen of malignant mesothelioma, demonstrating typical dense thickening of the pleura by firm gray-white tissue, which may show areas of cystic degeneration and mucinous material containing hyaluronic acid. The tumor usually arises in the parietal pleura but quickly involves the visceral pleura, causing a fusion of these two layers into a dense, white encasement of the lung. The tumor extends into the lung via the major and minor fissures and interlobular septae and commonly extends into and through the diaphragm. The underlying lung is characteristically atelectatic, but otherwise unremarkable. Pleural effusions are common. (*See* Color Plate.) **B,** Microscopic specimen of malignant mesothelioma. Malignant mesotheliomas are classified histologically by the World Health Organization as belonging in one of three groups: epithelial, fibrous (spindle cell), and biphasic or mixed. *Panel B* is an example of epithelial mesothelioma, which has a tubopapillary architecture with cuboidal tumor cells with one eccentric nucleolus and ample eosinophilic cytoplasm. (*See* Color Plate.) **C,** Example of fibrous mesothelioma, composed of atypical spindlelike cells with hyperchromatic nuclei of varying nuclear pleomorphism and mitotic activity. The cells are surrounded by a varying amount of collagen. (*See* Color Plate.)

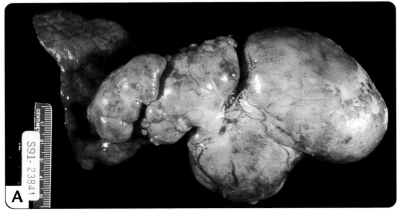

Figure 10-10.
Localized fibrous tumor of the pleura. **A,** Gross specimen of a pleural tumor. Most tumors are nodular, whorled, or lobulated. On cut section, they are composed of firm, gray-white tissue with focal cystic degeneration. They are attached to the pleura by a single pedicle, which contains vessels, or are broad-based with a sessile attachment. (*See* Color Plate.) **B,** Microscopic specimen of a pleural tumor. The tumor is composed of spindlelike

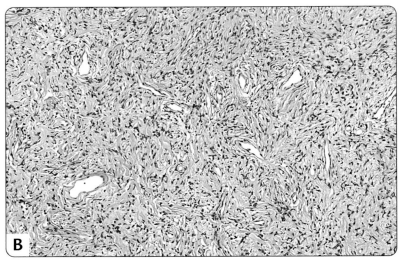

cells with collagen arranged in a variety of patterns, which include a storiform pattern, a hemangiopericytoma-like pattern, and a disorderly or random pattern of fibroblast-like cells. Dense, wirelike bands of collagen can be seen, and small vessels with hyalinized walls are common. (*See* Color Plate.)

PATHOLOGY OF CHEST WALL TUMORS

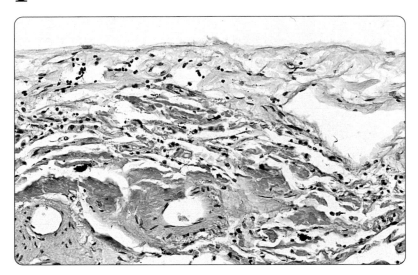

Figure 10-11.
Microscopic specimen demonstrating amyloid of the pleura. This Congo red stain reveals congophilic deposits of amyloid within the visceral pleura. The amyloid has a characteristic acellular eosinophilic appearance that reveals apple-green birefringence. (*See* Color Plate.)

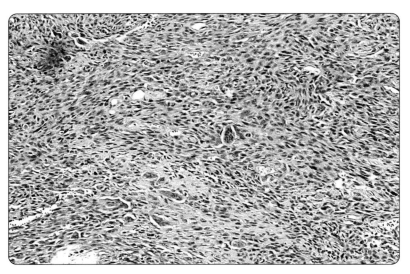

Figure 10-12.
Microscopic specimen demonstrating malignant fibrous histiocytoma. This neoplasm contains a polymorphous population of spindled cells arranged in a storiform and fascicular pattern. The tumor cells include fibroblasts and myofibroblasts, histiocytic-like cells, and multinucleated giant cells. A variable number of chronic inflammatory cells, including lymphocytes and plasma cells, are usually present. Increased mitotic activity and necrosis indicate a poor prognosis. (*See* Color Plate.)

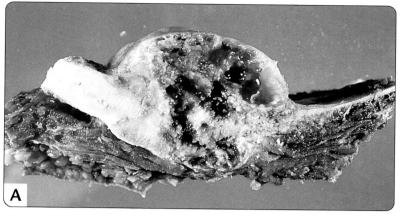

Figure 10-13.

Chondrosarcoma. **A,** Gross specimen of chondrosarcoma, which usually presents as a soft to firm, lobulated mass that is well-circumscribed, often with a distinct fibrous capsule. On cut section, it is gelatinous and gray to brown with varying amounts of hemorrhage. The tumor size varies from 1 to 15 cm. (See Color Plate.) **B,** Microscopic specimen, demonstrating that the tumor

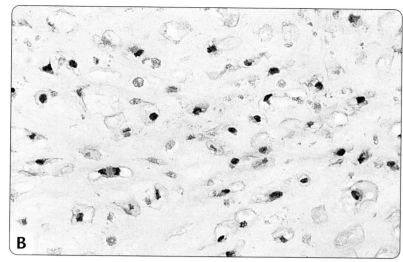

consists of chondrocytes and intervening cartilage. The cells contain small, dark nuclei with varying degrees of cellularity and pleomorphism, which distinguish these lesions from benign cartilage. (See Color Plate.)

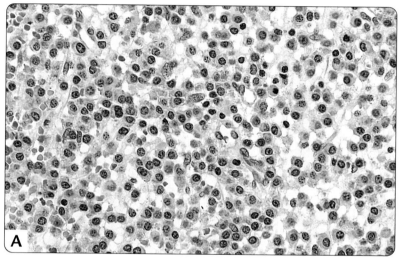

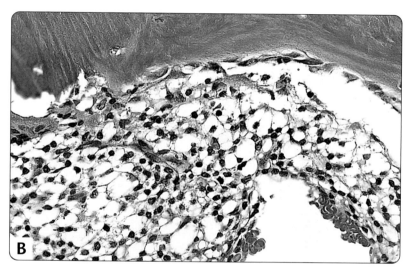

Figure 10-14.

Plasmacytoma. **A,** Microscopic specimen, demonstrating that the tumor is composed of a homogeneous population of plasma cells with varying degrees of cytologic atypia with little or no intervening stroma.

Occasionally, amyloid deposition is present. (See Color Plate.) **B,** The tumor cells erode adjacent bone, resulting in a reparative-lining of osteoblasts along with osseous border.

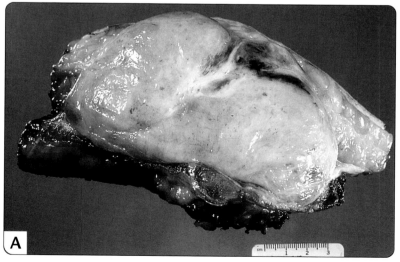

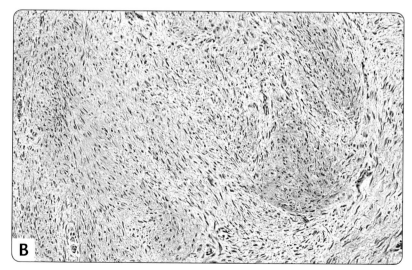

Figure 10-15.

Desmoid. **A,** Gross specimen, demonstrating that the tumor consists of a firm, glistening white mass with a trabeculated surface resembling scar tissue. Desmoids commonly reach 5 to 10 cm in greatest dimension and tumors as large as 20 cm can be found. (See Color Plate.) **B,** Micro-

scopic specimen of a tumor consisting of spindle-shaped cells with a relatively uniform appearance with interspersed collagen. Cellular atypia or hyperchromasia is rare. The cells and collagen are arranged in long, rather ill-defined bundles with a poorly circumscribed and infiltrative border. (See Color Plate.)

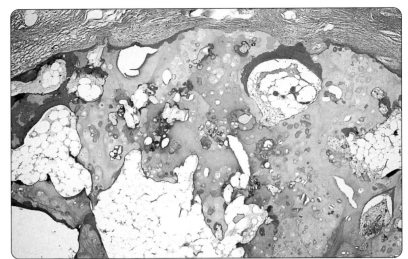

Figure 10-16.
Microscopic specimen of osteochondroma showing a lesion with a thick proliferating cartilage cap overlying poorly organized cancellous bone. Irregular endochondral ossification at the base of the cartilage cap can be seen. (*See* Color Plate.)

RADIOLOGY OF PLEURAL TUMORS

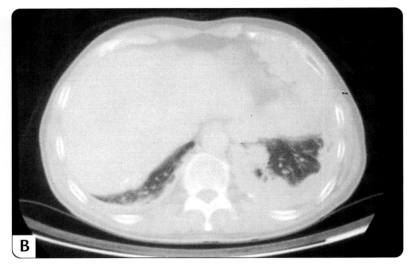

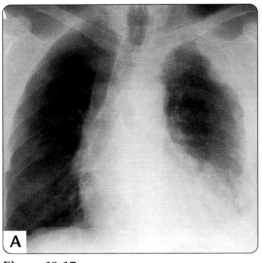

Figure 10-17.
Radiographic findings of malignant mesothelioma. **A,** Posteroanterior chest radiograph of a 70-year-old white man with a 7-month history of cough and exertional dyspnea. Recently the patient experienced left-sided chest discomfort. He worked as a railroad worker and pipe fitter for 40 years. Posteroanterior and lateral views of his chest radiograph demonstrate extensive left pleural nodular thickening encasing the left lung compatible with a malignant pleural mesothelioma. There are also bilateral calcified pleural plaques indicative of pleural changes related to prior asbestos exposure. **B,** A computed tomographic scan of the chest demonstrates extensive pleural disease involving the entire left hemithorax with involvement of the medial and lateral aspects of the pleura compatible with a malignant mesothelioma. The bulkiest portion of the tumor is seen in the anterior aspect of the left middle and lower pleural space, best demonstrated near the origin of the left hemidiaphragm. There is no definite extension through the diaphragm, but there is evidence of extension into the left major fissure. There are multiple bilateral calcified pleural plaques indicative of prior asbestos exposure.

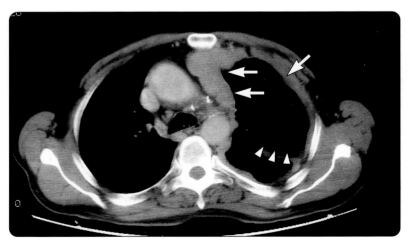

Figure 10-18.
Malignant mesothelioma. Axial computed tomographic scan through the upper chest of a 62-year-old man demonstrates diffuse nodular thickening of the left pleura (*arrows*) extending into the major fissure (*arrowheads*) due to a malignant mesothelioma.

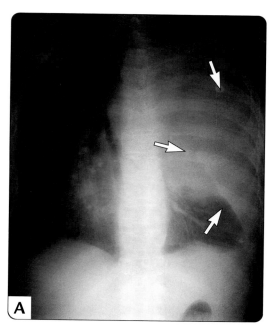

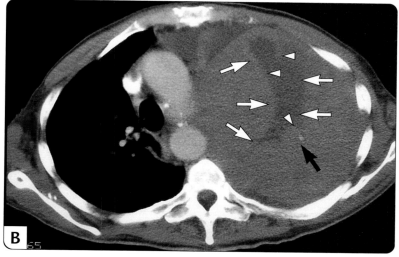

Figure 10-19. Localized fibrous tumor of the pleura. **A,** Posteroanterior chest radiograph of a 78-year-old man with progressive shortness of breath and slowly growing large left chest density (*arrows*). **B,** Computed tomographic scan of the midthorax demonstrates a large well-defined soft-tissue pleural mass (*white arrows*) with a central cleft (*arrowheads*) and calcification (*black arrow*) compatible with a localized fibrous tumor of the pleura.

RADIOLOGY OF CHEST WALL TUMORS

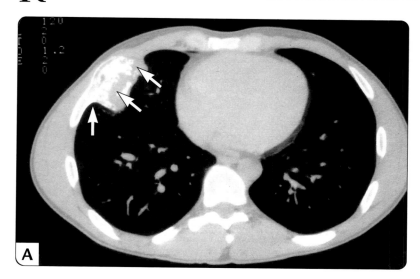

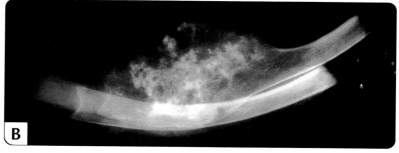

Figure 10-20. Costal chondrosarcoma. **A,** A 27-year-old man with a slowly enlarging right lower-chest wall mass. An axial computed tomographic scan through the lower chest demonstrates an expansile lesion involving the posterior aspect of the right sixth rib at the costochondral junction (*arrows*). **B,** Resected specimen confirms the presence of a low-grade chondrosarcoma of the rib.

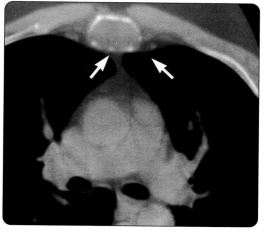

Figure 10-21. Plasmacytoma in a 48-year-old man with sternal pain. Axial scans through the body of the sternum demonstrate a soft-tissue mass (*arrows*) infiltrating and expanding the sternum. Biopsy specimens confirmed the presence of a plasmocytoma.

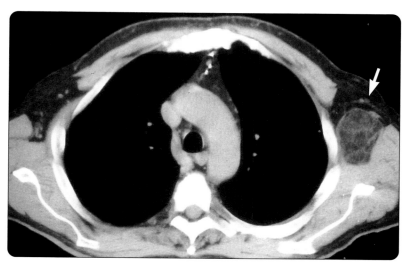

Figure 10-22. Liposarcoma in an 82-year-old man with a palpable left axillary mass. Axial computed tomographic scan obtained at the level of the aortic arch demonstrates a well-defined fatty lesion in the left axilla (*arrow*) with multiple septae through the lesion, compatible with a liposarcoma.

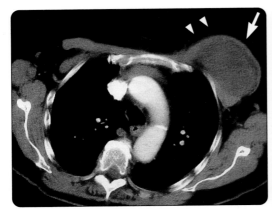

Figure 10-23.
Soft-tissue sarcoma in an 80-year-old man with left chest wall swelling. Axial computed tomographic scan obtained at the level of the aortic arch demonstrates a large soft-tissue mass (*arrow*) seen in the left chest wall below the left pectoralis major muscle (*arrowheads*) due to a soft-tissue sarcoma.

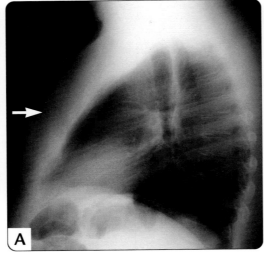

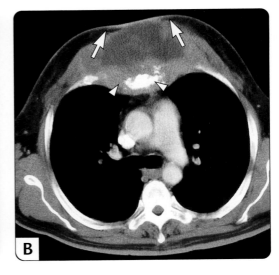

Figure 10-24.
Chest wall lymphoma. **A,** Lateral view of the chest in a 48-year-old man (aged 48 years presenting) with non-Hodgkin's lymphoma and chest wall swelling demonstrates marked soft-tissue thickening in the presternal region (*arrow*). **B,** Axial computed tomographic scan at the level of the carina demonstrates a large necrotic chest wall mass (*arrows*) with involvement of the sternum (*arrowheads*).

REFERENCES

1. International Mesothelioma Interest Group: A proposed new international TNM staging system for malignant pleural mesothelioma. *Chest* 1995, 108:1122–1128.

2. Patz EF, Shaffer K, Piwnica-Worms DR, *et al.*: Value of CT and MR imaging in predicting resectability. *AJR Am J Roentgenol* 1992, 159:961–966.

3. Harris RJ, Kavuru MS, Rice TW, Kirby TJ: The diagnostic and therapeutic utility of thoracoscopy: a review. *Chest* 1995, 108:828–841.

4. Pisani RJ, Colby TV, William DE: Malignant mesothelioma of the pleura. *Mayo Clin Proc* 1988, 63:1234–1244.

5. Antman KH: Natural history and epidemiology of malignant mesothelioma. *Chest* 1993, 103:373–376.

6. Vogelzang NJ: Malignant mesothelioma: diagnostic and management strategies for 1992. *Semin Oncol* 1992, 19:64–71.

7. Hammar SP: The pathology of benign and malignant pleural disease. *Chest Surg Clin N Am* 1994, 4:405–431.

8. Roggli VL, Pratt PC, Brody AR: Asbestos fiber type in malignant mesothelioma: an analytical scanning electron microscopic study of 94 cases. *Am J Ind Med* 1993, 23:605–614.

9. Alberts AS, Falkson F, Goedhals L, *et al.*: Malignant pleural mesothelioma: a disease unaffected by current therapeutic maneuvers. *J Clin Oncol* 1988, 6:527–535.

10. Antman K, Shemin R, Ryan L, *et al.*: Malignant mesothelioma: prognostic variables in a registry of 180 patients, the Dana-Faber Cancer Institute and Brigham and Women's Hospital experience over two decades, 1965–1985. *J Clin Oncol* 1988, 6:147–153.

11. Chailleux E, Dabouis G, Pioche D, *et al.*: Prognostic factors in diffuse malignant pleural mesothelioma: a study of 167 patients. *Chest* 1988, 93:159–162.

12. Ball DL, Cruickshank DG: The treatment of malignant mesothelioma of the pleura: review of five-year experience, with special reference to radiotherapy. *Am J Clin Oncol* 1990, 13:4–9.

13. Allen KB, Faber LP, Warren WH: Malignant pleural mesothelioma: extrapleural pneumonectomy and pleurectomy. *Chest Surg Clin N Am* 1994, 4:113–126.

14. Sugarbaker DJ, Heher EC, Lee TH, *et al.*: Extrapleural pneumonectomy, chemotherapy, and radiotherapy in the treatment of diffuse malignant pleural mesothelioma. *J Thorac Cardiovasc Surg* 1991, 101:10–15.

15. England DM, Hochholzer L, McCarthy MT: Localized benign and malignant fibrous tumors of the pleura: a clinicopathological review of 223 cases. *Am J Surg Path* 1989, 13:640–658.

16. Briselli M, Mark EJ, Dickersin GR: Solitary fibrous tumors of the pleura: eight new cases and review of 360 cases in the literature. *Cancer* 1981, 47:2678–2689.

17. Saifuddin A, Da Costa P, Chalmers AG, *et al.*: Primary malignant localized fibrous tumors of the pleura: clinical, radiological and pathological features. *Clin Pathol* 1992, 45:13–17.

18. Hartmann CA, Schutze H: Mesothelioma-like tumors of the pleura: a review of 72 autopsy cases. *J Cancer Res Clin Oncol* 1994, 120:331–347.

19. Kavuru MS, Adamo JP, Ahmad M, *et al.*: Amyloidosis and pleural disease. *Chest* 1990, 98:20–23.

20. Rizkalla K, Ahmad D, Garcia B, *et al.*: Primary malignant fibrous histiocytoma of the pleura: a case report and review of the literature. *Respir Med* 1994, 88:711–714.

21. Kavuru MS, Tubbs R, Miller ML, Wiedemann HP: Immunocytometry and gene rearrangement analysis in the diagnosis of lymphoma in an idiopathic pleural effusion. *Am Rev Respir Dis* 1992, 145:209–211.

22. Bailey SC, Head HD: Pleural chondrosarcoma. *Ann Thorac Surg* 1990, 49:996–997.

23. Anderson BO, Burt ME: Chest wall neoplasms and their management. *Ann Thorac Surg* 1994, 58:1774–1781.

24. Eng J, Sabanathan S, Pradhan GN, Mearns AJ: Primary bony chest wall tumors. *J R Coll Surg Edinb* 1990, 35:44–47.

25. Burt M: Primary malignant tumors of the chest wall: the Memorial Sloan-Kettering Cancer Center Experience. *Chest Surg Clin N Am* 1994, 4:137–153.

26. King RM, Pairolero PC, Trastek VF, Bernatz PE: Primary chest wall tumors: factors affecting survival. *Ann Thorac Surg* 1986, 41:597–601.

27. Burt M, Fulton M, Wessner-Dunlap S, *et al.*: Primary bony and cartilaginous sarcomas of chest wall: results of therapy. *Ann Thorac Surg* 1992, 54:226–232.

28. Burt M, Karpeh M, Ukoha O, *et al.*: Medical tumors of the chest wall. Solitary plasmacytoma and Ewing's sarcoma. *Cardiovasc Surg* 1993, 105:89–96.

29. Grosfeld JL: Primary tumors of the chest wall and mediastinum in children. *Semin Thorac Cardiovasc Surg* 1994, 6:235–239.

30. Pezzelle AT, Fall SM, Pauling FW, Sadler TR: Solitary plasmacytoma of the sternum: surgical resection with long-term follow-up. *Ann Thorac Surg* 1989, 48:859–862.

MEDIASTINAL MASSES

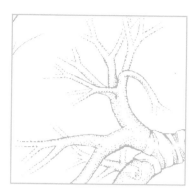
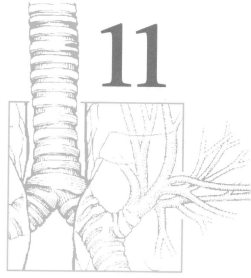

Rodolfo C. Morice &
Carlos A. Jimenez

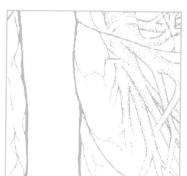

The mediastinum is the region of the chest bounded laterally by the mediastinal pleural reflections of both lungs, anteriorly by the undersurface of the sternum, and posteriorly by the vertebral bodies of the thoracic vertebrae. Longitudinally, it extends from the thoracic inlet to the diaphragm. Because of the variety of tissues it contains, tumors that originate in the mediastinum are numerous and diverse.

Clinical manifestations of these tumors range from vague or asymptomatic to a multiplicity of endocrine or systemic syndromes. The tumors can invade or compress airways and vital cardiovascular structures. In such cases, dramatic, life-threatening clinical presentations can occur [1].

ANATOMIC CONSIDERATIONS

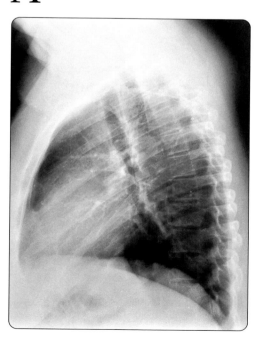

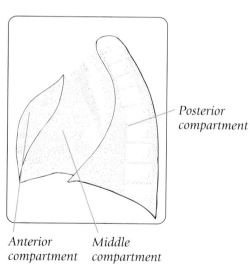

Posterior compartment

Anterior compartment *Middle compartment*

Figure 11-1.
Radiograph showing mediastinal compartments. The mediastinum is divided into anterior, middle, and posterior compartments. The anterior compartment is bounded anteriorly by the sternum and posteriorly by the anterior surface of the pericardium, aorta, and brachiocephalic vessels. This compartment contains the thymus gland, lymph nodes, connective tissue, internal mammary arteries and veins, and ectopic parathyroid glands or thyroid tissue. The middle compartment contains the heart and pericardium, the ascending and transverse sections of the aorta, the brachiocephalic vessels, and the superior and inferior vena cava. It also contains the thoracic portion of the trachea and proximal main stem bronchi, and the pulmonary arteries and veins. The phrenic and upper portion of the vagus nerves, as well as numerous lymphatics and connective tissue, are also within this compartment. The posterior compartment is bounded anteriorly by the dorsal surface of the pericardium, caudally by the diaphragm, laterally by the mediastinal pleural reflections, and posteriorly by the vertebral bodies of the thoracic spine. The paravertebral or costovertebral regions, although not truly within the mediastinum, generally are considered as part of the posterior mediastinal compartment. The latter contains the esophagus, the descending aorta, azygos and hemiazygos veins, the thoracic duct, autonomic nerves, adipose and connective tissue, and lymph nodes.

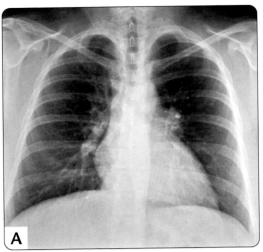

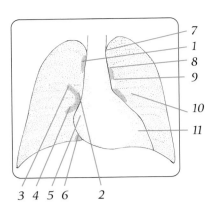

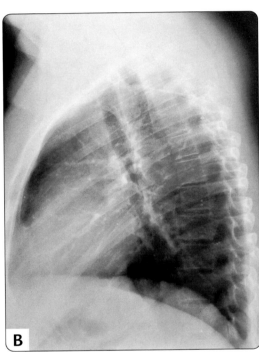

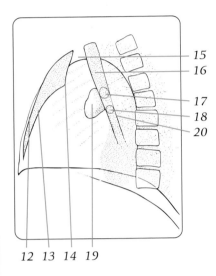

Figure 11-2.
Radiographs showing normal mediastinal borders and lines. Recognition of the normal structures that make up the mediastinal contours and lines on a posteroanterior and lateral chest radiograph remains the fundamental method for detecting mediastinal abnormalities. **A,** On the posteroanterior chest radiograph, the right mediastinal border is defined by the superior vena cava (*1*), azygos vein (*2*), right hilum—formed by the juxtaposed shadows of the right upper lobe pulmonary vein (*3*) and right interlobar pulmonary artery (*4*), the right atrium (*5*), and pericardial fat pad (*6*) at the diaphragmatic-pericardial junction. On the left side, the upper mediastinal contour is formed by the left subclavian artery (*7*), the aortic arch (*8*), and the aortopulmonary window (*9*)—a space occupied largely by mediastinal fat between the aortic arch and the left pulmonary artery (*10*). The shadow of the left ventricle (*11*) forms the remainder of the left infrahilar mediastinal border. Normally, the left atrium is rarely visualized. **B,** On a lateral chest radiograph, the anterior mediastinal space is well-demarcated by the undersurface of the sternum (*12*), the ventral border of the pericardium (*13*), the ascending portion of the aortic arch (*14*), and the brachiocephalic vessels (*15*). In the middle compartment, the air column of the trachea (*16*), as well as the openings of the right upper lobe bronchi (*17*) and left upper lobe bronchi (*18*) are visualized. The more dense shadows located anteriorly and posteriorly to the bronchial openings correspond to the right interlobar artery (*19*) and the confluence of pulmonary veins (*20*), respectively.

Diagnostic Techniques

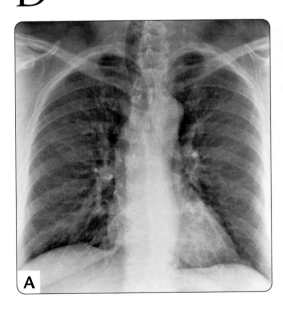

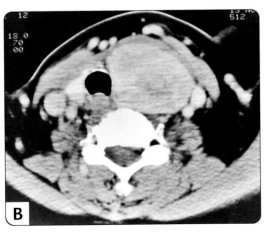

Figure 11-3.
A, Frontal chest radiograph showing displacement of the trachea from left to right in the lower neck and upper mediastinal area. On a standard chest radiograph, the distortion or obliteration of normal mediastinal lines is key to the initial identification of mediastinal disease. The correlation of the radiographic findings with presence or absence of symptoms and clinical examination is sufficient in some cases to establish a diagnosis. In most cases, however, further evaluation is necessary [2]. **B,** Computed tomographic scan of the chest shows lateral tracheal displacement and outward displacement of brachiocephalic vessels. It defines the mass as solid and contained anteriorly by the pretracheal fascia with no invasion of adjacent tissues. A computed tomographic scan of the chest has a much higher sensitivity for smaller lesions than does a conventional radiograph and allows for a better definition of superimposed structures. It also clarifies the association between adjacent tissues and the presence or absence of invasion and differentiates between tissue densities.

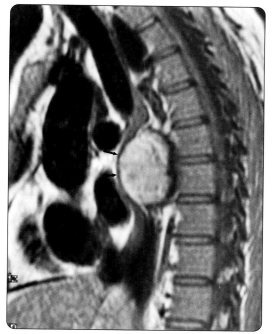

Figure 11-4.
Magnetic resonance image (MRI) of the mediastinum. An advantage of MRI over computed tomography is its ability to visualize vascular structures without requiring intravenous contrast enhancement. It also displays sagittal and coronal planes of mediastinal structures without requiring cumbersome patient repositioning or reformatting of transverse sections, as is the case with computed tomography. This image of a patient with a primary mediastinal pleomorphic sarcoma shows the location of the mass, and anterior displacement of the esophagus (*arrows*) is well-visualized from the perspective of the sagittal view. Blood flowing within cardiovascular structures is perceived as a radiolucency. No known significant biologic risks are associated with the use of the magnetic field at current imaging levels. However, magnetic field interference prevents the use of MRI in patients who have internal metallic devices, such as a pacemaker or a prosthesis.

MEDIASTINAL TUMOR MARKERS

Tumor	Marker
Germ cell tumors	Placental alkaline phosphatase, β-human chorionic gonadotropin, α-fetoprotein
Thymic carcinoid and small cell carcinoma	ACTH, neuron-specific enolase, bombesin, synaptophysin
Parathyroid adenoma	Parathyroid hormone
Neurogenic tumors Pheochromocytoma	Metanephrine, normetanephrine, epinephrine, norepinephrine
Neuroblastoma and ganglioneuroblastoma	Homovanillic acid, vanyllilmandelic acid, neuron-specific enolase

Figure 11-5.
Mediastinal tumor markers. Some mediastinal neoplasms express functional molecules that may serve as tumor markers and are useful for diagnosis and management. The mediastinal tumors with serum or urine tumor markers are shown in this table. In addition, several tissue tumor antigens are used in various immunohistochemical techniques for anatomic and functional tumor identity [3].

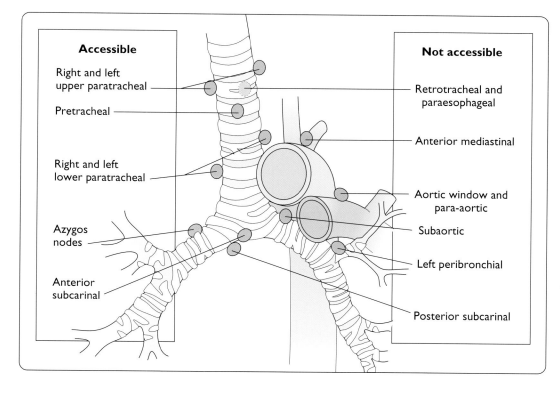

Figure 11-6.
Accessibility of lymph nodes for biopsy with standard mediastinoscopy. Most of the paratracheal, pretracheal, and anterior subcarinal lymph nodes are accessible through standard cervical mediastinoscopy. Nodes in the anterior or posterior compartments, as well as the hilar, para-aortic, subaortic, and lower left paratracheal regions cannot be accessed through this procedure. Extended cervical mediastinoscopy or anterior mediastinotomy would be required for tissue biopsy of these areas [5]. Positron-emission tomography (PET) with ^{18}F-fluorodeoxyglucose is a metabolic imaging technique used in the staging of non small cell lung cancer. It relies on the increased glucose metabolic activity by tumor cells relative to normal tissues. Its specificity is hampered by the fact that inflammatory conditions may also exhibit increased radioactive glucose uptake [6].

COMPARTMENTAL DISTRIBUTION OF MEDIASTINAL MASSES

Anterior compartment	Middle compartment	Posterior compartment
Thymic tumors	Metastasis to lymph nodes	Neurogenic tumors
Germ cell tumors	Benign lymphadenopathy	Meningoceles
Thyroid masses	Lymphomas	Thoracic spine neoplasms
Lymphomas	Bronchogenic cysts	Hiatal hernia
Parathyroid masses	Pleuropericardial cysts	Bochdalek hernia
Mesenchymal tumors	Vascular masses	Neurenteric cysts
	Morgagni hernia	Gastroenteric cysts
		Thoracic duct cysts

Figure 11-7.
Compartmental distribution of mediastinal masses. A practical classification of mediastinal masses based on the usual location of the mass within a mediastinal compartment is useful. However, tumors may extend across compartmental boundaries or have a wide distribution throughout several compartments, such as lymphoma. Tumors arising from the heart or esophagus are usually not categorized as mediastinal tumors.

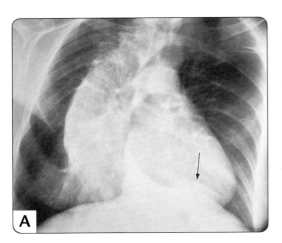

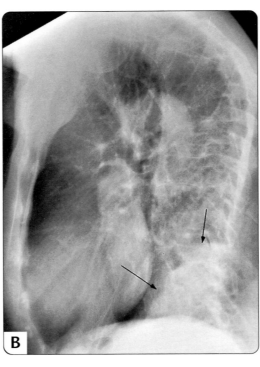

Figure 11-8.
Radiographs showing lesions extending into the mediastinum similar to mediastinal tumors. **A,** Frontal view shows severe scoliosis of the thoracic spine and a retrocardiac density over the left hemidiaphragm (*arrow*). **B,** On the lateral view, the smooth density that overlies the lower thoracic spine represents a hernia (*arrows*) through the foramen of Bochdalek. Foramen of Morgagni hernias present as a mass on the right side of the cardiophrenic angle [7].

ANTERIOR MEDIASTINAL MASSES

THYMIC TUMORS

Benign	Malignant
Benign thymoma (encapsulated)	Malignant thymoma (invasive)
Thymic hyperplasia	Thymic carcinoma
Thymolipoma	Thymic carcinoid
Thymic cysts	Small cell carcinoma of the thymus
Benign germ cell tumors of the thymus	Lymphoma of the thymus
	Malignant germ cell tumors of the thymus
	Metastatic neoplasms

Figure 11-9.
Thymic tumors. Thymic neoplasms constitute approximately 50% of tumors found in the anterior mediastinal compartment in adults but are rare in children. The primary forms of these tumors originate from normal thymic tissue components: epithelial cells, lymphoid tissue, germ cells, neuroendocrine cells, and adipose tissue. Although atypia is occasionally found in some of the epithelial cells, cytologic characteristics do not differentiate between benign or malignant thymomas. Their classification as malignant or benign depends on the presence or absence of encapsulation and invasion to adjacent tissue [8]. Most often, malignant thymomas invade locally, but widespread intrathoracic and sometimes transdiaphragmatic invasion can occur.

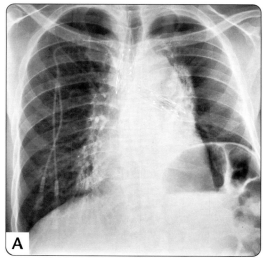
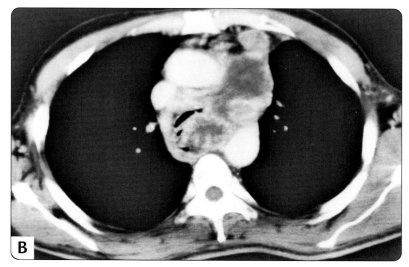

Figure 11-10.

Radiographs of thymic carcinoma. **A,** Frontal chest radiograph shows obliteration of the right mediastinal contour and right upper chest by confluent and multilobulated masses. **B,** Computed tomography at the level of the aortic arch shows neoplastic invasion of the anterior mediastinal compartment with extension into the chest wall. Histologic examination revealed a thymic carcinoma (lymphoepithelioma-like variant). These rare tumors of the thymus are radiologically and macroscopically indistinguishable from invasive thymomas. They spread locally across lymph nodes of various mediastinal compartments, pleura, and pericardium. Extrathoracic metastases are also common. Two main histologic varieties exist: squamous cell and lymphoepithelioma-like carcinomas.

CLASSIFICATION OF GERM CELL TUMORS

Benign
  Benign teratoma (dermoid cyst)
Malignant
  Seminoma
  Nonseminomatous tumors
    Malignant teratoma
    Choriocarcinoma
    Teratocarcinoma
    Endodermal sinus tumor
    Embryonal carcinoma
    Mixed histologic types

Figure 11-11.

Classification of germ cell tumors [9]. Primary mediastinal germ cell tumors account for approximately 10% of all mediastinal tumors. In the adult, approximately 80% of these tumors are benign. Benign teratomas are slow-growing tumors, are equally distributed among men and women, and usually do not produce symptoms. Rarely, they may rupture into the pleural or pericardial space or form bronchial fistulae. Primary malignant mediastinal germ cell tumors occur most frequently in men of 20 to 35 years of age. Pure seminomas are slow-growing and often asymptomatic. Nonseminomatous varieties are more aggressive; most patients have symptoms caused by compression, invasion, or metastatic disease. In addition, several hematologic malignancies are associated with nonseminomatous germ cell tumors [10]. Tissue and serologic markers present in malignant germ cell neoplasms (*see* Fig. 11-5) are helpful in the differential diagnosis from benign teratomas [11].

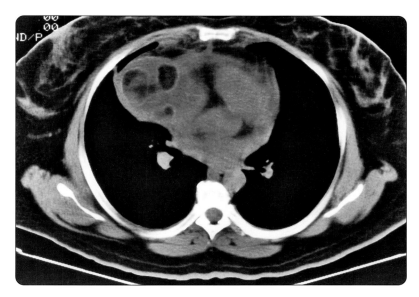

Figure 11-12.

Computed tomographic scan of a benign teratoma. This computed tomographic image reveals a well-circumscribed tumor, with partial calcific rim and heterogenous density contents. Numerous cysts are seen within the mass. These contain various adipose and soft-tissue densities that are characteristic of benign teratoma. Multicystic spaces were lined with various fully differentiated epithelia. Hair, fat, and cartilaginous tissue were present within the cysts. These tumors, also known as dermoids or epidermoid cysts, have an excellent prognosis after complete surgical removal [12].

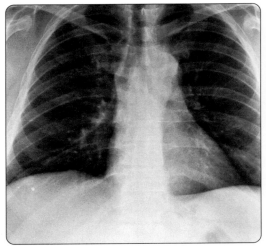

Figure 11-13.
Posteroanterior radiograph of the chest of a young man showing widening of the mediastinal borders as a result of seminoma. Although relatively slow growing, seminomas invade adjacent tissues and most often present with symptoms. Unless metastases have occurred, systemic manifestations are rare. Serum human chorionic gonadotropin is elevated in approximately 10% of patients with primary mediastinal seminomas. Surgical removal is rarely indicated because most seminomas are locally invasive and metastases are present in more than 50% of patients at time of diagnosis. (*From* Morice [13]; with permission.)

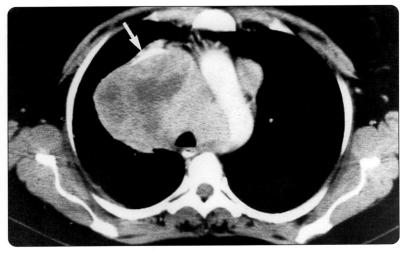

Figure 11-14.
Computed tomographic scan of a nonseminomatous mediastinal tumor (choriocarcinoma). This image shows a large mass on the right side of the upper thorax. It is located predominantly in the anterior mediastinum, but it encroaches into the middle mediastinum. The mass is partially necrotic and invades the perivascular structures. The superior vena cava (*arrow*) appears distorted and compressed. In comparison to other mediastinal tumors, choriocarcinomas grow very rapidly. These tumors present almost invariably with signs and symptoms of local invasion. More than two thirds of patients present with gynecomastia associated with elevated serum levels of human chorionic gonadotropin [14].

PRIMARY MEDIASTINAL MASSES OF MESENCHYMAL ORIGIN

Adipose tissue
  Lipoma
  Liposarcoma
  Mediastinal lipomatosis
Vascular tissue
  Hemangioma
  Angiosarcoma
  Hemangiopericytoma
  Lymphangioma
Muscle tissue
  Leiomyoma
  Leiomyosarcoma
  Rhabdomyoma
  Rhabdomyosarcoma

Fibrous tissue
  Fibroma
  Fibrosarcoma
  Benign fibrous histiocytoma
  Malignant fibrous histiocytoma
Mesodermal tissue
  Benign mesenchymoma
  Malignant mesenchymoma
Miscellaneous
  Osteosarcoma
  Granulocytic sarcoma
  Synovial sarcoma
  Pleomorphic adenoma

Figure 11-15.
Primary mediastinal masses of mesenchymal origin. Such masses are rare—they account for approximately 6% of all mediastinal masses in adults and 10% in children [15]. Given its broad distribution, tumors derived from mesenchymal tissue can occur in all mediastinal compartments [16]. Lipomas are the most common of all mesenchymal tumors in the mediastinum and are easily identifiable by their characteristic density on computed tomograms. Primary mediastinal liposarcomas are extremely rare and almost always present with symptoms caused by compression or inva-

sion of neural or bronchovascular structures [17]. Mesenchymal tumors of vascular origin are very rare. Hemangiomas are the most common and comprise less than 0.5% of all mediastinal masses [18]. Rather than true neoplasms, hemangiomas are developmental vascular proliferations. They present as rounded or lobulated, well-defined densities. Occasionally, phleboliths can be seen within the mass. These can be isolated or multifocal, as in patients with Rendu-Osler-Weber syndrome. Hemangiosarcomas are rare, aggressive tumors with dismal prognosis. Mediastinal lymphangiomas, most often seen in children, represent developmental abnormalities and are sometimes associated with chylothorax [19]. Mediastinal tumors of muscle origin, other than those arising from esophageal smooth muscle, are infrequent. They arise from vascular muscle component or, in cases of rhabdomyosarcomas, can originate from teratomas that undergo single tissue differentiation. Mediastinal fibrous tumors are most often primaries of pleura and neural structures with secondary extension into the mediastinum. Few cases of primary mediastinal benign and malignant fibrous histiocytomas have been reported [20]. Tumors of pluripotential mesodermal tissue that occur in the mediastinum are thought to arise from teratomatous differentiation. Other tumors, such as pleomorphic adenoma, originate from ectopic glandular bronchial epithelium within mediastinal lymph nodes.

MEDIASTINAL LYMPH NODE ENLARGEMENT

Benign, infectious

Granulomatous
    Tuberculosis
    Fungi
Mononucleosis
Reactive lymphadenitis

Benign, noninfectious

Granulomatous
    Sarcoidosis
    Silicosis
    Hypersensitivity pneumonitis
    Wegener's granulomatosis
    Associated with neoplasms
Angioimmunoblastic lymphadenopathy
    Amyloidosis
    Drug induced (*eg,* diphenylhydantoin)
    Lymphoid hamartoma
    Angiofollicular hyperplasia (*eg,* Castelman's disease)

Malignant

Primary large cell lymphoma of the mediastinum
lymphoblastic, Hodgkin's lymphoma, extathoracic and mediastinal
Metastasis to mediastinal lymph nodes

Figure 11-16.
Mediastinal lymph node enlargement. Lymph node enlargement, which is usually caused by systemic infections, noninfectious inflammatory conditions, and extramediastinal malignancy, is the most common cause of mediastinal abnormality. Although most mediastinal lymph nodes are located in the middle compartment, numerous nodal chains exist throughout the mediastinum. Therefore, conditions that cause lymph node enlargement most often affect several mediastinal compartments simultaneously. Specific diagnosis of mediastinal lymph node abnormalities usually requires tissue or bacteriologic confirmation. However, various patterns in the distribution of the lymphadenopathy may provide clues to help guide the patient work-up based on possible causes. Symmetrical, bilateral hilar lymphadenopathy is a feature of sarcoidosis. Asymmetric hilar distribution with involvement of substernal and cervical nodes is often seen in lymphomas. Granulomatous infections tend to cause a more focal and unilateral distribution.

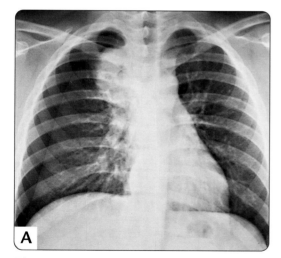 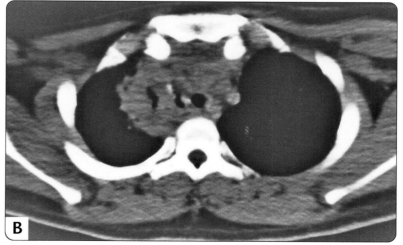

Figure 11-17.
Wegener's granulomatosis presenting as a mediastinal mass. **A,** Frontal chest radiograph shows widening of upper mediastinal profile by a right paratracheal mass that extends down to the azygous area. The trachea appears compressed and deviated to the left. There is a right pneumothorax after needle biopsy of the mass. **B,** Computed tomographic scan confirms the presence of a solid mass with obliteration of soft-tissue planes of trachea and vascular structures. The main diagnostic categories considered in this case of a man 21 years of age, who had a history of fever, weight loss, and mild hemoptysis, included lymphoma and granulomatous infections. Bronchoscopic examination in this patient showed extensive tracheal and right main stem bronchial narrowing with mucosal infiltration and partial necrosis. The diagnosis of "limited" Wegener's granulomatosis was made by tissue analysis obtained via mediastinoscopy and corroborated by the presence of positive serology tests for antineutrophil cytoplasmic autoantibodies [21].

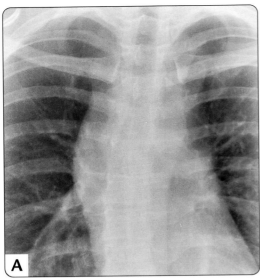

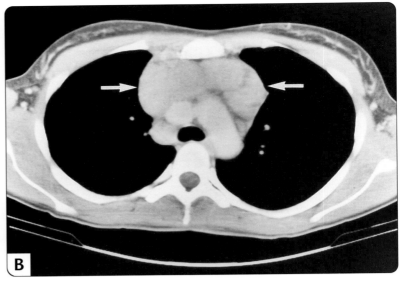

Figure 11-18.
Nodular sclerosing Hodgkin's lymphoma. **A,** Frontal radiograph shows a large mediastinal mass protruding on both sides of the mediastinal borders. **B,** Computed tomographic scan reveals several confluent, lobulated, solid masses that fill the anterior mediastinal space entirely and wrap around the middle mediastinal vascular structures (*arrows*). Lymphomas constitute approximately 20% of all mediastinal neoplasms in adults [22]. Most lymphomas that occur in the mediastinum also appear in extrathoracic sites. However, three lymphoma types are known for their preferential mediastinal location: Hodgkin's disease, lymphoblastic lymphoma [23], and large cell lymphoma [24]. Of these, the nodular sclerosing form of Hodgkin's disease is by far the most common of the mediastinal lymphomas. Constitutional symptoms, rather than local compressive manifestations, are usually observed with mediastinal Hodgkin's disease. The other two non-Hodgkin's varieties—lymphoblastic lymphoma and large cell lymphoma—are more aggressive, usually cause compressive symptoms, and have a worse prognosis [25].

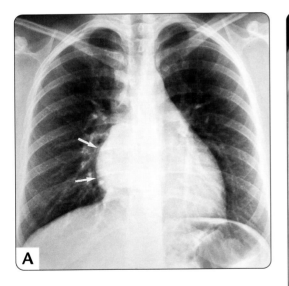

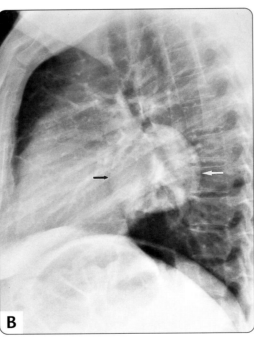

Figure 11-19.
Mediastinal bronchogenic cyst. **A,** Posteroanterior chest radiograph discloses a homogeneous, infracarinal, soft-tissue mass superimposed on the cardiac shadow (*arrows*). **B,** The lateral radio-graph identifies a round, sharply defined mass in the retrocardiac area (*arrows*). These radiologic features are characteristic of bronchogenic cyst. These cysts are congenital and often detected during childhood or adolescence. Compressive airway manifestations occur particularly in infants: more than 50% of them are asymptomatic. Some may remain undiagnosed into adulthood. Occasionally, fistula formation and drainage of the cystic contents into the bronchial tree can occur. Development of fever, pain, and change in the size of the cyst are indications of infection or intracystic bleeding. Nearly two thirds of the bronchogenic cysts are located near the main carina. Less often, they may be associated with a lobar or segmental bronchus and have an intrapulmonary rather than mediastinal location [26].

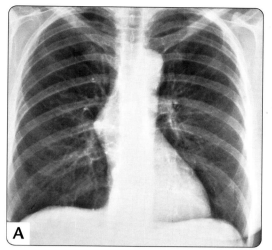

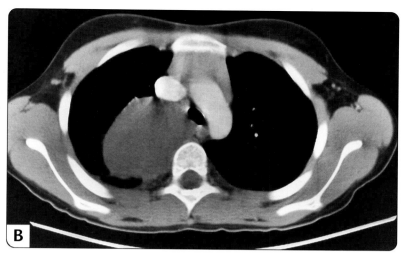

Figure 11-20.

Aneurysm of the ascending aorta. **A,** Posteroanterior radiograph of an asymptomatic woman aged 63 years shows a smooth, abnormal density that overlaps the right hilar area. **B,** Computed tomographic scan confirms a fusiform aneurysm of the ascending aorta with dense calcification of its wall. Aortic aneurysms are the most common cause of mediastinal vascular masses. These can have multiple causes, but most are atherosclerotic. Among various other causes, aortic aneurysms can be related to Marfan syndrome, trauma, mycotic infection, rheumatic aortitis, and syphilis. Sixty percent of thoracic aortic aneurysms affect the descending aorta; the rest affect the ascending portion and transverse arch.

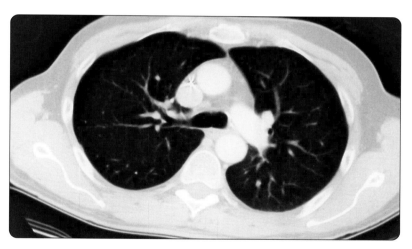

Figure 11-21.

Computed tomographic scan showing the presence of two aortic arches surrounding the trachea. In most cases, this form of congenital malformation becomes evident in childhood [27]. Dyspnea, occasionally confused with asthma, can occur when the trachea is significantly compressed [28]. Other forms of congenital abnormalities of the thoracic aorta include right aortic arch, aortic diverticula, cervical aortic arch, and pseudocoarctation of the aorta.

POSTERIOR MEDIASTINAL MASSES

CLASSIFICATION OF NEUROGENIC MEDIASTINAL TUMORS

Nerve sheath origin
  Benign
    Neurofibroma
    Neurilemoma
    (benign schwannoma)
    Granular cell tumor
    Melanotic schwannoma
  Malignant
    Malignant schwannoma
    (neurogenic sarcoma)

Autonomic ganglia origin
  Benign
    Ganglioneuroma
  Malignant
    Ganglioneuroblastoma
    Neuroblastoma

Paraganglionic origin
  Benign
    Pheochromocytoma
    Benign paraganglioma
    (chemodectoma)
  Malignant
    Malignant pheochromocytoma
    Malignant paraganglioma
    (chemodectoma)

Figure 11-22.

Classification of neurogenic mediastinal tumors. Neurogenic tumors of the mediastinum account for approximately 20% of all mediastinal tumors in adults and 40% in children. The clinical presentation and prognosis of these tumors varies with the age of the population. In children, most derive from autonomic ganglia, more than 50% are malignant, and most cause compressive or invasive manifestations. In adults, most are of nerve sheath origin, benign, and asymptomatic. Tumors of nerve sheath origin present as paraspinal masses [29]. Of these, neurilemomas present as solitary and well-encapsulated tumors. Occasionally, they can degenerate into malignant schwannomas [30]. Neurofibromas are most often multiple and seen in patients with von Recklinghausen's disease. Neoplasms derived from autonomic ganglia represent a continuum of various levels of differentiation. These range from the benign and mature ganglioneuroma to the malignant and most anaplastic neuroblastoma. In addition to local compressive or invasive manifestations, these tumors can secrete a variety of hormones that result in gastrointestinal and vasoactive systemic syndromes. Paraganglionic tumors can occur in all mediastinal compartments. They can be catecholamine-secreting pheochromocytomas or nonfunctioning paragangliomas. In addition to catecholamines, some paraganglionic tumors can secrete a variety of substances, eg, vasoactive intestinal peptide and parathyroid-like and corticotrophin hormones [31].

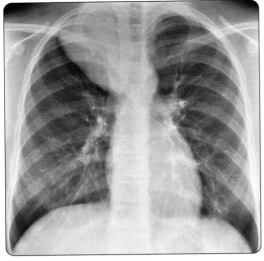

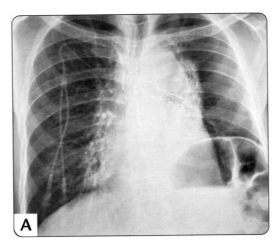

Figure 11-24.
Malignant paraganglioma. Paragangliomas or chemodectomas originate from chemoreceptor-autonomic tissue. Thus, most arise from and are located in the ascending or transverse portion of the aortic arch, where normal chemoreceptor aortic bodies are usually found [32]. **A,** Frontal radiograph shows an ill-defined mass that obliterates the aortopulmonary window and left hilum. The left hemidiaphragm is elevated because of paralysis, which indicates neoplastic phrenic nerve invasion. Endoluminal stents have been placed in the trachea and right main stem bronchus. **B,** Computed tomographic image shows extensive, necrotic mass at the level of the aortic arch with extension throughout all mediastinal spaces at this level. The tracheal lumen is severely reduced and displaced.

Figure 11-23.
Radiograph of a ganglioneuroma. This frontal radiograph shows a well-demarcated opacity that occupies the right upper paramediastinal area and apical lung field. These tumors are primarily a disease of young children. They are most often large and of paravertebral location. In contrast to tumors of nerve sheath origin, foraminal intraspinal extension is rare.

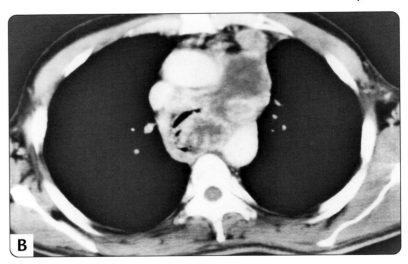

REFERENCES

1. Robie DK, Gursoy MH, Pokorny WJ: Mediastinal tumors: airway obstruction and management. *Semin Pediatr Surg* 1994, 3:259–266.

2. Laurent F, Latrabe V, Lecesne R, *et al.*: Mediastinal masses: diagnostic approach. *Eur Radiol* 1998, 8:1148–1159.

3. Ritter JH, Wick MR: Primary carcinomas of the thymus gland. *Semin Diagn Pathol* 1999, 16:18–31.

4. Klemm KM, Moran CA: Primary neuroendocrine carcinomas of the thymus. *Semin Diagn Pathol* 1999, 16:32–41.

5. McNeil TM, Chamberlain JM: Diagnostic anterior mediastinotomy. *Ann Thorac Surg* 1966, 2:532–539.

6. Pieterman RM, van Putten JW, Meuzelaar JJ, *et al.*: Preoperative staging of non-small-cell lung cancer with positron-emission tomography. *N Engl J Med* 2000, 343:254–261.

7. Shields TW, Lees WM, Fox RT: Anterior cardiophrenic angle tumors. *Q Bull Northwestern Univ Med Sch* 1962, 36:363–366.

8. Marx A, Muller-Hermelink HK: From basic immunobiology to the upcoming WHO-classification of tumors of the thymus. The Second Conference on Biological and Clinical Aspects of Thymic Epithelial Tumors and related recent developments. *Pathol Res Pract* 1999, 5:515–533.

9. International Germ Cell Cancer Collaborative Group: International Germ Cell Consensus Classification: a prognostic factor-based staging system for metastatic germ cell cancers. *J Clin Oncol* 1997, 15:594–603.

10. Weidner N: Germ-cell tumors of the mediastinum. *Semin Diagn Pathol* 1999, 16:42–50.

11. Collins KA, Geisinger KR, Wakely PR Jr, Olympio G, Silverman JF: Extragonadal germ cell tumors: a fine needle aspiration biopsy study. *Diagn Cytopathol* 1995, 12:223–229.

12. Moran CA, Suster S: Primary germ cell tumors of the mediastinum: I. Analysis of 322 cases with special emphasis on teratomatous lesions and a proposal for histopathologic classification and clinical staging. *Cancer* 1997, 80: 681–690.

13. Morice RC: Mediastinal disease. In *Pulmonary and Critical Care Medicine,* edn 3 (vol II). Edited by Bone RC. St Louis: Mosby-Year Book; 1995: 1–25.

14. Cohen BA, Needle MA: Primary mediastinal choriocarcinoma in a man. *Chest* 1975, 67:106–108.

15. King RM: Primary mediastinal tumors in children. *J Pediatr Surg* 1982; 17:512–520.

16. Mack TM: Sarcomas and other malignancies of soft tissue, retroperitoneum, peritoneum, pleura, heart, mediastinum, and spleen. *Cancer* 1995, 75:211–244.

17. Burt M, Ihde JK, Hajdu SI, *et al.*: Primary sarcomas of the mediastinum: results of therapy. *J Thorac Cardiovasc Surg* 1998, 115:671–680.

18. Moran CA, Suster S: Mediastinal hemangiomas: a study of 18 cases with emphasis on the spectrum of morphological features. *Hum Pathol* 1995, 26:416–421.

19. Pachter MR, Lattes R: Mesenchymal tumors of the mediastinum: III. Tumors of Lymph vascular origin. *Cancer* 1963, 16:108–111.

20. Pachter MR, Lattes R: Mesenchymal tumors of the mediastinum: I. Tumors of fibrous tissue, smooth muscle, and striated muscle. *Cancer* 1963, 16:23–26.

21. Jennette JC, Falk RJ: Small-vessel vasculitis. *N Engl J Med* 1997, 337:1512–1523.

22. Grosfeld JL, Skinner MA, Rescorla FJ, West KW, Scherer LR III: Mediastinal tumors in children: experience with 196 cases. *Ann Surg Oncol* 1994, 1:121–127.

23. Shepherd SF, A'Hern RP, Pinkerton CR: Childhood T-cell lymphoblastic lymphoma: does early resolution of mediastinal mass predict for final outcome? The United Kingdom Children's Cancer Study Group (UKCCSG). *Br J Cancer* 1995, 72:752–756.

24. Aisenberg AC: Primary large cell lymphoma of the mediastinum. *Semin Oncol* 1999, 26:251–258.

25. Rodriguez J, Pugh WC, Romaguera JE, Cabanillas F: Primary medistinal large cell lymphoma. *Hematol Oncol* 1994, 12:175–184.

26. Salyer DC, Salyer WR, Eggleston JC: Benign developmental cysts of the mediastinum. *Arch Pathol Lab Med* 1977, 101:136–139.

27. Kersting-Sommerhoff BA, Sechtem UP, Fisher MR, *et al.*: MR imaging of congenital anomalies of the aorta. *Am J Roentgenol* 1987, 149:9–13.

28. Bevelaqua F, Schicchi JS, Haas F, *et al.*: Aortic arch anomaly presenting as exercise-induced asthma. *Am Rev Respir Dis* 1989, 140:805–808.

29. Marchevsky AM: Mediastinal tumors of peripheral nervous system origin. *Semin Diagn Pathol* 1999, 16:65–78.

30. Fukai I, Masaoka A, Yamakawa Y, Niwa H, Eimoto T: Mediastinal malignant epithelioid schwannoma. *Chest* 1995, 108:574–575.

31. Trump DL, Livingston JL, Baylin SB: Watery diarrhea syndrome in an adult with ganglioneuroma-pheochromocytoma. *Cancer* 1977, 40:1526–1532.

32. Nwose P, Galbis JM, Okafor O, Torre W: Mediastinal paraganglioma: a case report. *Thorac Cardiovasc Surg* 1998, 46:376–379.

METASTASES TO THE LUNGS

Carlos A. Jimenez &
Rodolfo C. Morice

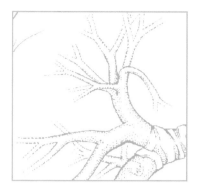
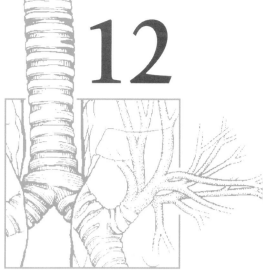
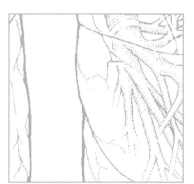

Secondary neoplastic involvement of the lungs is clinically important because of its prognostic implication and common occurrence. As a group, pulmonary metastases represent the most common form of pulmonary malignancies. Lung metastases are diagnosed in 30% to 40% of all patients with cancer [1]. Most patients lack significant respiratory symptoms at the time of initial presentation; the diagnosis is often made by abnormal findings on a chest roentgenogram. The primary site is often clinically apparent before symptoms of pulmonary involvement develop. Clinical manifestations such as dyspnea and cough are ominous signs of advanced disease. Wheezing, hemoptysis, hoarseness, and respiratory distress may also occur due to malignant invasion of tracheobronchial tree, mediastinal structures, or pleura. Despite the overall grave prognosis, surgical resection of pulmonary metastases and newer chemotherapy regimens have led to improved outcomes in selected patients.

Extrapulmonary tumors may reach the lungs by several routes: hematogenous, lymphogenous, direct invasion, and endobronchial dissemination. Of these, metastatic spread through the pulmonary or bronchial arteries is the most common. Retrograde extension into lymphatic channels from pulmonary and hilar lymph nodes can occur, but this presentation is most commonly the result of lymphatic penetration from hematogenous peripheral tumor implants. A combination of several mechanisms of tumor spread may also occur in a patient. The location of the primary tumor, access to the vascular system, and tumor or local tissue factors are important determinants for the development and progression of pulmonary metastases.

Patterns of Metastases

COMMON PATTERNS OF PULMONARY METASTASES

Micronodular	Coarse nodules	Cannon ball	Lymphatic/interstitial	Tumor emboli	Tracheobronchial
Thyroid	Head and neck	Sarcomas	Breast	Hepatoma	Renal
Renal	Gastric	Germ cell	Stomach	Renal	Thyroid
Choriocarcinoma	Gynecologic	Renal	Pancreas	Choriocarcinoma	Melanoma
Breast	Lymphoma	Colorectal	Prostate	Gastric	Colorectal
Bone sarcomas	Choriocarcinoma	Melanoma	Lymphoma	Atrial myxoma	Breast

Figure 12-1.

Common patterns of pulmonary metastases. Any neoplasm can invade the lungs, but some tumors have a particular predilection for pulmonary dissemination. Various appearances of pulmonary metastases on the chest radiograph may offer clues as to the origin of the primary neoplasm [2]. The primary neoplasms listed on this table are ranked based on their likelihood to produce a particular configuration of pulmonary metastases.

Pulmonary Nodules

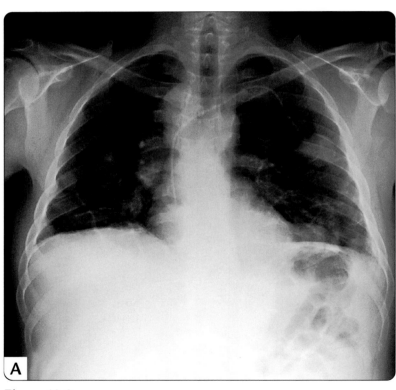

A

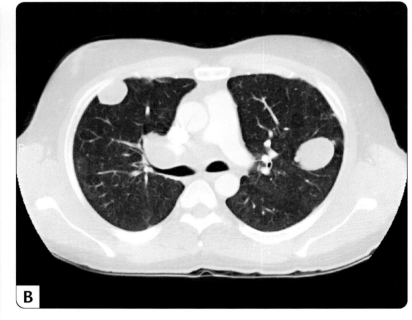

B

Figure 12-2.

A–D, Pulmonary metastases. Most commonly, pulmonary metastases present as multiple pulmonary nodules. The pattern of nodules ranges from diffuse micronodular (miliary) to large, well-defined single or multiple masses ("cannon ball"). The uniformity and small size of the pulmonary nodules suggests a simultaneous dissemination from a highly vascular tumor. Irregular size of nodular metastases indicates sequential embolic inoculations and different growth patterns. Nodules are preferentially located in the periphery and lower lung regions corresponding to zones of higher pulmonary blood flow. Characteristically, these nodules are smooth and well circumscribed. Hemorrhage in the periphery of the nodule or posttreatment changes may induce irregular margins. Calcification within the nodules can occur, which should not be misinterpreted as a manifestation of benign disease. This calcification can be found after chemotherapy or irradiation of tumors and in metastases from sarcomas of bone, cartilage, and synovial tissues. Calcium deposits can also occur in adenocarcinomas from ovary, thyroid, breast, and gastrointestinal tract. Computed tomography (CT) is the preferred method for evaluation of pulmonary metastases. High-resolution scanners are sensitive and can detect nodules as small as 2 to 3 mm in diameter. Posteroanterior (*panel A*) and CT roentgenograms (*panel B*) of a patient with metastatic germ cell tumor.

(Continued on next page)

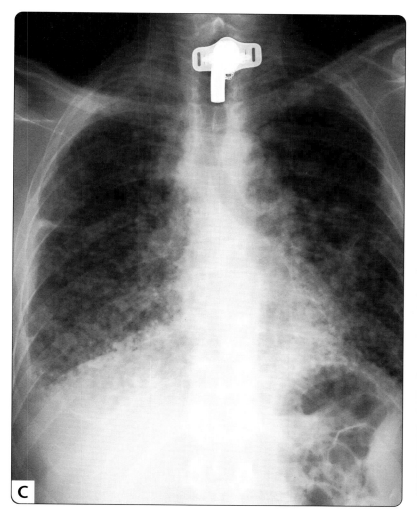

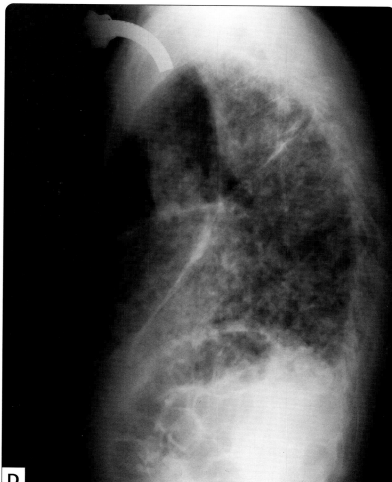

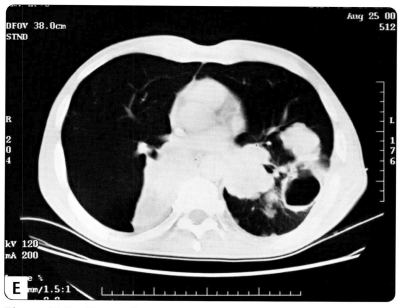

Figure 12-2. *(Continued)*
These images reveal multiple nodules of homogenous density ranging in size from 5 mm to 3 cm, distributed throughout both lungs. These lesions predominate in the bases and mid-lung zones. Hilar and mediastinal lymphadenopathy are also present. Posteroanterior (*panel C*) and lateral roentgenogram (*panel D*) of a 42-year-old man reveal widespread micronodular metastases from a papillary thyroid carcinoma. In some areas, the small nodules are well circumscribed. In other areas, they become coales cent and less defined. This pattern has been described as "snow storm." Note the presence of a metal tracheostomy cannula after radical neck surgery and a right pleural effusion. **E**, CT scan through the upper thorax shows large nodules from a metastatic adenoid cystic carcinoma of the parotid gland. One of the nodules is cavitated. Intranodular cavitation is most common in metastatic sarcomas and squamous cell carcinomas of the head and neck.

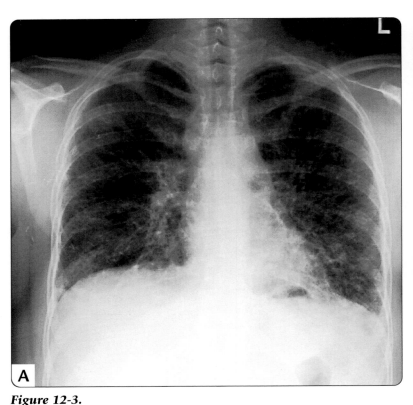

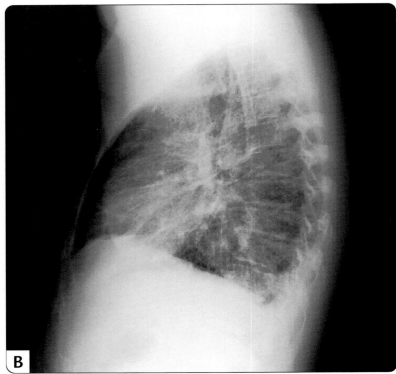

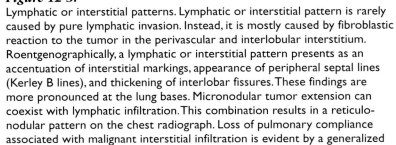

Figure 12-3.

Lymphatic or interstitial patterns. Lymphatic or interstitial pattern is rarely caused by pure lymphatic invasion. Instead, it is mostly caused by fibroblastic reaction to the tumor in the perivascular and interlobular interstitium. Roentgenographically, a lymphatic or interstitial pattern presents as an accentuation of interstitial markings, appearance of peripheral septal lines (Kerley B lines), and thickening of interlobar fissures. These findings are more pronounced at the lung bases. Micronodular tumor extension can coexist with lymphatic infiltration. This combination results in a reticulonodular pattern on the chest radiograph. Loss of pulmonary compliance associated with malignant interstitial infiltration is evident by a generalized reduction of lung volumes. Pleural effusion and mediastinal adenopathy are frequently present in association with a lymphatic pattern of pulmonary

metastases. The most common clinical manifestation of lymphangitic metastases is dyspnea of gradual onset. In some cases, cough and wheezing suggestive of airway disease may be the prominent symptoms. Posteroanterior (*panel A*) and lateral chest (*panel B*) roentgenograms reveal a bilateral, coarse linear, and reticular interstitial pattern. Well-formed Kerley B lines are also evident. There is bilateral enlargement of hilar lymph nodes. This 27-year-old woman with invasive ductal carcinoma of the breast had been treated with a modified radical right mastectomy and a prophylactic simple left mastectomy. She also received combined chemoradiation therapy. At the time the chest roentgenograms were obtained, the patient complained of a 1-month history of progressive dyspnea. Lymphatic spread of adenocarcinoma was confirmed by transbronchial lung biopsies.

TRACHEOBRONCHIAL METASTASES

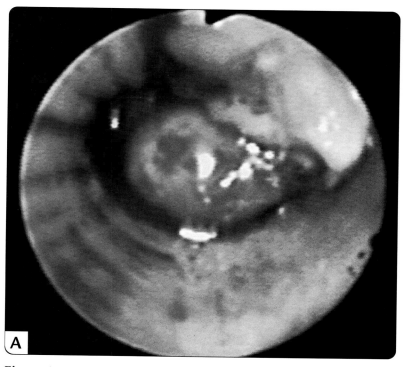

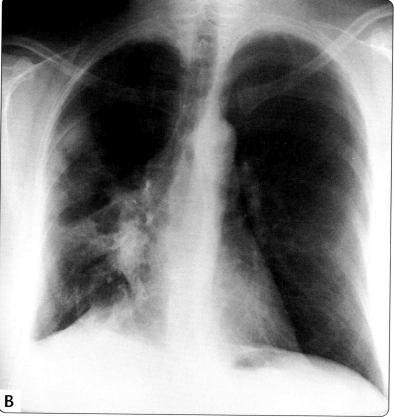

Figure 12-4.

Metastatic malignant invasion. Metastatic malignant invasion of the tracheal or bronchial wall is often the result of contiguous penetration from adjacent metastases to mediastinal lymph nodes or from submucosal lymphatic infiltration. Occasionally, tracheobronchial metastases can occur as isolated forms of endoluminal airway invasion in the absence of demonstrable pulmonary or mediastinal involvement. **A,** Bronchoscopic image of the left mainstem bronchus. It shows a friable, fungating mass that originates from the left upper lobe and extends into the left mainstem bronchus. This 59-year-old man with metastatic renal adenocarcinoma was diagnosed with dyspnea and hemoptysis. **B,** Computed tomographic scan of the left hilar area shows a very large mass with endobronchial extension, causing left upper lobe atelectasis.

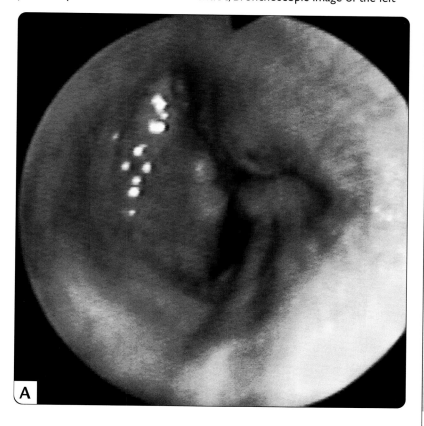

Figure 12-5.

A, Endobronchial photograph of the right bronchus intermedius of a 64-year-old woman with metastatic choriocarcinoma. Bronchoscopic findings indicate concentric submucosal and endobronchial malignant infiltration of the right bronchus intermedius and right middle lobe. **B,** Posteroanterior roentgenogram reveals middle lobe collapse and a right hilar mass. There are also adjacent parenchymal nodular densities due to focal pulmonary metastases.

TUMOR EMBOLI

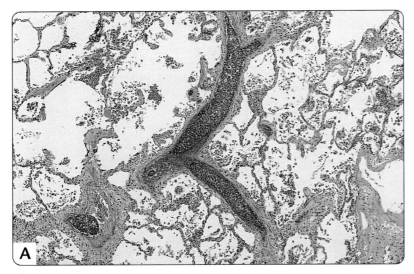

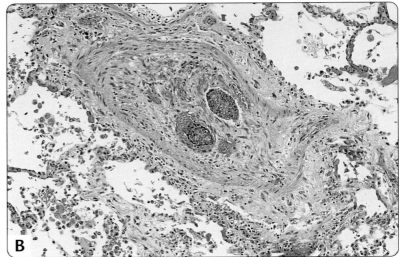

Figure 12-6.
Tumor emboli. Tumor emboli are common autopsy findings in patients with malignancies. Symptoms from this form of dissemination are usually absent. When present, clinical manifestations are similar to other forms of pulmonary thromboembolism: acute onset of dyspnea, hypoxemia, and cor pulmonale. In most cases, these tumors affect arterioles and small arteries. Tumor cells usually do not invade the vessel walls, but intimal fibrosis is often present. Occasionally, tumor emboli originating from primary neoplasms that invade the inferior vena cava, such as renal carcinomas and hepatomas, may be large. These can cause occlusion of the main pulmonary artery or its segmental branches resulting in sudden death. **A**, Low power view photomicrograph of an autopsy specimen from a patient with salivary gland carcinoma. Small arterial branches contain aggregates of metastatic carcinoma. **B**, Higher power microscopy of the same specimen. There is a complete occlusion of a small artery caused by plugs of carcinoma surrounded by organizing thrombus and intimal proliferation.

TREATMENT AND PROGNOSIS OF PULMONARY METASTASES

SELECTION OF PATIENTS FOR RESECTION OF PULMONARY METASTASES

Primary tumor is under control

Metastases can be resected completely

Absence of extrapulmonary metastases; if present, they can be completely resected

Adequate pulmonary function to allow resection

Effective systemic therapy is unavailable or has been administered before resection

Figure 12-7.
Selection of patients for resection of pulmonary metastases. Most pulmonary metastases in adults cannot be cured. With appropriate selection, surgical resection of lung metastases can lead to prolonged survival and quality of life [3]. In addition, metastasectomy with curative intent is an option in some types of cancers, such as germ cell tumors, neuroblastoma, and gestational trophoblastic neoplasms. Surgical resection is indicated when residual disease is present in the lung after systemic chemotherapy.

FACTORS ASSOCIATED WITH IMPROVED OUTCOME AFTER PULMONARY METASTASECTOMY

Complete resection
Unilateral involvement
Single metastasis
Smaller metastasis
Longer disease-free interval
Longer tumor-doubling time
Absence of lymph node involvement
Asymptomatic
Type of tumor
No recurrence after metastasectomy

Figure 12-8.

Factors associated with improved outcome after pulmonary metastasectomy. Complete resection of the entire tumor is the most important factor associated with long-term survival after metastasectomy. Other factors, listed in this figure, have shown variable significance as prognostic indicators. Patients with germ cell tumors have the best overall survival rate: 68% at 5 years and 63% at 10 years [4]. Disease-free interval refers to the time since the resection of the primary tumor to the time of diagnosis of lung metastases. Surgical approaches attempt to remove all disease with maximal preservation of viable lung parenchyma. Metastases are most often located in the periphery and can be excised with mechanical stapling, laser, or electrocautery. Bilateral metastases can be approached by median sternotomy, staged thoracotomies, or bilateral thoracosternotomy ("clamshell") incision). The role of video-assisted thoracoscopy (VATS) for treatment of metastatic disease has not been fully defined. Inability to palpate the lung during VATS may result in incomplete resection [5].

MANAGEMENT OF TRACHEOBRONCHIAL METASTASES

Indications	Therapies
Dyspnea related to tracheobronchial malignancy, not to systemic disease	Laser
	Argon plasma coagulation (APC)
Tracheobronchial obstruction with:	Electrocautery
Functional lung distal to obstruction, or	Stents
postobstructive pneumonia	Brachytherapy
	Balloon or mechanical dilation
	Photodynamic therapy
	Cryotherapy
	Gene therapy

Figure 12-9.

Management of tracheobronchial metastases. Neoplastic airway invasion is common among patients with metastatic malignancies. These patients may have symptoms related to tracheobronchial tumor extension such as dyspnea, bleeding, intractable cough, and postobstructive pneumonia. In selected cases, bronchoscopic interventions can prevent imminent death, offer clinical stability that will allow additional cancer treatment, or palliate symptoms. Proper patient selection for endobronchial therapy is crucial. For patients with hemoptysis, the bleeding source must be endobronchial and within the reach of the bronchoscope. Arterial embolization may be considered when the source of bleeding is extrabronchial. Obstructive airway lesions should be ablated to regain significant lung function or relieve postobstructive pneumonia. In the absence of postobstructive pneumonia, there will be no benefit from endobronchial therapy if the lung distal to the obstruction is nonfunctional. Patients selected for endobronchial therapies should have respiratory rather than systemic symptoms of widespread malignancy. Argon plasma coagulation is a form of noncontact electrocoagulation [6]. It offers the simplicity and low cost of an electrocoagulator with the noncontact approach of an Nd:YAG laser. Patients with diffuse, concentric malignant infiltration and with significant distortion of anatomic landmarks are best treated with endobronchial brachytherapy [7]. Similarly, obstructions caused by lesions that extrinsically compress the airway are best palliated with endoluminal stents and dilation.

PROGNOSTIC GROUPING OF PATIENTS WITH LUNG METASTASES

Group	Resectable	Disease-free interval, *mo*	No. of metastases	Median survival, *mo*
I	Yes	≥36	Single	61
II	Yes	≥36	Multiple	34
II	Yes	<36	Single	34
III	Yes	<36	Multiple	24
IV	No	—	—	14

Figure 12-10.

Prognostic grouping of patients with lung metastases. Three parameters of prognostic significance were included by the International Registry of Lung Metastasis: resectability, disease free interval (DFI), and number of metastases. DFI and number of metastases were independent risk factors in patients with resectable disease. Patients with germ cell and Wilms' tumors, which have the best prognosis, were not included in these groups. The median survival rate for all others was 33 months, with a 5-year survival of 34% and 10-year survival of 23%. According to the major tumor types, epithelial tumors (37% survival at 5 years and 21% at 10 years, median 40 months) and sarcomas (31% survival at 5 years and 26% at 10 years, median 29 months) behaved similarly. Melanomas had the worst prognosis (21% survival at 5 years and 14% at 10 years, median 19 months). Other studies have reported 5-year survival for single histologies of 27% to 49% for breast carcinoma, 39% to 53% for colorectal carcinoma, and 43% for head and neck malignancies [8]. (*Adapted from Pastorino et al. [4].*)

REFERENCES

1. Burt M: Pulmonary metastases. In *Fishman's Pulmonary Diseases and Disorders,* edn 3. Edited by Fishman AP, Elias JA, Fishman JA, *et al.* New York: McGraw-Hill, 1998:1851–1860.

2. Fraser RS, Müller NL, Colman N, Paré PD: Neoplastic secondary neoplasms. In *Fraser and Pare's Diagnosis of Diseases of the Chest,* edn 4. Edited by Fraser RS, Müller NL, Colman N, Paré. Philadelphia: WB Saunders; 1999:1381–1417.

3. Robert JH, Vala D, Sayegh Y, Spiliopoulos A: The surgical treatment of lung metastases: an update. *Crit Rev Oncol Hematol* 1998, 28:91–96.

4. Pastorino U, Buyse M, Friedel G, *et al.,* and the International Registry of Lung Metastases: Long-term results of lung metastasectomy: prognostic analysis based on 5206 cases. *J Thorac Cardiovasc Surg* 1997, 11:37–49.

5. Ferson P, Keenan RJ, Luketich JD: The role of video-assisted thoracic surgery in pulmonary mestases. *Chest Surg Clin North Am* 1998, 8:59–76.

6. Morice RC, Ece T, Ece F, Keus F: Endobronchial argon plasma coagulation for treatment of hemoptysis and neoplastic airway obstruction. *Chest* 2001, in press.

7. Kelly JF, Delclos ME, Morice RC, Huaringa A, Allen PK, Komaki R: High-dose-rate endobronchial brachytherapy effectively palliates symptoms due to airway tumors: the 10-year M. D. Anderson Cancer Center experience. *Int J Radiat Oncol Biol Phys* 2000, 48:697–702.

8. Downey RJ: Surgical treatment of pulmonary metastases. *Surg Oncol Clin North Am* 1999, 8:341–354.

LOWER RESPIRATORY TRACT INFECTIONS: ACUTE EXACERBATION OF CHRONIC BRONCHITIS

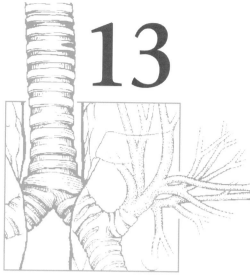
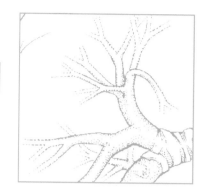
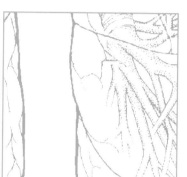

Antonio Anzueto &
G. Douglas Campbell, Jr

Acute exacerbation of chronic bronchitis (AECB) is a common cause of morbidity and mortality in the adult population. This is a complex condition that occurs in patients with underlying lung disease, especially with chronic obstructive pulmonary disease (COPD). The cost of AECB is very high, not only because of the economic impact, but also because of the increased morbidity and early mortality rate. In 1992, approximately 430,000 hospitalizations in the United States occurred with primary discharge diagnosis of COPD, making it the leading cause of hospitalization. In a prospective cohort of 1016 adults hospitalized with AECB who had hypercapnia, Connors et al. [2] found that only 25% of patients were alive and able to report a good, very good, or excellent quality of life 6 months after discharge. These investigators also found that the mortality rate after AECB was 11% during the initial hospitalization, 33% after 180 days, and 49% at 2 years.

SIGNIFICANCE OF COPD IN THE UNITED STATES

Number of diagnoses have increased by 41.5% since 1982

Affects 14 million people

    12.5 million with chronic bronchitis

    1.65 million with emphysema

Caused 85,544 deaths in 1991

    Fourth leading cause of death

    Increased 32% from 1979

Approximately $16 billion/y in direct and indirect costs

Figure 13-1.
COPD has been estimated to affect up to 25 million patients in the United States. COPD is a disease with world-wide distribution that has a high morbidity and mortality rate [1]. Patients with COPD suffer recurring episodes of exacerbations, which may be caused by infection, industrial pollutants, environmental allergies, and other factors.

SIGNS AND SYMPTOMS OF AECB

Symptoms	Patients, % Anthonisen et al. [3] (n = 173)	Ball et al. [5] (n = 471)
Increased dyspnea	90	45
Increased sputum production	69	77
Purulent sputum	60	66
Increased cough	82	NR
Fever	29	12
Average number of exacerbations	2.56/y	3/y

Figure 13-2.
The clinical presentation with acute exacerbation of AECB is variable. Anthonisen et al. [3] classified the severity of exacerbation based on three major signs: increase in dyspnea, increase in sputum production, and the presence of purulent sputum. Three levels of exacerbation were recognized. Type I is most severe; worsening dyspnea with increased sputum volume and purulence. Type II is less severe; any two of the previously mentioned symptoms. Type III is least severe; one of the symptoms associated with fever or upper respiratory tract infections. There is a wide variability in the presence of these symptoms in clinical trials. In a recent publication by Stockley et al. [4], the presence of purulent sputum suggests an infectious process and is associated with positive gram stain, positive culture, and many microorganisms isolated in the culture of the sputum sample. (*Adapted from* Anthonisen et al. [3] and Ball et al. [5].)

MOST FREQUENTLY ISOLATED PATHOGENS IN AECB

Study	Number of isolates	Total isolates accounted for, % S. pneumoniae	H. influenzae	M. catarrhalis
Basran, 1990	60	25.0	43.3	3.3
Aldons, 1991	53	15.0	70.0	13.0
Bachand, 1991	84	21.4	30.0	10.7
Lindsay, 1992	398	17.0	49.7	19.0
Chodosh, 1992	214	22.4	37.9	22.4
Ball, 1994	85	16.5	52.0	13.0
Anzueto, 1998	673	7.0	28.0	18.0
De Abate, 1998	647	7.0	47.0	10.0

Figure 13-3.
The presence of pathogenic bacteria in the sputum of patients with AECB suggests that microorganisms may play an important role in this condition. The predominant organisms have been identified as *H. influenzae*, *M. catarrhalis*, and *S. pneumoniae*. *M. pneumoniae*, and *C. pneumoniae* may be associated with 5% to 15% of the overall exacerbation, but the true incidence of these pathogens is not well known because of limitations in diagnosis [7–9]. (*Adapted from* Ball et al. [10], Anzueto et al. [11], and De Abate et al. [12].)

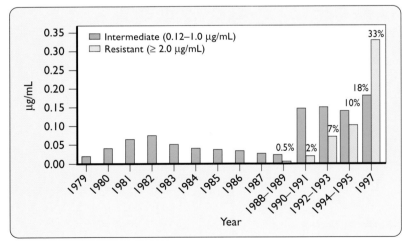

Figure 13-4.
Increasing prevalence of penicillin-resistant *S. pneumonia* in the United States (1979–1997). It has been estimated that 20% to 40% of *H. influenzae* and more than 75% of *M. catarrhalis* are beta-lactamase-producing organisms [13,14]. Another important feature to be taken into consideration is the emergence of the multidrug-resistant *S. pneumoniae*. Multidrug-resistant isolates of *S. pneumoniae* has progressively increased and reaches approximately 40% to 50% in the United States [15,16]. Half of these *S. pneumoniae* strains will exhibit high levels of resistance. Furthermore, resistance to other commonly used antibiotics to treat these conditions is also high in these isolates. (*Adapted from* Doern [14].)

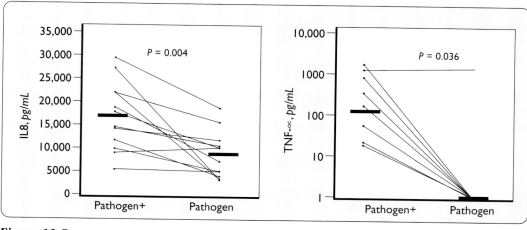

Figure 13-5.

Interleukin-8 (IL8) and TNF-alpha in AECB-paired samples. The role of infection has been controver-sial in patients with acute exacerbation of chronic bronchitis. Recent work by Manso *et al.* [17] and other investigators [8–20] using fiberoptic bronchoscopies to sample the lower airways of patients with COPD has demon-strated that potential respiratory bacterial pathogens are present in the airway in these patients up to 50% of the exacerbations. Several investigators have demonstrated that the pres-ence of pathogens in the airways is associated with a significant inflammatory response. Sethi *et al.* [21] demonstrated that neutrophil airway infiltration is greater during exacerbations asso-ciated with the isolation of bacteria than during exacerbations with negative sputum. These investigators have demonstrated an increase of inflammatory cytokines, primary tumor necrosis factor-alpha and IL8.

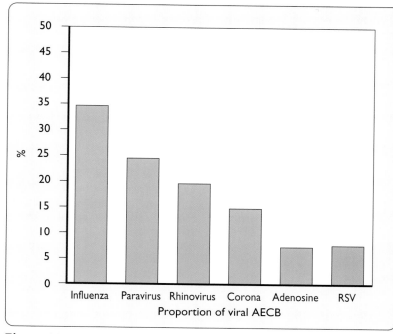

Figure 13-6.

Viral etiology of AECB. The role of viral infection in acute exacerbation of chronic bronchitis is controversial. Several investigators have reported a viral infection associated with AECB; this has been manifested mainly by an increase in antibody titers or culture of respiratory secretions [22]. Furthermore, patients infected with the influenza virus have a threefold increase in the bacteria infection later. Secondary bacterial infections have been reported after other viral infections including herpes virus and rhinovirus [22]. The relationship between the viral infection and the bacterial infection requires further investigation, but it is clear in some patients that a viral process will precede the presence of a bacterial infection. Viral infection is associated with 30% of AECB—there is a fourfold increase in antibody titer.

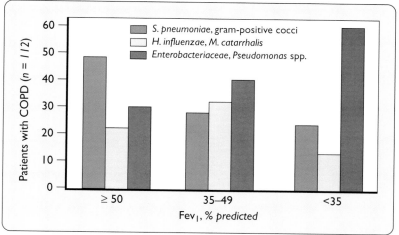

Figure 13-7.

Relationship between disease severity and respiratory pathogens. There have been several studies showing that patients with more severe obstruc-tive lung disease have a significantly higher prevalence of gram-negative organisms during an acute exacerbation [23,24]. Eller *et al.* [23] evaluated sputum cultures from 112 inpatients with AECB. Sixty-four percent of patients with an FEV₁ of 35% or less predicted versus only 30% of those with FEV₁ of 50% or more (*P* = 0.16) had evidence of gram negative organ-isms in the sputum. The most commonly isolated organisms included *Enterobacteriaceae* and *Pseudomonas*, *Proteus vulgaris*, *Serratia marcescens*, *Stenotrophomonas maltophilia*, and *Escherichia coli*. Miravitlles *et al.* [24] recently published a study with similar results that supports these findings. These investigators evaluated the relationship between FEV₁ and the isola-tion of diverse pathogens indisputable from 91 patients with COPD who had type I (severe) or type II (moderate) symptoms of AECB. Patients were separated into groups by FEV₁ (>50% or <50% of predicted). There were significantly more *H. influenzae* and *P. aeruginosa* in the group of FEV₁ of less than 50% of predicted (*P*=0.05). In contrast, there were significantly more potentially non-pathogenic microorganisms in the group with FEV₁ of 50% or greater (*P* < 0.5). These investigators also performed a multivaried logistic analysis and found that *H. influenzae* was cultured significantly more commonly on patients who were actively smoking (odds ratio [OR] 8.2; confidence interval [CI] 1.9–43) and whose FEV₁ was less than 50% of predicted (OR 6.85; CI 1.6-52). *P. aeruginosa* was also cultured significantly more frequently in those with poor lung function, FEV₁ less than 50% (OR 6.6; CI 1.2–124).

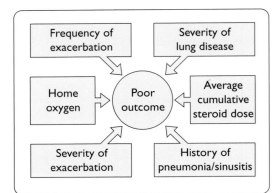

Figure 13-8.

AECB factors associated with poor treatment outcome. Because the morbidity and mortality for AECB are high, many investigators have attempted to describe clinical characteristics that could be used to stratify patients with AECB. The clinical parameters that are implicated as possible risk factors for treatment failure in AECB are as follow: 1) older age (>65 years), 2) severe underlying COPD (FEV₁ <35% of predicted), 3) frequent exacerbations (>4/y), 4) more severe symptoms at diagnosis (Anthonisen types I and II), 5) comorbidities (especially in cardiopulmonary disease, but also congestive heart failure, diabetes mellitus, chronic renal failure, chronic liver disease), and 6) prolonged history of COPD (>10 y) [25,26]. Recently, Dewan *et al.* [27] reported the study of 107 patients with 232 exacerbations over 2 years. The treatment failure rate of these exacerbations was 15%. The investigators noted that the patients who had more than four exacerbations during the 2-year period had more than a 100% failure rate. These investigators also described that the use of home oxygen and maintenance corticosteroid therapy was associated with a significant relapse rate. (*Adapted from* Dewan [27].)

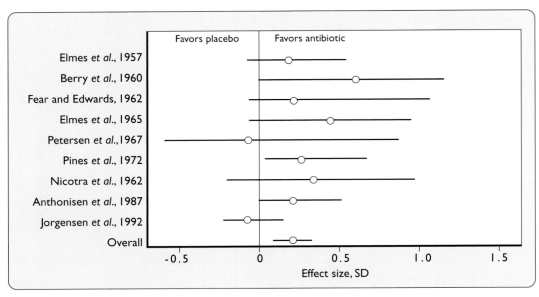

Figure 13-9.

Clinical improvement with antibiotics: meta-analysis of placebo-controlled clinical trials. One way to assess the efficacy of antibiotic therapy in the treatment of AECB is to evaluate clinical outcome. Saint *et al.* [28] reported the result of a meta-analysis of the role of antibiotics in the treatment of AECB. These investigators analyzed nine placebo-controlled, randomized studies published between 1957 and 1992 that were conducted in outpatient settings. The study showed statistically significant overall benefit for antibiotic-treated patients. Analysis of the studies that provided data on expiratory flow noted an improvement of 10.75 L/min in the antibiotic-treated group. The authors concluded that these antibiotic-associated improvements may be clinically significant, particularly in patients with low baseline peak flow rates and limited respiratory reserve. The classic study that has addressed the use of antibiotics in AECB was reported by Anthonisen *et al.* [3]. These investigators conducted a large-scale, placebo-controlled trial designed to determine the effectiveness of antibiotics in the treatment of AECB. In this study, 173 patients with chronic bronchitis were followed up for 3.5 years during which time they had 362 episodes of exacerbations. The patients were randomized to antibiotics or placebo in a double-blind, crossover fashion. Three oral antibiotics were used for 10 days (amoxicillin, trimethoprim sulfamethoxazole, and doxycycline). Approximately 40% of exacerbations were type I (severe), 40% were type II (moderate), and only 20% were type III (mild). Patients with the most severe exacerbations (type I) received a significant benefit from antibiotics, whereas there was no significant difference between antibiotics and placebo in patients who had only one of the defined symptoms (type III). Overall, the patients treated with antibiotics showed a more rapid improvement in peak flow, a greater percentage of clinical success, and a smaller percentage of clinical failure than those who received placebo. The length of illness decreased to 2 days shorter for the antibiotic-treated group. The major criticisms of this study were that no microbiology was performed and that all antibiotics were assumed to be equivalent. Allegra and Grassi [29] found significant benefits for the use of amoxicillin-clavulanate therapy compared with placebo in patients with severe disease. Patients who received these antibiotics had a higher success rate (86.4% vs 50.3% in the placebo group, P < 0.1) and fewer recurring exacerbations.

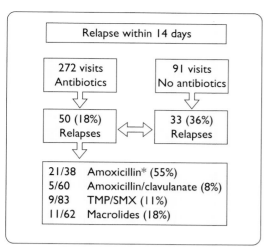

```
Relapse within 14 days

272 visits          91 visits
Antibiotics         No antibiotics

50 (18%)            33 (36%)
Relapses   <──>     Relapses

21/38   Amoxicillin* (55%)
5/60    Amoxicillin/clavulanate (8%)
9/83    TMP/SMX (11%)
11/62   Macrolides (18%)
```

Figure 13-10.

If antibiotics have an effect on the outcome of acute exacerbation of chronic bronchitis, the next step is to determine if there are differences within the antibiotics. Most of the recently published antibiotic clinical trials were designed to compare a new antibiotic with an established compound for the purpose of new registration

and licensing. Equivalency is the desired outcome of such trials; therefore, the agent chosen for comparison is considered unimportant. In addition, these trials frequently include patients with poorly defined severity (often without any obstructive lung disease) and acute illness of minor severity. The recent retrospective study of outpatients with documented COPD evaluated the risk factors for therapy failure at 14 days after an acute exacerbation [30]. The participating patients had a total of 362 exacerbations over an 18-month period. One group received antibiotics (270 visits) and the second group (92 visits) did not. Both groups had similar demographics and severity of underlying COPD. The patients' mean age was 67 ± 10 years, 100% of patients smoked more than 50 packs/year, and 45% were active smokers. Based on the American Thoracic Society COPD classification, 39% had mild disease, 47% had moderate disease, and 14% had severe disease. The majority (45%) with severe symptoms at diagnosis (Type I) received antibiotics versus 40% with mild symptoms. The overall relapse rate (defined as a return visit within 14 days with persistent or worsening symptoms) was 22%. In the multivariate analysis, the major risk factors for relapse was the lack of antibiotic therapy (32% vs 19%, P < 0.01 compared with the antibiotic-treated group). The type of antibiotic used was also an important variable associated with the 14-day treatment failure. Patients treated with amoxicillin had a 54% relapse rate with only 13% of other antibiotics (P < 0.1). Furthermore, treatment with amoxicillin resulted in higher incidence of failure, even when compared with those who did not receive antibiotics (P = 0.06). Other variables, such as COPD severity, types of exacerbations, prior or concomitant use of corticosteroids, and use of oxygen therapy were not significantly associated with the 14-day relapse. This study showed that the use of antibiotics was associated with a significantly lower rate of therapy failure. Furthermore, patients who received antibiotics and failed within 14 days had a significantly higher rate of hospital admission than those who did not receive antibiotics. These data emphasize that it is important to give antibiotics and that appropriate therapy is necessary. A likely explanation of this failure could be that the pathogens were resistant to amoxicillin. (*Adapted from* Adams et al. [30].)

DIFFERENCES IN CHARACTERISTICS BASED ON ANTIBIOTIC SELECTION

	First-line	Second line	Third line
Days of therapy	8.9 ± 3.3	8.3 ± 2.3	7.5 ± 2.5*
Weeks between AECB	17.1 ± 22	22.7 ± 30	34.3 ± 35.5*
14-day failure rate (n = 36)	19%	16%	7%*
Hospitalizations (% of total failures)	53%	14%	8%*
Cost per episode, $	942 ± 2173	563 ± 2296	542 ± 1946

Data are presented in percentages (as indicated) and otherwise in mean ± standard deviation.
*P ≤ 0.05 third line versus first line.

Figure 13-11.

Recently, Destache et al. [31] reported the impact of antibiotics selection, antimicrobial efficacy, and related cost in AECB. This study was a retrospective review of 60 outpatients from a pulmonary clinic at a teaching institution who were diagnosed with COPD and chronic bronchitis. The participating

patients had a total of 224 episodes of AECB requiring antibiotic treatment. The antibiotics were divided arbitrarily into three groups: first-line (amoxicillin, cotrimoxazole, and tetracycline), second-line (cephradine, cefuroxime, cefaclor, cefprozil), and third-line (amoxicillin-clavulanate, azithromycin, and ciprofloxacin) agents. The failure rates were significantly higher (at 14 days) for the first-line compared with the third-line agents (19% vs 7%, P < 0.5). When compared with the patients who received the first-line agents, those treated with third-line agents had a significantly longer time between exacerbations (34 weeks vs 17 weeks, P < 0.2), lower days of therapy (8.9 ± 3.3 days vs 17.5 ± 2.5, P < 0.02), and fewer hospitalizations (3 of 26 [12%] vs 18 of 26 [69%], P < 0.2). The initial pharmaceutical cost was higher in the third-line agents ($8.3 ± $8.7.6 vs $45.4 ± $11.11, P < 0.0001), the total cost of therapy was lower ($542 vs $942). (*Adapted from* Destache et al. [31].)

COST OF TREATMENT OF ACUTE EXACERBATION OF CHRONIC BRONCHITIS

Age group	Hospital costs (millions of dollars)	Outpatient costs (millions of dollars)
≥65 years	1141	34
<65 years	408	14
All ages	1549	48

Figure 13-12.

It has been suggested that many infections in AECB are noninvasive or are produced by a variety of agents and therefore will resolve spontaneously and do not require antibiotic therapy. Work

by Adams et al. [30] and Destache et al. [31] have shown that the failure of therapy is associated with a very high cost. Niederman et al. [32] recently reported that age older than 65 years and inpatient treatment are the major determinants contributing to the overall cost of AECB. The cost was estimated at $1.2 billion for the 27,540 inpatients 65 years of age or older versus $452 million for 5.8 million outpatients in the same group. The mean length of stay was longer and the in hospital mortality rate was significantly higher for those older than 65 years of age. (*Adapted from* Niederman et al. [32].)

CHARACTERISTICS OF AN IDEAL ANTIBIOTIC

Activity against most likely organisms: *S. pneumoniae, H. influenzae, M. catarrhalis*

Resistant to destruction by beta-lactamase

Good penetration into bronchial tissue

Well-tolerated/conveniently dosed

Cost effective

Figure 13-13.
The most important characteristics that should be taken into consideration when selecting antimicrobial agents for the treatment of AECB should include the following questions. 1) How active is the agent against the most common pathogens isolated in AECB and are there significant gaps in the coverage of these organisms? 2) Does the antibiotic cover the spectrum of causative organisms based on clinical risk factors? 3) How likely are the pathogens to be resistant to the agents chosen? 4) How much of the antibiotics can penetrate the sputum, bronchial mucosa, and epithelial lining fluid? 5) How difficult is it to take the medication and what are the major side effects? 6) How cost-effective is the agent? The ideal antibiotic should satisfy all of these criteria. However, because all antimicrobial agents possess only portions of these characteristics, the goal for the treating physician is to weigh the importance of these factors for each and every patient with AECB. After all these factors are considered, it is possible to make an informed choice about the most appropriate antibiotic to administer for a patient with acute symptoms of exacerbation.

PERCENTAGE OF SERUM CONCENTRATIONS OF ANTIBIOTIC ACHIEVED IN SPUTUM, EPITHELIAL LINING FLUID, AND BRONCHIAL MUCOSA

	Antibiotic	Sputum, %	ELF, %	Bronchial mucosa, %
Penicillin	Amoxicillin		13	40
	Piperacillin	10 to 14		27 to 40
Cephalosporins	Cefixime			34 to 36
	Ceftazidime	2 to 15		51
	Cefuroxime	14		
	Doxycycline	18		
Macrolides	Erythromycin	5	114	
	Azithromycin		3200 to 5700	
	Clarithromycin		3900 to 10,300	
Quinolones	Ciprofloxacin	200	140 to 185	240
	Gatifloxacin	125	170	170
	Sparfloxacin		1250	360
	Moxifloxacin		870	170
Aminoglycosides	Amikacin	10		
	Gentamicin	20		
	Tobramycin		50	

Figure 13-14.
Good antibiotic penetration into sputum, bronchial mucosa, and epithelial lining fluid (ELF) is the ideal. The goal of antimicrobial therapy is to deliver the appropriate drug to the specific site of infection. In AECB, the bacteria is found predominantly in the airway lumen, along the mucosa cell surfaces, and within the mucosa tissue. Various antibiotic classes exceeded markedly different degrees of penetration into the tissues and secretions of the respiratory tract. Although no studies show that the concentration of antibiotics at one particular intrapulmonary site is better than any other site, the concentration of antibiotics in sputum, bronchial mucosa, and macrophages are thought to be predictive of clinical efficacy. These antibiotics exhibited concentration-effect relationship in bacteria eradication [33,34]. (*Adapted from* Nix [33] and Fick and Stillwell [34].

PATIENT PROFILES FROM THE CANADIAN CHRONIC BRONCHITIS GUIDELINES

Acute bronchitis (group 1)
  Healthy people without previous respiratory problems
"Simple" chronic bronchitis (group 2)
  Age ≤ 65 years **and**
  Fewer than four exacerbations per year **and**
  Minimal or no impairment in pulmonary function **and**
  No comorbid conditions
"Complicated" chronic bronchitis (group 3)
  Age > years **or**
  Four or more exacerbations per year
"Complicated" chronic bronchitis with comorbid illness (group 4)
  Criteria for group 3 **and**
  Congestive heart failure **or**
  Diabetes **or**
  Chronic renal failure **or**
  Chronic liver disease **or**
  Other chronic disease

Figure 13-15.
Based on the concept for risk classification of patients by clinical parameters, a target approach for treatment of AECB has been proposed by the Canadian Bronchitis Symposium [35]. This group if investigators developed a classification for patients with symptoms of acute bronchitis by using the following factors: 1) number and severity of acute symptoms, 2) age, 3) severity of airflow obstruction (measured by FEV_1), 4) frequency of exacerbations, and 5) history of comorbid conditions. This symposium suggested that patients could be profiled adequately into different categories. Acute bronchitis (group 1) includes healthy people without previous respiratory problems. Simple AECB (group 2) includes patients younger than 65 years, those who have had four or fewer exacerbations per year, those with minimal or no impairment in lung function (by pulmonary function test), and those without any comorbid conditions. Complicated AECB (group 3) includes patients older than 65 years, those with FEV_1 of 50% or less of predicted value, or those with four or fewer exacerbations per year. Finally, complicated AECB with associated comorbid illness (group 4) includes patients with congestive heart failure, liver disease, diabetes, or chronic renal failure plus all the factors associated with the other groups. (*Adapted from* Balter *et al.* [35].)

OUR RECOMMENDATIONS FOR ANTIBIOTIC THERAPY

Category	Probable pathogens	Oral therapy
Acute bronchitis (group 1)	Viral	Symptomatic
"Simple" AECB (group 2)	*Haemophilus* spp. (*H. influenzae*) *M. catarrhalis, S. pneumoniae,* atypical organisms (possibly)	Doxycycline or newer macrolide (azithromycin/clarithromycin) or newer cephalosporins
"Complicated" AECB (groups 3 & 4)	As above, with the possible addition of *Pseudomonas* spp., *Enterobacteriaceae,* and other gram-negative organisms	Fluoroquinolones* Amoxicillin-clavulanate

If at risk for Pseudomonas infection, use ciprofloxacin.

Figure 13-16.
Based on the antibiotic characteristics and the patient profiles, we recommend that patients with acute bronchitis without underlying lung disease are more likely to have a viral pathogen and they should not receive antibiotic therapy. In these patients, the treatment of the condition should be the use of the congestiveness, antipyretics, hydration, and observation. If the patient's symptoms do not improve or if they persist for more than 7 to 10 days, the presence of atypical microorganisms, mainly mycoplasma, is likely and should be treated appropriately. In patients with simple acute exacerbation of chronic bronchitis, the core organisms (*H. influenzae, M. catarrhalis*, and *S. pneumoniae*) are more likely to be present and also likely not to be resistant to common antibiotics. In these patients, we recommend the use of new generation macrolides and doxycycline. The new fluoroquinolones should be used if the viruses are resistant pathogens. In patients who have more complicated exacerbations, it is more likely that the pathogens will be resistant to standard antibiotics, therefore the new fluoroquinolones or amoxicillin-clavulanate should be the first-line therapy. In patients who have bronchiectasis or who are at risk for infectious *P. aeruginosa*, the only available oral therapy is ciprofloxacin. (*Adapted from* Balter *et al.* [35].)

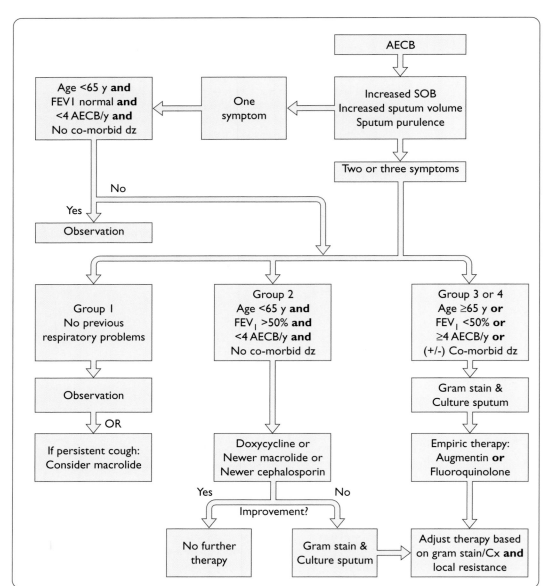

THERAPEUTIC STRATEGIES FOR AECB

Agents	Comments
Corticosteroids	Improves flow rates
Ipratropium	Bronchodilator effects
Beta-agonists	Effects may be additive to ipratropium
Albuterol	Decreased bacterial burden
Metaproterenol	
Salmeterol	
Antibiotics	May improve flow rates
	May decrease length of hospital stay

Figure 13-18.
Antibiotic therapy is part of the different treatment modalities in patients with AECB. The use of parenteral corticosteroids is not defined clearly. A recent randomized, double-blind, placebo-controlled trial with the use of systemic corticosteroids during acute exacerbation [36] suggests that if corticosteroids are going to be administered, they should be given for a short period of time. Short-acting beta$_2$-agonist is another important therapy in this patient population. Recent reports have raised the possibility that the overuse of short-acting beta$_2$-agonists can be associated with significant morbidity and cardiovascular-related mortality rates. If beta$_2$-agonists are going to be used, our recommendation is that they be used by MDI with spacer every 2 to 4 hours and not as a continuing nebulization. (*Adapted from* the American Thoracic Society [1].)

PREVENTION OF RESPIRATORY TRACT INFECTIONS

Cessation of smoking [37]

Influenza immunization [38]

Pneumococcal immunization

Figure 13-19.

Preventive therapy should be the mainstem in the treatment of patients with COPD. Aggressive smoking cessation should be emphasized in all the patients who are active smokers. Smoking cessation is the only therapy that has been shown to be associated with a decrease in the reduction in spirometry. Yearly influenza immunizations have been demonstrated to have a significant impact on the incidence of viral infections and the overall mortality rate. The role of pneumococcal administration remains controversial; however, in patients with significant COPD, pneumococcal vaccine has been shown to be composed of the most frequent isotypes that are associated with highly resistant strains. Therefore, all patients with COPD should have pneumococcal immunizations.

REFERENCES

1. American Thoracic Society: Standards for the diagnosis and care of patients with chronic obstructive pulmonary disease. *Am J Respir Crit Care Med* 1995, 152:S77–S121.

2. Conners AF, Dawson NV, Thomas C: Outcomes following acute exacerbations of severe chronic obstructive lung disease. The SUPPORT Investigators (Study to Understand Prognosis and Preferences for Outcome and Risk of Treatment). *Am J Respir Crit Care Med* 1996, 154:959–967.

3. Anthonisen NR, Manfreda J, Warren CP, et al.: Antibiotic therapy in acute exacerbation of chronic obstructive pulmonary disease. *Ann Intern Med* 1987, 106:196–204.

4. Stockley R, O'Brien C, Pye A, Hill S: Relationship of sputum color to nature and outpatient management of acute exacerbations of COPD. *Chest* 2000, 117:1638–1645.

5. Ball P, Tillotson G, Wilson R: Chemotherapy for chronic bronchitis controversies. *Presse Med* 1995, 24:189–194.

6. Ball P: Epidemiology and treatment of chronic bronchitis and its exacerbations. *Chest* 1995, 108(suppl 2):43S–52S.

7. Chodosh S: Bronchitis and asthma. In *Infectious Disease*. Edited by Gorbach SL, Barlett JG, Blacklow NR. Philadelphia: WB Saunders; 1992:476–485.

8. Bachard RT J: Comparative study of clarithromycin and ampicillin in the treatment of patients with acute bacterial exacerbation of chronic bronchitis. *J Antimicrob Chemother* 1991, 27:91–100.

9. Lindsay G, Scorer HJ, Carniage CM: Safety and efficacy of temafloxacin versus ciprofloxacin in lower respiratory tract infections: a randomized, double-blind trial. *J Antimicrob Chemother* 1992, 30:89–100.

10. Ball P: Efficacy and safety of cefprozil versus other beta-lactam antibiotics in the treatment of lower respiratory tract infections. *Eur J Microbiol Infect Dis* 1994, 13:851–856.

11. Anzueto A, Niederman MS, Tillotson G, et al.: Etiology, susceptibility and treatment of acute bacterial exacerbations for complicated chronic bronchitis in the primary care setting: ciprofloxacin 750 mg b.i.d. versus clarithromycin 500 mg b.i.d. *Clin Ther* 1998, 20:885–890.

12. De Abate AC, Henry D: Sparfloxacin vs ofloxacin in the treatment of acute bacterial exacerbations of chronic bronchitis: a multicenter, double-blind, randomized, comparative study. *Chest* 1998, 114:120–130.

13. De Groot R, Dzoljic-Danilovic G, van Klingeren B, et al.: Antibiotic resistance in *Haemophilus influenzae*: mechanisms, clinical importance, and consequences of therapy. *Eur J Pediatr* 1991, 150:534–546.

14. Doern GV, Jones RN, Pfaller A, et al.: *Haemophilus influenzae* and *Moraxella catarrhalis* from patients with community-acquired respiratory tract infections: antimicrobial susceptibility patterns from the SENTRY antimicrobial surveillance program (United States and Canada, 1997). *Antimicrob Agents Chemother* 1999, 43:385–389.

15. Doern GV, Brueggemann AB, Huynh H, et al.: Antimicrobial resistance with Streptococcus pneumoniae in the United States, 1997–98. *Emerg Infect Dis* 1999, 5:757–765.

16. Gotfried MG, Neuhauser MM, Garey KW, et al.: In vitro Streptococcus pneumoniae (SP) resistance: correlation with outcomes in patients with respiratory infections. *J Antimicrob Chemother* 1999, 44:83.

17. Mansó JR, Rosell A, Manterola J, et al.: Bacterial infection in chronic obstructive pulmonary disease. Study of stable and exacerbated outpatients using the protected specimen brush. *Am J Respir Crit Care Med* 1995, 152:1316–1320.

18. Fagon JY, Chastre J, Trouillet JL, et al.: Characterization of distal bronchial microflora during acute exacerbation of chronic bronchitis. *Am Rev Respir Dis* 1990, 142:1004–1008.

19. Martinez JA, Rodriguez E, Bastida T, et al.: Quantitative study of the bronchial bacterial flora in acute exacerbations of chronic bronchitis. *Chest* 1994, 105:976.

20. Soler N, Torres A, Ewig S, et al.: Bronchial microbial patterns in severe exacerbations of chronic obstructive pulmonary disease (COPD) requiring mechanical ventilation. *Am J Respir Crit Care Med* 1998, 157:1498–1505.

21. Sethi S, Muscarella K: Airway inflammation and etiology of acute exacerbations of chronic bronchitis. *Chest* 118:1557-1565, 2000.

22. Hogg JC: Chronic bronchitis: the role of viruses. *Semin Respir Infect* 2000, 15:32–40.

23. Eller J, Ede A, Schaberg T, et al.: Infective exacerbations of chronic bronchitis. Relation between bacteriologic etiology and lung function. *Chest* 1998, 13:1542–1548.

24. Miravitlles M, Espinosa C, Fernandez-Laso E, et al.: Relationship between bacterial flora in sputum and functional impairment in patients with acute exacerbations of COPD. *Chest* 1999, 116:40–46.

25. Murata GH, Gorby MS, Kapsner CO, et al.: A multivariate model for the prediction of relapse after outpatient treatment of decompensated chronic obstructive pulmonary disease. *Arch Intern Med* 1992, 152:73–77.

26. Ball P, Harris JM, Lowson D, et al.: Acute infective exacerbations of chronic bronchitis. *Q J Med* 1995, 88:61–68.

27. Dewan NA, Rafique S, Kanwar B, et al.: Acute exacerbation of COPD: factors associated with poor treatment outcome. *Chest* 2000, 117:662–671.

28. Saint S, Bent S, Vittinghoff E, et al.: Antibiotics in chronic obstructive pulmonary disease exacerbations: a meta-analysis. *JAMA* 1995, 273:957–960.

29. Allegra L, Grassi C: Ruolo degli antibiotici nel trattamento delle riacutizza della bronchite cronica. *Ital J Chest Dis* 1991, 45:138–148.

30. Adams S, Melo J, Anzueto A: Effect of antibiotics on the recurrence rates on chronic obstructive pulmonary disease exacerbations. *Chest* 2000, 117:1345–1352.

31. Destache CJ, Dewan N, O'Donohue WJ, et al.: Clinical and economic considerations in the treatment of acute exacerbations of chronic bronchitis. *J Antimicrob Chemother* 1999, 43:107–113.

32. Niederman MS, McCombs JS, Unger AN, et al.: Treatment cost of acute exacerbations of chronic bronchitis. *Clin Ther* 1999, 21:576–592.

33. Nix DE: Intrapulmonary concentrations of antimicrobial agents. *Infect Dis Clin North Am* 1998, 12:631–646.

34. Fick RB, Stillwell PC: Controversies in the management of pulmonary disease due to cystic fibrosis. *Chest* 1989, 95:1319–1327.

35. Balter MS, Hyland RH, Low DE, et al.: Recommendations on the management of chronic bronchitis: a practical guide for Canadian physicians. *Can Med Assoc J* 1994, 151:5–23.

36. Niewoehner DE: Effect of systemic glucocorticoids on exacerbation of chronic obstructive pulmonary disease. *N Engl J Med* 2000, 340:1941–1947.

37. Anthonisen NR: Effects of smoking intervention and the use of inhaled anticholinergic bronchodilator on the rate of decline of FEV1. *JAMA* 1994, 272:1497–1505.

38. Centers for Disease Control and Prevention: Prevention and control of influenza: recommendations of the advisory committee on immunization practices. *MMWR* 1995, 44(No. RR-3):1–22.

NOSOCOMIAL INFECTIONS

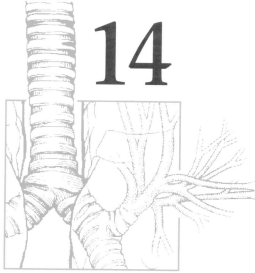
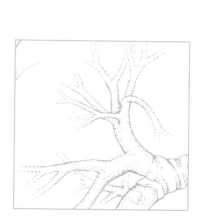
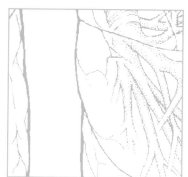

David W. Hines

Nosocomial infections are established by hospital pathogens 48 to 72 hours after admission. These infections are becoming increasingly difficult to treat because the organisms in the hospital are developing resistance to antibiotics faster than new ones can be developed. Strains of bacteria, fungi, mycobacteria, and viruses resistant to all known therapies are becoming more common. Because they can be transported through hospitals quickly on the surfaces of inanimate objects and on the hands of health care workers, multiresistant organisms are usually associated with a high mortality rate. Hospital-acquired infections can involve every organ system. Some infections are unavoidable due to underlying diseases and host factors. Other infections are preventable if standard antiseptic procedures (especially handwashing) and isolation procedures are used, injudicious use of antibiotics are avoided, and meticulous attention is paid to protocols for the insertion of indwelling lines and catheters. Hospital physicians should familiarize themselves with antibiotic resistance patterns and the antibiotic formulary and treatment guidelines established for their institutions.

URINARY TRACT INFECTIONS

EPIDEMIOLOGY OF URINARY TRACT INFECTIONS

33 million patients are admitted to hospitals in the United States yearly

3–6 million patients have indwelling urinary catheters

900,000 episodes of nosocomial UTIs will occur

35,000 bacteremias are from nosocomial UTIs

4500 deaths are attributable to nosocomial UTIs

85% of nosocomial UTIs are related to indwelling catheters

10%–15% of nosocomial UTIs are from urologic procedures

UTIs—urinary tract infections.

Figure 14-1.
Epidemiology of urinary tract infections. Nosocomial urinary tract infections account for 40% of all hospital-acquired infections and for excess charges of $500 million every year [1]. Most of these infections are catheter-related and therefore potentially avoidable.

NORMAL HOST DEFENSE MECHANISMS AGAINST URINARY TRACT INFECTIONS

Defense	Mechanism
Urethra	Maintains distance between exogenous organisms and bladder
Urination	Clears 99.9% of the bacteria that ascend into the bladder
Tamm-Horsfall protein and oligosaccharides	Bind bacteria; aid in their elimination
Glycosaminoglycan	Lines bladder epithelium; helps prevent attachment to underlying cells
Inflammatory response	Polymorphonuclear cells ingest microbes; exfoliation moves infected cells into the urine to be eliminated

Figure 14-2.

Normal host defense mechanisms against urinary tract infections. Numerous defense mechanisms protect us from urinary tract infections; indwelling catheters interfere with many of them. Catheters may damage the urethral epithelium, provide a direct route for bacteria to ascend into the bladder, and become a nidus for these organisms, which, despite antibiotic therapy, can never be cleared. Within 30 days, all patients with catheters have bacteriuria. Glycocalyx (biofilm) coating the catheters may cover and protect these bacteria, which then adhere to the catheter surface.

RISK FACTORS FOR NOSOCOMIAL URINARY TRACT INFECTIONS

Increased duration of indwelling catheter
Female gender
Diabetes mellitus
Renal insufficiency
Older age
Severity of underlying illness
Improper insertion or care of indwelling catheter

Figure 14-3.

Risk factors for nosocomial urinary tract infections. Host-related risk factors for nosocomial urinary tract infections include diabetes, renal insufficiency, older age, female gender, and severity of underlying illness. Factors over which there is more control include duration of indwelling catheters and their proper care.

ORGANISMS ISOLATED FROM CATHETER-INDUCED BACTERIURIA

	Catheterization, n (%)	
Organism	Short-term (incidence)	Long-term (weekly prevalence)
Providencia stuartii	—	384 (24)
Proteus spp	8 (6)	232 (15)
Escherichia coli	33 (24)	228 (14)
Pseudomonas aeruginosa	12 (9)	188 (12)
Enterococcus spp	9 (7)	179 (11)
Morganella morganii	—	118 (7)
Klebsiella spp	11 (8)	68 (4)
Coagulase-negative staphylococci	11 (8)	53 (3)
Other gram-negative bacilli	10 (7)	93 (6)
Other gram-positive bacteria	6 (4)	56 (4)
Yeast	35 (26)	—
Total	**135 (99)**	**1599 (100)**

Figure 14-4.

Organisms isolated from catheter-induced bacteriuria. Short-term catheters are more likely than long-term catheters to be associated with *Escherichia coli*, coagulase-negative staphylococci, and yeast. Long-term catheters are more often colonized and infected with *Pseudomonas* species and various members of the Enterobacteriaceae group [1]. Asymptomatic bacteriuria in the absence of significant pyuria should be left untreated unless the patient is about to undergo a urologic procedure. (*Adapted from* Warren [1].)

COMPLICATIONS OF BACTERIURIA FROM INDWELLING URINARY CATHETERS

Acute	Chronic
Fever	Nephrolithiasis
Pyelonephritis	Chronic pyelonephritis
Bacteremia	Interstitial nephritis
Death	Renal failure
	Periurinary trauma/infection
	Bladder cancer

Figure 14-5.
Complications of bacteriuria from indwelling urinary catheters. Most episodes of bacteriuria associated with short-term catheters are asymptomatic, and less than 5% become bacteremic. Long-term catheters are more likely to become obstructed and infected and are associated with renal stones, renal insufficiency, and bladder infections [1].

PREVENTION OF URINARY TRACT INFECTIONS IN THE HOSPITAL

Use a closed sterile drainage system with aseptic care

Use proper handwashing techniques

Reduce the number of days the catheter remains in place, when possible

Avoid prophylactic antibiotic therapy

Consider other methods of antiseptic care, such as condom catheters, intermittent catheterization, suprapubic catheters, and intraurethral catheters (for men with prostatic obstruction)

Figure 14-6.
Prevention of urinary tract infections in the hospital. The most important interventions for preventing nosocomial catheter-related urinary tract infections are a closed system, removing the catheter as soon as possible, and strict compliance with handwashing and generally accepted infection control practices.

CATHETER-RELATED INFECTIONS

DEFINITIONS OF CATHETER-RELATED INFECTIONS

Colonized catheter

Growth of >15 CFUs (semiquantitative culture) or >10^3 CFUs (quantitative culture) from a proximal or distal catheter segment in the absence of accompanying symptoms

Exit-site infection

Erythema tenderness, and induration or purulence within 2 cm of the exit site of the catheter

Pocket infection

Erythema and necrosis of the skin over the reservoir of a totally implantable device, or purulent exudate in the subcutaneous pocket containing the reservoir

Tunnel infection

Erythema, tenderness, and induration in the tissues overlying the catheter and >2 cm from the exit site

CR-BSI

Isolation of the same organism from a semiquantitative or quantitative culture of a catheter segment and from the blood of a patient with accompanying clinical symptoms of BSI and no other apparent source of infection

In the absence of laboratory confirmation, defervescence after an implicated catheter is removed from a patient with BSI may be considered indirect evidence of CR-BSI

Infusate-related BSI

Isolation of the same organism from the infusate and from separate percutaneous blood cultures, with no other identifiable source of infection

BSI—bloodstream infection; CFUs—colony-forming units; CR-BSI—catheter-related bloodstream infection.

Figure 14-7.
Definitions of catheter-related infections. An estimated 200,000 nosocomial bloodstream infections develop every year in the United States, and most are related to an intravascular device. Bloodstream infections are associated with increased mortality (10% to 20%) and morbidity rates, prolonged hospitalization, and increased medical costs. Complications include septic thrombophlebitis, endocarditis, and metastatic infections to joints, eyes, and bones [2].

FACTORS ASSOCIATED WITH INFUSION-RELATED PHLEBITIS AND INFECTION AMONG PATIENTS WITH CATHETERS

Peripheral catheters	Central catheters
Catheter material and size	Number of lumens (multiple > single)
Site of catheter	Site (subclavian < intrajugular < femoral)
Experience of personnel	Experience of personnel
Duration of catheter	Duration of catheter
Composition of infusate	Presence of infection elsewhere
Frequency of dressing changes	Bacteremia
Skin preparation	Type of dressing
Host factors	Host factors
Emergency room insertion	

Figure 14-8.
Factors associated with infusion-related phlebitis and infection among patients with catheters. Between January 1990 and April 1995, catheter-related bloodstream infections (per 1000 central catheter days) reported by National Nosocomial Infection Surveillance hospitals ranged from 4.9 in medical intensive care units to 15.6 in burn units. How the patients become infected is always debatable. Important predisposing factors for these infections include the number of catheterized lumens, how often they are accessed, where the catheters are placed, and how long they remain in place. Some portals of entry are illustrated in Figure 14-9 [2].

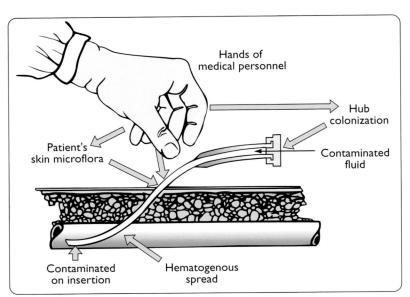

Figure 14-9.
Potential sources for contamination of intravascular devices. Intravascular catheters can become colonized or infected with a variety of organisms from various sites, including the normal flora of the skin, pathogens introduced on the hands of health care workers, and—less likely—contaminated devices and infusates.

MICROBIOLOGY OF CATHETER-RELATED BLOODSTREAM INFECTIONS

Coagulase-negative staphylococci account for 28% of all bloodstream infections

Staphylococcus aureus is the next most common pathogen

Enterococci, especially vancomycin-resistant strains, are emerging as important pathogens

Candida spp, especially *Candida albicans*, have increased almost fivefold from 1980 (1/10,000 discharges) to 1990 (4.9/10,000 discharges)

Gram-negative rods (*eg, Klebsiella, Enterobacter, Citrobacter,* and *Serratia* spp), common causes of bloodstream infections before 1980, are mainly associated with pressure-monitoring systems and contaminated intravenous fluids

Figure 14-10.
Microbiology of catheter-related bloodstream infections. The past two decades have witnessed the emergence of gram-positive organisms and fungi as the most important pathogens of catheter-related bloodstream infections. Reasons for their dominance include the increasing use of indwelling catheters, increasing survival of very low birthweight infants, and recognition of coagulase-negative *Staphylococcus* species as a pathogen. Vancomycin-resistant enterococci are reaching epidemic proportions at many hospitals, presumably due to antibiotic pressures (cephalosporins and vancomycin), gastrointestinal colonization with vancomycin-resistant enterococci, prolonged hospitalizations, and severe illness [3,4]. Other pathogens are listed in the figure.

STRATEGIES FOR PREVENTING CATHETER-RELATED BLOODSTREAM INFECTIONS

Use proper handwashing and antiseptic techniques

Choose sites appropriate for catheter insertion

Use barrier precautions while inserting catheters

Select catheters carefully (*eg*, Teflon/polyurethane catheters are associated with fewer infections than polyvinyl chloride/polyethylene catheters)

Replace peripheral lines every 48–72 h

Use silver-impregnated cuffs with temporary central lines

Establish infusion therapy teams or designate experienced staff for catheterization procedures

Factors that have *not* been shown conclusively to reduce the risk for catheter-related infections include:

Topical antibiotic ointments

In-line membrane filters

Dressing materials (transparent semipermeable vs gauze)

Frequent changing (<48 h) of intravenous set-ups

Figure 14-11.
Strategies for preventing catheter-related bloodstream infections. Most, if not all, foreign bodies invading the bloodstream will eventually become infected, even when the patient is given meticulous care. A few strategies that will delay the inevitable are listed in the figure.

NOSOCOMIAL GASTROINTESTINAL DISEASE

INFECTIONS CAUSED BY *CLOSTRIDIUM DIFFICILE*

Characteristics/parameters	Finding in *C. difficile* disease
Epidemiology	Found in 3% of healthy adults and ≥10% of hospitalized adults
	A spore-forming organism that may persist in the environment for months [5]
Presenting symptoms/findings	Crampy abdominal pain and fever; often a history of using antibiotics or stool softeners, or a history of procedures
	Some patients have peritonitis symptoms without diarrhea
Diagnosis	Culture of organism, cytotoxin assay, enzyme immunoassay
Treatment	Metronidazole, 500 mg orally 3×/d for 7–10 d, or vancomycin, 125 mg orally 4×/d for 7–10 d
Outcome	~10%–20% of patients relapse
Approach to relapse	Re-treat

Figure 14-12.
Infections caused by *Clostridium difficile*. The many causes of diarrhea in hospitalized patients include noninfectious entities such as drugs, inflammatory bowel disease, malabsorption syndromes, endocrine disorders, malignancies, and mechanical bowel problems. Of all the infectious causes of diarrhea, *C. difficile* is the most common, followed by rotavirus, *Salmonella* species, and foodborne staphylococcal disease. *C. difficile* is so common that the initial evaluation of diarrhea in the hospitalized patient should be limited to tests for this pathogen, unless the patient is immunocompromised or a large outbreak of another type of infection has occurred [5]. Severe cases of diarrhea may mimic appendicitis or accompany toxic megacolon. Colectomy may be necessary in particularly severe cases [6]. Nearly all cases improve with treatment. If symptoms persist, tests for other pathogens should be done. Oral therapy is more effective than parenteral therapy and is the preferred route of administration. Relapse is common and does not suggest drug resistance or an abnormal host. Metronidazole is the preferred first-line agent over vancomycin (which may lead to increased colonization with vancomycin-resistant enterococci).

THE COMPROMISED HOST

Cause of host immunodeficiency	Pathogen(s)/ underlying disorder
Transplantation	Cytomegalovirus
AIDS	*Cryptosporidium* spp, Microsporidia, *Clostridium difficile*, *Mycobacterium avium* complex, *Salmonella* spp
Neutropenia	Typhlitis
Wound colonization/ infection	Toxic shock syndrome

Figure 14-13.
The pathogens most often associated with specific host immune defects. Although these infections may be community acquired, symptoms may manifest during hospitalization for other illnesses. An acute bloody diarrhea may develop several months after a bone marrow transplantation, suggesting cytomegalovirus infection. The diagnosis is made endoscopically with biopsy. Gastrointestinal symptoms are common in patients with AIDS. The pathogens listed in the figure are among many that may cause symptoms in this setting. When symptoms are moderate to severe, a stool examination should be performed that includes routine bacterial culture, ova and parasite examination, *Clostridium difficile* testing, and special stains (eg, modified acid-fast stain) for *Cryptosporidium* species and Microsporidia. In the neutropenic patient, typhlitis or neutropenic enterocolitis may present with right-sided pain, mimicking appendicitis. Many patients with neutropenia can be managed with antibiotics alone. *Pseudomonas* coverage is also recommended. Diarrhea is a common symptom in patients with toxic shock syndrome. The associated findings of rash, reddened oral mucosa, and hypotension should suggest this diagnosis.

SURGICAL SITE INFECTIONS

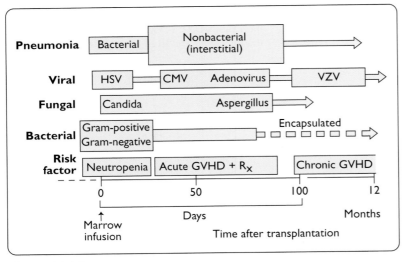

Figure 14-14.
Common infections by time after bone-marrow transplantation.
CMV—cytomegalovirus; GVHD—graft-versus-host disease; HSV—herpes
simplex virus; R_x—therapy; VZV—varicella zoster virus. (*Adapted from*
Meyers [7].)

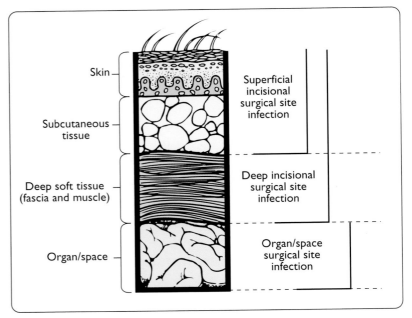

Figure 14-15.
The anatomy and classification of surgical site infections. The Centers for
Disease Control and Prevention has revised the definition of a surgical
wound infection. It is referred to as a surgical site infection, and the
anatomic depth of the wound is included in its classification [8].

EPIDEMIOLOGY OF SURGICAL SITE INFECTIONS

24% of all nosocomial infections

Occur in 2%–5% of patients undergoing surgery (16 million/year
in the United States)

Prolong hospitalization by an average of 7 days

Annual cost of $130–$845 million (asssuming a cost of
$400–$2600/wound)

Figure 14-16.
Epidemiology of surgical site infections. Surgical site infections occur in only
2% to 5% of all surgical procedures, but they account for almost 25% of all
nosocomial infections. They prolong hospital stays by an average of 1 week,
and costs nationwide run in the hundreds of millions of dollars.

MICROBIOLOGY OF SURGICAL SITE INFECTIONS

Staphylococcus aureus and coagulase-negative staphylococci are the
most common pathogens

Polymicrobial—aerobes and anaerobes are seen in patients
undergoing surgery involving the respiratory, gastrointestinal,
and genitourinary tracts

Candida spp are common in immunosuppressed patients

Vancomycin-resistant *Escherichia coli* is an emerging pathogen

Figure 14-17.
Microbiology of surgical site infections. The organisms responsible for
surgical wound infections include normal skin flora most commonly,
followed by organisms that colonize the particular surgical site.

Figure 14-18.
Risk factors for surgical site infections. There are numerous predisposing
factors for surgical wound infections. The risk for infection increases with
the number of coexisting risk factors.

RISK FACTORS FOR SURGICAL SITE INFECTIONS

Prolonged preoperative hospitalization

Preoperative shaving

Length of the operation

Surgical technique

Presence of remote infections

Host factors (age, diabetes, obesity, nutrition, malignancy)

TRANSFUSION-RELATED INFECTIONS

NONVIRAL TRANSFUSION-RELATED INFECTIONS

Bacterial

Environmental: staphylococci; other gram-positive and -negative contaminants

Endogenous: syphilis; Lyme disease; brucellosis; infection with *Yersinia, Salmonella,* and *Campylobacter* spp

Rickettsial

Rocky Mountain spotted fever

Q fever

Parasitic

Malaria, babesia

Toxoplasmosis

Trypanosomiasis

Leishmaniasis

Figure 14-19.

Nonviral transfusion-related infections. Nonviral transfusion-related infections are uncommon in the United States. The only one routinely screened for is syphilis. Accepted safety measures generally are based on medical history and knowledge of potentially transmissible local agents. No case of transfusion-related Lyme disease has been reported yet; however, because *Borrelia burgdorferi* can survive for 6 weeks in stored blood, the potential for transfusion-related infection exists. Environmental contaminants that are present during blood donation or storage can cause bacteremias with staphylococci or *Serratia* or *Pseudomonas* species. Platelet transfusions seem to be responsible for most of these infections [9].

VIRAL TRANSFUSION-RELATED INFECTIONS

Hepatitis A

Hepatitis B

Hepatitis C

Hepatitis D

HIV-1 and -2

Cytomegalovirus

Epstein-Barr virus

Parvovirus B-19

Figure 14-20.

Viral transfusion-related infections. Each year 12 million units of blood are donated in the United States. Before routine screening of donations was implemented, one third of the recipients developed some form of viral hepatitis. Now, less than 5% of recipients develop hepatitis, 90% of which is caused by the hepatitis C virus. Posttransfusion infection by hepatitis A virus, which is transmitted during the donor's asymptomatic incubation period, has been well documented. Nosocomial transmission infections by hepatitis B virus are most common among patients receiving hemodialysis and blood transfusions and by perinatal transmission. Less common modes of transmission include spring-loaded lancets, jet injectors, endoscopies, and multidose vials. Even though blood is screened for the HIV antibody, there is still a defined risk for transfusion-acquired HIV (*eg*, from a recently infected donor, before antibodies have reached detectable levels). Estimates of the risk of HIV transmission from a screened unit of blood is between 1:450,000 and 1:660,000 [10].

RESISTANT ORGANISMS OF SPECIAL CONCERN

TRENDS IN NOSOCOMIAL ANTIMICROBIAL RESISTANCE PROBLEMS

1950s–1970s	Penicillin-resistant staphylococci
1960s–1980s	Methicillin-resistant staphylococci
	Aminoglycoside-resistant gram-negative bacilli
Present	Methicillin-resistant staphylococci
	Multiresistant gram-negative bacilli
	Vancomycin-resistant enterococci
	Multidrug-resistant tuberculosis
	Resistant viruses (cytomegalovirus, herpes simplex virus)
	Azole-resistant yeasts
Future	Vancomycin-resistant staphylococci
	Pan-resistant gram-negative bacilli
	Multiresistant enterococci

Figure 14-21.

Trends in nosocomial antimicrobial resistance problems. Antibiotic resistance is a major concern in hospitals today. Knowing the resistance patterns at a particular hospital is crucial for patient care issues (*eg*, selection of appropriate empiric antibiotics in a critically ill patient) and more administrative concerns (*eg*, pharmacy restrictions, isolation policies, and development of therapy guidelines). Infections with antibiotic-resistant strains are likely to prolong hospitalization, increase the risk of death, and require therapy with more toxic and expensive antimicrobials. The intensive care unit may serve as a breeding ground for multiresistant organisms for several reasons: patients in the intensive care unit are often ventilator-dependent for long periods of time, are given large amounts of broad-spectrum antibiotics, and are placed in close contact with other critically ill patients in whom resistant organisms are likely to be present. Once resistance emerges, the organisms can spread throughout the hospital rather quickly, either directly (*ie*, by contact with the patient) or indirectly on the hands of health care workers or on environmental sites and devices that become contaminated. These organisms include methicillin-resistant *Staphylococcus aureus*, vancomycin-resistant *Enterococcus* species, gram-negative bacilli resistant to most antibiotics, and multidrug-resistant *Mycobacterium tuberculosis* [11].

Precautions	When used	Examples of diseases	Instructions
Standard	All patients	All patients	Use barrier precautions as needed to prevent contact with blood, body fluids, excretions, secretions, and contaminated items
			Wash hands after contact or glove removal
			Wash hands between patients
Airborne	Diseases spread by small droplets	Measles Varicella* Tuberculosis	Private room, negative air pressure ≥6 air exchanges/h, discharge air to the outside or filter air appropriately Respiratory protection for all persons entering the room
Droplet	Diseases spread by larger droplets	Invasive *Haemophilus influenza* Invasive *Neisseria meningitidis* Drug-resistant pneumococcus[†] Pharyngeal diphtheria Mycoplasma pneumonia Pertussis, rubella Streptococcal pharyngitis, pneumonia, scarlet fever Adenovirus, influenza Mumps, parvovirus	Private room, if possible Wear masks if working within 3 ft of the patient
Contact	Diseases spread by contact with intact skin or surfaces	Multidrug-resistant bacteria *Clostridium difficile* *Escherichia coli* O157:H7, hepatitis A, *Shigella* spp, rotavirus[‡] Respiratory syncytial virus Parainfluenza, enterovirus Herpes simplex virus Impetigo, furunculosis Wound infections, cellulitis Lice, scabies Scalded skin syndrome Conjunctivitis	Wear gloves when entering the room Change gloves after contact with infective material Wear a gown for substantial contact with the patient or environmental surfaces

*Also use contact precautions.
[†]*Invasive disease including meningitis, pneumonia, sinusitis, otitis media.*
[‡]*For diarrhea, if fecally incontinent.*

Figure 14-22.
Overview of new isolation guidelines. The Centers for Disease Control and Prevention isolation guidelines [12] separate diseases by mode of transmission (airborne, droplet, or contact) and are meant to limit horizontal transmission of multiresistant or contagious organisms by reinforcing hand-washing, barrier precautions, cohorting patients, and glove precautions (changing gloves between patients) when patients are known to have or are at high risk of acquiring multiresistant organisms (eg, all patients in intensive care units and nursing homes). (*Adapted from* the Centers for Disease Control and Prevention [12].)

ESTABLISHING HOSPITAL GUIDELINES FOR ANTIBIOTICS ADMINISTRATION

Select a formulary based on bacterial resistance patterns

Restrict agents with special indications, excessive toxicities, or high cost

Audit use of specific antibiotics

Monitor antibiotic susceptibility patterns and usage periodically and give feedback to the medical staff

Establish prophylactic, empiric, and therapeutic guidelines

Figure 14-23.
Establishing hospital guidelines for antibiotics administration. On a macrobiologic scale, we cannot ignore the resident flora of the hospital. Like a long-term intensive care unit patient on broad-spectrum antibiotics who acquires multiresistant organisms, the hospital becomes colonized with its own particular flora. Physicians must be aware of these potential pathogens and their antibiotic sensitivities to prescribe antibiotics effectively. Unrestricted antibiotic use and misuse has a profound effect on the hospital flora and efforts to optimize antibiotic therapy should be pursued.

REFERENCES

1. Warren JW: Nosocomial urinary tract infections. In *Principles and Practice of Infectious Diseases*, edn 4. Edited by Mandell GL, Bennett JE, Dolin R. New York: Churchill Livingstone; 1995:2607–2616.

2. Pearson ML and the Hospital Infection Control Practices Advisory Committee: Guideline for prevention of intravascular device-related infections. *Infect Control Hosp Epidemiol* 1996, 17:438–473.

3. Henderson DK: Bacteremias due to percutaneous intravascular devices. In *Principles and Practice of Infectious Diseases*, edn 4. Edited by Mandell GL, Bennett JE, Dolin R. New York: Churchill Livingstone; 1995:2587–2598.

4. Hospitals Infection Program, Centers for Disease Control and Prevention: National nosocomial infections surveillance report, May 1995: a report from the NNIS system. *Am J Infect Control* 1995, 23:377–385.

5. McFarland LV, Mulligen ME, Kwok RYY, et al.: Nosocomial acquisition of *C. difficile* infection. *N Engl J Med* 1989, 320:204–210.

6. Present DH: Toxic megacolon. *Med Clin North Am* 1993, 7:1129–1148.

7. Meyers JD: Infections in marrow transplant recipients. In *Principles and Practice of Infectious Diseases*, edn 3. Edited by Mandell GL, Douglas R, Bennett JE. New York: Churchill Livingstone; 1990:2291–2294.

8. Wong ES: Surgical site infections. In *Hospital Epidemiology and Infection Control*. Edited by Mayhall CG. Baltimore, MD: Williams & Wilkins; 1996:154–174.

9. Kitchen AD, Barbara JA: Transfusion-transmitted nonviral infections. *Curr Opin Infect Dis* 1994, 7:493–498.

10. Lackritz EM, Satten GA, Aberle-Grasse J, et al.: Estimated risk of transmission of HIV by screened blood in the United States. *N Engl J Med* 1995, 333:1721–1725.

11. Flaherty JP, Weinstein RA: Nosocomial infection caused by antibiotic-resistant organisms in the intensive care unit. *Infect Control Hosp Epidemiol* 1996, 17:236–248.

12. Centers for Disease Control and Prevention: Guidelines for isolation precautions in hospitals. *Am J Infect Control* 1996, 24:24–52.

TUBERCULOSIS

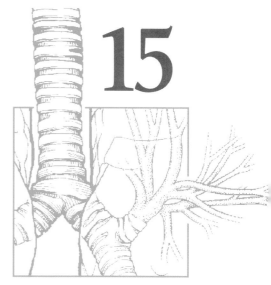

Joseph H. Bates

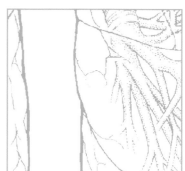

Tuberculosis was a relatively unimportant disease worldwide until the beginning of the industrial revolution. In the early 1600s in England, when people began to move to the city to live and work in more crowded conditions, the incidence of tuberculosis began to increase. By the 1700s, the disease reached epidemic proportions in England and Western Europe, killing one in four and infecting almost all persons. This epidemic, coined the great white plague, spread slowly, reaching Eastern Europe in the late 1700s, Russia and Asia in the 1800s, sub-Saharan Africa in the early part of the 1900s, New Guinea in the 1940s, and the upper reaches of the Amazon in the latter part of the 20th Century. In the 1970s, tuberculosis morbidity and mortality rates were declining in almost all the countries. Since the 1980s, the spread of HIV, together with major upheavals in established governmental and social support infrastructures, caused a marked increase in tuberculosis morbidity and mortality rates. These changes have been noted most in sub-Saharan Africa, Russia, and Southeast Asia. In some of these regions, the emergence of multidrug-resistant tuberculosis has vastly complicated treatment programs and tuberculosis control efforts.

Tuberculosis is under control in the United States and the number of new cases has decreased each year since emphasis on proper control measures was reestablished in 1992. However, tuberculosis is a global concern; the United States must participate with other economically advanced countries to bring tuberculosis under control everywhere.

Major advances are being made in understanding the molecular pathogenesis of tuberculosis, in the development of rapid diagnostic tests, and in the search for new antituberculosis drugs. The best long-range solution for tuberculosis control worldwide will be the development of a highly effective and safe vaccine, but such a development seems years away.

EPIDEMIOLOGY

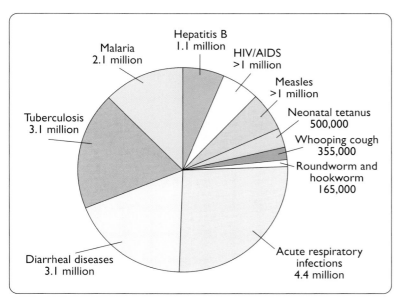

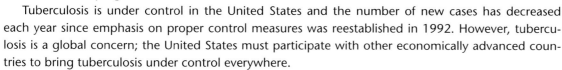

Figure 15-1.
Tuberculosis is the second leading cause of death from an infectious disease worldwide, ranking behind HIV infection. Tuberculosis is the most common cause of death for patients dying of AIDS worldwide. Tuberculosis case rates are increasing rapidly in most countries in sub-Saharan Africa and in many European countries. Russia has experienced an alarming increase in case rates over the period of 1990 to 2000 with drug-resistant tuberculosis also increasing rapidly. Long-term projections for tuberculosis case rates for Africa, Eastern Europe, and Southeast Asia indicate a continuing increase in morbidity and mortality [1].

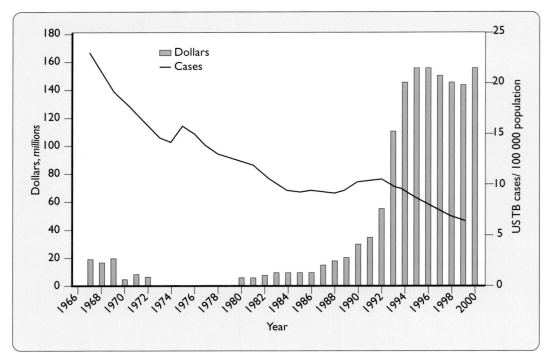

Figure 15-2.
Tuberculosis case rates and categorical spending for tuberculosis control. Tuberculosis case rates decreased approximately 5% a year every year it was measured, beginning in the 1950s until the mid-1980s (when the slope of the annual decline reached a plateau) and then increased over the next several years until it peaked in 1991 to 1992. Since then, the yearly decrease has been reestablished, decreasing at a faster rate than that observed previously. The greatest increases were noted in a few large states, particularly New York, New Jersey, Florida, Texas, and California. The unexpected increase resulted primarily from a failure of the public health infrastructure for tuberculosis control that developed as a result of a major cutback in government funding for this purpose. Other contributing factors included the HIV epidemic, the increase in the prevalence of drug and alcohol abuse, the expanding homeless population, and the marked increase in size of the prison population nationwide [2–4].

ETIOLOGY AND DIAGNOSIS

MICROBIOLOGY OF TUBERCULOSIS

Pathogen characteristics	Implications
Grows best under aerobic conditions	Grows best when PO_2 is high
Slow grower (generation time 18 to 22 hours)	Diagnosis is time consuming
High cell wall lipid content	Basis for acid-fast staining
Does not live outside the host	Transmission via droplet nuclei
Only a few susceptible hosts—man, guinea pig, monkey, and elephant	*Mycobacterium bovis* virulent for most mammals
Lives within human macrophage where it may remain viable for decades	Latent infection

Figure 15-3.
Mycobacterium tuberculosis grows best under aerobic conditions but remains viable and metabolically active under microaerophilic conditions. It grows slowly; cultures may require 6 to 8 weeks to show growth on solid media, whereas liquid media reveal growth in 2 to 3 weeks. Rapid diagnostic technique using DNA amplification can make laboratory diagnosis with great accuracy in those patients who have smear-positive sputum. *M. tuberculosis* mutates in the laboratory to show resistance to all known antituberculosis drugs in a predictable manner [5].

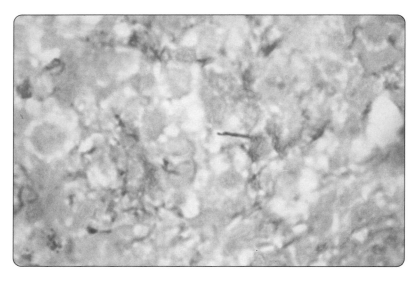

Figure 15-4.
Acid-fast stain (Ziehl-Neelson) showing *Mycobacterium tuberculosis*. Stained smears of sputum become positive when the microbial count equals or exceeds 10,000 organisms/mL. When one organism is seen per oil emersion field the microbial concentration is approximately 100,000/mL. DNA amplification techniques can be used to detect M. tuberculosis in smear-positive sputum. When the smear is negative for bacilli DNA, amplification gives about 30% false-negative results. These methods are also available for histologic specimens that have been fixed in formalin and are applied to other body fluids such as urine and pleural and cerebrospinal fluids [6,7]. (See Color Plate.)

A. PRESENTATION OF *MYCOBACTERIUM TUBERCULOSIS* INFECTION VERSUS ACUTE DISEASE

Criteria	Infection	Disease
PPD+	Yes	Yes
Symptoms	No	Yes
Chest radiograph	Normal (patients may have an abnormal chest radiograph unrelated to tuberculosis)	Abnormal
Communicable	No	Yes

PPD+—positive PPD + - positive purified protein derivative (skin test for tuberculosis).

B. FACTORS THAT LEAD TO DISEASE PROGRESSION

HIV
Substance abuse
Diabetes mellitus
Silicosis
Cancer
Chemotherapy
Malnutrition

Figure 15-5.

A, Presentation of *Mycobacterium tuberculosis* infection versus active disease. After exposure to *M. tuberculosis* and the development of an immune response (positive tuberculin skin test), patients have a 5% chance of developing active disease in the next 2 years. Over the rest of their lifetime, there is an additional 5% risk of disease. **B**, In the presence of any of the risk factors listed in this figure, the odds of developing active disease are much higher. An person infected with HIV exposed to *M. tuberculosis* has a 10% chance per year of developing active disease, unless adequate prophylactic measures are taken.

RISK FACTORS ASSOCIATED WITH LATENT TUBERCULOSIS INFECTION

>5 mm induration	>10 mm induration	>15 mm induration
Contacts with patients with tuberculosis	Residents of countries with high prevalence rates	No risk factors
HIV infection and other forms of immunosuppression	Residents of prisons, nursing homes, and homeless shelters	
Abnormal chest radiograph results	Intravenous drug use	
	Some low income populations	
	Medical risk factors, (*eg*, diabetes, renal failure, steroids, malignancies, transplantation, malnutrition, silicosis)	
	Locally defined high-risk populations	
	Children in close contact with persons with active disease	

PPD—purified protein derivative.

Figure 15-6.

Approximately 75% of newly diagnosed cases of tuberculosis are tuberculin skin test (TST) positive when first diagnosed, although almost all cases become TST-positive after approximately 2 months of successful chemotherapy. Vaccination with bacille Calmette-Guerin (BCG) produces a positive TST in most subjects, but this reaction tends to wane over time. After 10 years, most subjects are TST-negative unless they have inhaled viable *M. tuberculosis* in the interim. For those at high risk of becoming infected with *M. tuberculosis*, such as some health care workers, prison employees, workers in homeless shelters, and those visiting countries that have a high prevalence of tuberculosis, annual TSTs are advised. For these patients, the initial skin test should be repeated in 2 to 4 weeks if the first reading shows less than 10 mL induration. The second TST may elicit a "booster reaction," giving a larger degree of induration on the second test; the second test reading should be recorded as the baseline measure of the skin test [8].

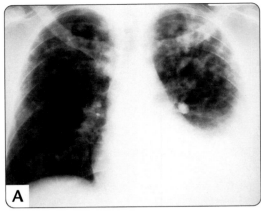

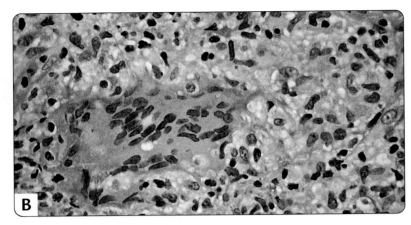

Figure 15-7.
A, Radiograph of an alcoholic patient aged 53 years, with progressive weight loss, fever, and sweats, admitted with acute dyspnea and left-sided pleuritic chest pain. Note the large pleural effusion on the left and bilateral patchy infiltrates. A thoracentesis revealed an exudative fluid that grew *Mycobacterium tuberculosis*. A bronchoscopy specimen was also positive for acid-fast bacillus. **B**, Hematoxylin-eosin stain of the pleural biopsy on the patient in *panel A*, revealing an epithelioid cell granuloma. Epithelioid cells are phagocytic cells of the monocyte-macrophage lineage as is the multinucleated giant cell. Most such granulomas stain negative for acid-fast bacilli because the bacilli are present in small numbers. Culture of the biopsied plural tissues is positive for *M. tuberculosis* in up to 60% of such cases.

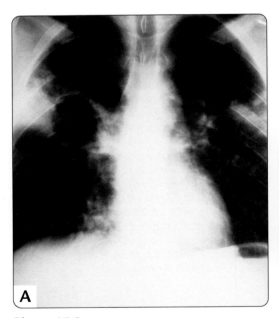

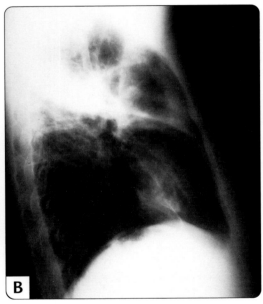

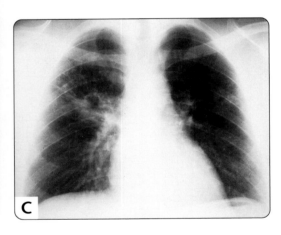

Figure 15-8.
A, Radiograph of a man aged 49 years with a chronic productive cough, fever, and night sweats. Note the large cavity in the superior segment of the right lower lobe and bilateral infiltrates. **B**, Lateral view of the patient in *panel A* whose sputum cultures were positive for *M. tuberculosis*. Patients with cavitary disease usually have many organisms present in their sputum samples; thus, patients with undiagnosed cavitary lung disease who have repeatedly negative sputum smears for acid-fast bacilli have a low probability of having tuberculosis. **C**, Radiograph of the patient in *panel A* after 6 months of therapy for tuberculosis, demonstrating almost complete resolution of the infiltrates and cavity. (Panel C *courtesy of* V. Yadava, MD.)

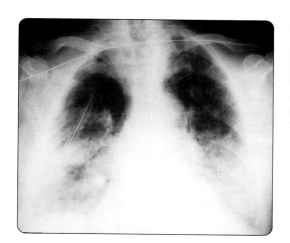

Figure 15-9.
Radiograph of an 80-year-old nursing home resident who was diagnosed with fever, shortness of breath, diffuse pulmonary infiltrates, and a spontaneous pneumothorax requiring chest tube placement. Sputum smears and cultures were positive for *Mycobacterium tuberculosis*. The lower lobe distribution without evidence of apical disease suggests a primary infection. Tuberculosis among nursing home residents may go unrecognized because lower lobe disease is a common presentation. All chronic or slow-to-resolve pneumonias among nursing home residents should be studied for the possibility of tuberculosis. (*Courtesy of* V. Yadava, MD.)

TREATMENT

A. FIRST-LINE ANTITUBERCULOSIS AGENTS

Drug	Dosage form	Daily dose	Twice-weekly dosage	Adverse reactions	Drug interactions
Isoniazid	Oral, intramuscular	5 mg/kg, up to 300 mg	15 mg/kg, up to 900 mg	Hepatic enzyme elevation, hepatitis, peripheral neuropathy, hypersensitivity	Phenytoin, disulfiram, corticosteroids
Rifampin	Oral	10 mg/kg, up to 600 mg	10 mg/kg, up to 600 mg	Orange discoloration of body fluids, nausea, vomiting, hepatitis, febrile reaction, purpura	Warfarin, nortriptyline, barbiturates, benzodi-azepines, oral contraceptives, corticosteroids, digitalis, halothane, oral hypo-glycemics, quinidine
Pyrazinamide	Oral	15–30 mg/kg, up to 2 g	15–70 mg/kg, up to 4 g	Hepatotoxicity, hyperuricemia arthralgia, rash, gastrointestinal upset	Allopurinol; diuretics may amplify uricemia
Ethambutol	Oral	15–25 mg/kg	50 mg/kg	Optic neuritis (decreased red-green color discrimination, decreased visual acuity), rash	Aluminum salts
Streptomycin	Intramuscular	15 mg/kg, up to 1 g in persons age < y; 10 mg/kg up to 750 mg in persons >60 y	25–30 mg/kg, up to 1.5 g	Ototoxicity, nephrotoxicity	Furosemide, ethacrynic acid, mannitol, cisplatin, indomethacin, acyclovir, amphotericin B, capreomycin, bacitracin, polymyxin B, vancomycin, aminoglycosides

Figure 15-10.
A, Treatment of active tuberculosis requires the use of at least two potent antituberculosis drugs to which the infecting isolate is sensitive. When there is a slight possibility of a resistant strain, three drugs are advised when therapy is begun. The most common combination used in the United States is isoniazid, rifampin, and pyrazinamide. When this combination is given and ingested in the proper doses, the cure rate can be as high as 98% for those who complete a full course of treatment lasting from 6 to 9 months. If drug resistance is unlikely, as is the case for some patients in select geographic areas of the United States, isoniazid and rifampin alone may be given as the initial regimen for newly diagnosed patients older than 60 years. When drug resistance is a possibility, four or more drugs should be selected for the initial regimen, with adjustments in the treatment regimen planned after results of drug susceptibility are reported.

(Continued on next page)

B. SECOND-LINE ANTITUBERCULOSIS AGENTS

Drug	Dosage form	Daily dose	Adverse reactions	Drug interactions
Capreomycin	Intramuscular	15–30 mg/kg, up to 1 g	Renal, auditory, and vestibular	Furosemide, ethacrynic acid, mannitol, cisplatin, indomethacin, amphotericin B, polymyxin B, vancomycin, other aminoglycosides
Kanamycin	Intramuscular	15–30 mg/kg, up to 1 g	Renal, auditory, and vestibular	Furosemide, ethacrynic acid, mannitol, cisplatin, indomethacin, amphotericin B, polymyxin B, vancomycin, other aminoglycosides
Amikacin	Intramuscular	15 mg/kg, 5 d/week	Renal, auditory, and vestibular	Furosemide, ethacrynic acid, mannitol, cisplatin, indomethacin, amphotericin B, polymyxin B, vancomycin, other aminoglycosides
Ethionamide	Oral	15–20 mg/kg, up to 1 g	Gastrointestinal, liver toxicity	Cycloserine
P-aminosalicylic acid (PAS)	Oral	150 mg/kg, up to 12 g	Gastrointestinal, liver toxicity	Rifampin, probenecid, digoxin, oral antigoagulants, ammonium chloride
Fluoroquinolones (use one)				
Ofloxacin	Oral	6–12 mg/kg	Gastrointestinal	Antacids, sucralfate
Ciprofloxacin	Oral	7–11 mg/kg	Gastrointestinal	Antacids, sucralfate
Sparfloxacin	Oral	400 mg first day, then 200 mg/d	Photosensitivity and gastrointestinal	Antacids, sucralfate
Levofloxacin	Oral	7–11 mg/kg	Gastrointestinal	Antacids, sucralfate
Rifabutin	Oral	300 mg	Liver toxicity, thrombocytopenia, fever, rash	Saquinavir, delavirdine

Figure 15-10. (Continued)
B, Second-line antituberculosis agents are used when there is multidrug resistance involving all or almost all first-line drugs. Second-line drugs are generally more toxic, less effective, and require careful monitoring by specialists fully familiar with their use.

THERAPEUTIC REGIMENS FOR ACTIVE TUBERCULOSIS

In communities where isoniazid or rifampin resistance is <4%

Isoniazid + rifampin + pyrazinamide until sensitivities are known

Isoniazid + rifampin daily for 9 mo (if isolate is susceptible to both)

Isoniazid + rifampin + pyrazinamide + ethambutol or streptomycin daily for 2 mo followed by isoniazid + rifampin for 4 mo

For patients requiring directly observed therapy

Isoniazid + rifampin + pyrazinamide + ethambutol daily for 2 wk then twice weekly for 4 mo or until sputum cultures are negative for 3 mo

Isoniazid + rifampin + pyrazinamide + ethambutol or streptomycin 3 times weekly for 6 mo or until sputum cultures are negative for 3 mo

Isoniazid, 900 mg, + rifampin, 600 mg twice weekly for 9 mo

In communities where isoniazid or rifampin resistance is >4%

Isoniazid + rifampin + pyrazinamide + ethambutol or streptomycin daily until sensitivities are known

For multidrug-resistant tuberculosis strains

Combinations of several first- and second-line agents, chosen based on susceptibility data, including at least 2 drugs to which the isolate is sensitive

Directly observed therapy

Figure 15-11.
Therapeutic regimens for active tuberculosis. Knowledge of the incidence of multidrug-resistant isolates of tuberculosis in the local community is important when deciding on initial therapy. If more than 4% of the tuberculosis isolates in a community are multidrug resistant, then a four-drug regimen is used until sensitivities are known. Directly observed therapy (DOT) is used increasingly throughout the United States. All patients who are alcoholic or who have other demonstrated behavioral disorders should be treated with DOT. Many experts advise treating most, if not all, patients with DOT. Cure rates in the United States using DOT have generally been better and the emergence of drug resistance has been less than for those patients who ingest medications without supervision.

TUBERCULOSIS AND HIV

Transmission

1 of 3 TB cases in HIV patients is recently acquired

Immunity is not conferred by previous exposure to TB organisms

Lack of cavitary disease with HIV may render patients less contagious

Spread of TB facilitated by grouping HIV patients together in health care facilities, homeless shelters, and prisons

Clinical manifestations

Positive purified protein derivative with early stages of HIV only

Usual symptoms (fever, sweats, cough, and weight loss) are usually more exaggerated

Rapid progression from exposure to active disease (from loss of cell-mediated immunity)

Higher rate (40%–80%) of extrapulmonary manifestations

Lymphadenitis with fistula formation and abscesses

Radiographic features

Nonapical distribution

Infiltrates in any lung zone

Cavitation rare late in the disease

Intrathoracic adenopathy in 1 of 3 cases

Miliary infiltrates and pleural effusions

Normal chest radiograph in early stages of pulmonary TB

TB—tuberculosis.

Figure 15-12.

Tuberculosis and HIV. All patients with tuberculosis should be screened for HIV, and conversely, all HIV positive patients should have a purified protein derivative (PPD) skin test. The sensitivity of the test is inversely proportional to the degree of immunosuppression. Anergy is common, so a negative PPD should be interpreted with caution. Prophylactic regimens should be continued for 12 months. Tuberculosis should be considered in any HIV-positive patient with unexplained fevers, cough, infiltrate, adenopathy, meningitis, brain abscess, pericarditis, pleural effusion, or an abscess anywhere in the body. The diagnosis is difficult because the symptoms are nonspecific, the PPD is often negative despite active disease, atypical radiographs are the rule, and extrapulmonary manifestations are common.

TREATMENT REGIMENS FOR HIV-INFECTED ADULTS WITH TB

Clinical circumstances and treatment considerations	Initial therapy*	Continuation phase of therapy
DOT	Isoniazid, rifampin, pyrazinamide, and ethambutol or streptomycin daily for 2 wk and then 2–3 ×/wk for 6 wk *or*	Isoniazid and rifampin 2–3 ×/wk to complete 6 mo of treatment
	Isoniazid, rifampin, pyrazinamide, and streptomycin or ethambutol 3 ×/wk for 6 mo	
DOT not considered necessary to ensure patient's compliance	Isoniazid, rifampin, pyrazinamide, and streptomycin or ethambutol daily (pending susceptibility data) and then isoniazid, rifampin, and pyrazinamide to complete 8 wk of therapy with these 3 drugs	Isoniazid and rifampin daily to complete 6 mo of treatment
Resistance (or intolerance) to isoniazid[†]	—	Rifampin, ethambutol, and pyrazinamide × 18 mo (and for ≥12 mo after culture conversion)
Resistance (or intolerance) to rifampin[†]	—	Isoniazid, ethambutol, and pyrazinamide × 18 mo (and for ≥12 mo after culture conversion)
Possible or confirmed resistance to both isoniazid and rifampin (cases of MDR TB)[†]	Isoniazid, rifampin, pyrazinamide, and streptomycin or ethambutol, plus additional 2nd-line drugs or a quinolone antibiotic, so that patient receives ≥3 drugs to which local MDR TB strains are likely to be susceptible	≥3 drugs to which patient's *Mycobacterium tuberculosis* strain is susceptible; appropriate duration of therapy is not known

In areas where surveillance for drug-resistant TB has documented drug resistance rates of <4%, isoniazid, rifampin, and pyrazinamide alone may be used for initial therapy.
[†]*All patients with drug-resistant TB should receive DOT; MDR TB should be treated in consultation with physicians experienced at treating such patients.*
DOT—directly observed therapy; MDR TB—multidrug-resistant tuberculosis.

Figure 15-13.

Treatment regimens for HIV-infected adults with tuberculosis. All patients should receive directly observed therapy (DOT). Rifampin can be used only if the patient is not receiving antiretroviral agents. Most patients receiving antiretroviral therapy should have rifabutin substituted for rifampin. Dosing of rifabutin should be determined by an expert regarding its use in combination with the various protease inhibitors, nonnucleoside reverse transcriptase inhibitors, and nucleoside reverse transcriptase inhibitors [9]. A 6-month treatment regimen may be followed in HIV-positive persons infected with a pansensitive strain when there is a good initial response to therapy and the sputum culture becomes negative within 2 months of treatment initiation [10].

TREATMENT REGIMENS IN SPECIAL CASES

Pregnancy

Isoniazid, rifampin, and ethambutol comprise the preferred initial regimen.

Pyrazinamide should be reserved for patients with multidrug-resistant tuberculosis because safety regarding teratogenetic effects has not been established.

Streptomycin is contraindicated because of congenital deafness.

Risk of TB in an infant is small if the mother was on therapy >2 weeks before delivery.

Encourage breastfeeding postpartum; levels of TB medications in breast milk are insufficient to rely on for therapy; bacille Calmette-Guerin vaccination is recommended for the child if the mother's compliance is doubtful.

The NPO patient

Isoniazid intramuscularly

Rifampin intravenously

Streptomycin intramuscularly

Ciprofloxacin and ofloxacin intravenously

Capremycon, kanamycin, and amikacin intramuscularly or intravenously

The pediatric patient

Forty percent of PPD-positive children progress to active disease; children with infectious household contacts are treated with isoniazid for 3 months and then the PPD is repeated; continue for 9 months if the PPD is positive.

If susceptibility data from the source are absent, aggressive diagnostic steps (*eg*, morning gastric aspirate or bronchoscopy) should be considered in children with active disease.

Hilar adenopathy may take 2 to 3 years to resolve.

Therapy and management are similar to that for adults, but ethambutol should be used with caution because ocular toxicity is more difficult to evaluate in children.

Figure 15-14.

Treatment regimens in special cases. Therapy for tuberculosis is complicated enough in the otherwise healthy host and is even more challenging in the pregnant, NPO (nothing by mouth), and pediatric populations. The figure lists some suggestions for dealing with these situations.

MULTIDRUG-RESISTANT TUBERCULOSIS

Description

Resistance to both isoniazid and rifampin

14% of patients with TB are resistant to either isoniazid or rifampin

Two thirds of MDR TB cases from New York, California, Texas, New Jersey, or Florida

Lethal outbreaks in the 1980s and 1990s in hospitals, prisons, and homeless shelters

Contributing factors

HIV

Close contact with patients with MDR TB

Noncompliance with TB therapy and inadequate follow-up

Increased immigration from areas of high prevalence (Asia, Africa, Latin America)

Increased numbers of the homeless, intravenous drug users, and institutionalized patients

Cutbacks in public funding of TB control programs

MDR—multidrug-resistant; TB—tuberculosis.

Figure 15-15.

Multidrug-resistant tuberculosis (MDR TB). Transmission of strains doubly resistant to isoniazid and rifampin was recognized in the late 1980s and increased in the 1990s. Such strains take their origin from patients who do not respond to treatment most likely because of inadequate ingestion of a prescribed regimen or as a result of physician error in prescribing. Probable treatment failure should be considered when a positive culture from a patient does not convert to a negative culture within 4 to 6 months of therapy initiation. Repeat drug sensitivity studies should be obtained at this point and at least two new drugs to which the infecting organism is sensitive should be added. If the patient is not on directly observed therapy (DOT), such supervised therapy should begin at this point. When only one new drug is added to a failing regimen, the probability of treatment failure is great and the persisting microbe will be resistant to the newly added drug.

CANDIDATES FOR TREATMENT OF LATENT TUBERCULOSIS INFECTION

Isoniazid treatment should be offered to adult tuberculin skin test positive reactors with the following risk factors:

HIV-positive

Recent tuberculin skin test conversion (within 2 years)

Close contact with an infectious patient

Therapy with immunosuppressive drugs

Immunosuppressed state such as diabetes, renal failure, and profound malnutrition

Chest radiograph abnormalities and clinical evaluation suggesting old tuberculosis fibrotic lesions

Silicosis

Immigrants who are recent arrivals from countries with high prevalence

Figure 15-16.

Candidates for treatment of latent tuberculosis infection. Isoniazid administered for 12 months reduces the risk for tuberculosis developing by more than 90% over the lifetime of the subject. Treatment for 6 months provides protection at a level of approximately 70%. Treatment for 9 months provides greater protection than does 6 months of treatment; 9 months of treatment is advised as a minimum for most patients. The dosage in adults is 300 mg once daily. Two- and 3-month regimens of daily rifampin with isoniazid or pyrazinamide may be as effective as longer courses of isoniazid given alone. For HIV-positive adults, 2-month regimens that include rifampin or rifabutin with isoniazid or pyrazinamide are advised [11].

BACILLE CALMETTE-GUÉRIN IN THE PREVENTION OF TB

Indicated for:

Children and adolescents who reside in areas where TB infection and transmission is high and where measures to protect them are likely to fail

Considered for:

Health care workers employed in areas where exposure to TB is great or multidrug-resistant strains of *Mycobacterium tuberculosis* are prevalent

Not recommended for:

Patients with symptomatic HIV infection or other forms of immunosuppression

Patients or health care workers with minimal exposure to TB as routine immunization

Adverse side effects (incidence/1 million vaccinations)

Local abscess, regional adenopathy (25–387)

Musculoskeletal lesions (0.06–0.89)

Multiple lymphadenitis (0.31–0.39)

Fatal disseminated lesions (0.06–1.59)

TB—tuberculosis.

Figure 15-17.

Bacille Calmette-Guérin (BCG) in the prevention of tuberculosis. BCG is the most commonly used vaccine worldwide, but its effectiveness is disputed. Trials in Europe have demonstrated strong protection, whereas trials in Asia show a very weak effect. Reasons for the variation in effectiveness are unknown, but it is known that there is genetic variability among the various BCG vaccines used [12]. BCG is seldom given to patients in the United States because the risk for acquiring new infection is low. Instead of BCG vaccination, persons at high risk of becoming infected are advised to have periodic tuberculin skin tests and when tuberculin conversion is observed to have a clinical evaluation and treatment for latent infection. For persons who are tuberculin-skin-test negative and at high risk of inhaling strains that are multidrug resistant, BCG may be recommended. Adverse side-effects are rare but increase in those who are immunosuppressed [12,14].

HOW TO ESTABLISH AN EFFECTIVE TB INFECTION CONTROL PROGRAM

Assign responsibility for the program to qualified person(s), who generally include practitioners in infection control, occupational health, and engineering

Develop a TB infection control plan that includes knowledge of local epidemiology, tuberculin skin test status of health care workers and patients at risk, and periodic review of surveillance data, infection control policies, and engineering controls

Rapidly identify, isolate, and treat all patients with TB

Establish engineering controls to ensure negative pressure rooms or adequate air recirculation through high-efficiency particulate air filters at all times in areas where TB patients receive care

Implement use of respiratory protective devices that filter out >95% of 1 μm particles by people entering the room of a patient known or suspected of having TB and provide training programs to ensure proficiency and compliance with their use

Provide health care workers with periodic TB training and education appropriate for their work responsibilities, as well as PPD testing and postexposure counseling

Coordinate efforts with the local public health departments

Install ultraviolet light fixtures in the upper part of isolation rooms, taking care to ensure against harmful effects to the skin and eyes

Figure 15-18.

How to establish an effective hospital and clinic infection control program. It is important to charge an infection control person to be responsible for the development of a comprehensive tuberculosis control program following guidelines published by the Centers for Disease Control and Prevention (CDC). In geographic areas where there is a significant incidence of tuberculosis, a high-degree of supervision should be fostered regarding perplexing pneumonias and pneumonias that are slow to resolve or are unresponsive to common antimicrobial drugs. All patients suspected of having pulmonary tuberculosis should be placed in a properly constructed isolation room having negative air pressure with respect to the hallway and ultraviolet light fixtures in place on the upper walls [15]. The use of properly fitted face masks approved by the CDC is also important [16]. The patients who are most infectious are those whose sputum smears are positive for acid-fast bacilli and are on no anti-tuberculosis drugs. After chemotherapy is started with two or more drugs to which the infecting organism is sensitive, the degree of infectiousness decreases sharply within 2 weeks. After 2 weeks of effective treatment, most patients can be removed from isolation.

PREVENTING AND CONTROLLING TUBERCULOSIS IN THE COMMUNITY

Major priorities

- Promptly identify and effectively treat all new cases of tuberculosis with a goal that 95% of patients will be cured by 1 year after diagnosis.

- Promptly identify all close contacts of each infectious case, provide tuberculin skin testing with careful clinical evaluation, and offer therapy as indicated

- Provide tuberculin skin testing for groups at high risk for latent tuberculosis infection and treat as indicated

- Provide laboratory and diagnostic service, including radiograph interpretation to all persons who need it. Laboratory support should include expert examination of biologic specimens for acid-fast bacilli with reports available within 24 hours. Culture for mycobacteria and drug susceptibility data should be available for all patients.

- Insure a functioning central registry is in place for collecting and collating data on all new cases of tuberculosis with epidemiologic, clinical, and laboratory reports tracked to allow monitoring of treatment outcome, contact investigation, and treatment of latent infection.

Figure 15-19.

Preventing and controlling tuberculosis in the community. Tuberculosis control for a community or state is the responsibility of the health department. When adequate resources are available, the case rate can be expected to decrease approximately 5% per year and 90% to 95% of newly diagnosed cases will be cured. Tuberculosis elimination is a reasonable goal for many tuberculosis control programs in the United States [17]. For those states that have many foreign-born residents, the task will be much more difficult. Approximately 40% of all new cases of tuberculosis in the United States occurs among foreign-born people [18]. Drug-resistant tuberculosis is a special concern for tuberculosis controllers. Drug resistance is becoming less of a problem in the United States, but it was increasing in the first half of the 1990s. Drug resistance is an increasing problem in Mexico, Russia, and some eastern European countries. Persons coming to the United States rom these countries who develop tuberculosis after arrival should be evaluated promptly for drug-resistant organisms.

REFERENCES

1. Raviglione MC, Snider DE Jr, Kochi A: Global epidemiology of tuberculosis, morbidity and mortality of a worldwide epidemic. *JAMA* 1995, 273:220–226.

2. Centers for Disease Control and Prevention: Reported tuberculosis in the United States 1999. Atlanta: Centers for Disease Control and Prevention. 2000.

3. Perelman MI: Tuberculosis in Russia. *Int J Tuber Lung Dis* 2000, 4:1097–1103.

4. Bizkin NJ, Vernon AA, Simone PM, et al.: Tuberculosis prevention and control activities in the United States: an overview of the organization of tuberculosis services. *Int J Tuber Lung Dis* 1999, 3:663–674.

5. Perry S, Catanzaro A: Clinical utility of rapid diagnostic test for TB based on clinical suspicion of disease. *Am J Respir Crit Care Med* 1999, 159:A195.

6. Salian NV, Rish JA, Eisenach KD, et al.: Polymerase chain reaction to detect mycobacterium tuberculosis in histological specimens. *Am J Respir Crit Care Med* 1998, 158:1150–1155.

7. Portillo-Gomez L, Morris SL, Panduro A: Rapid and efficient detection of extrapulmonary Mycobacterium tuberculosis by PCR analysis. *Int J Tuber Lung Dis* 2000, 4:361–370.

8. Centers for Disease Control and Prevention: Essential components of a tuberculosis prevention and control program. *MMWR* 1995, 44(RR-11):1–34.

9. Centers for Disease Control and Prevention: Prevention and treatment of tuberculosis among patients infected with human immunodeficiency virus: principles of therapy and revised recommendations. *MMWR* 1998, 47(RR-20):1.

10. Centers for Disease Control and Prevention: *Core Curriculum on Tuberculosis*, edn 4; 2000:118–119.

11. American Thoracic Society and Centers for Disease Control and Prevention: Targeted tuberculin testing and treatment of latent tuberculosis infection. *Am J Respir Crit Care Med* 2000, 161:221.

12. Colditz GA, Brewer TF, Berkey CS, et al.: Efficacy of BCG vaccine in the prevention of tuberculosis: meta-analysis of the published literature. *JAMA* 1994, 271:698–702.

13. Rodrigues ZC, Diwan VK, Wheeler JG: Protective effect of BCG against tuberculosis meningitis and military tuberculosis: a meta-analysis. *Int J Epidemiol* 1993, 22:1154–1158.

14. Centers for Disease Control and Prevention: The role of BCG vaccination in the prevention and control of tuberculosis in the United States. *MMWR* 1996, 45(RR-4):1–18.

15. First MW, Nardell EA, Chaission W, et al.: Guidelines for the application of upper-room ultraviolet germicidal irradiation for preventing transmission of airborne contagion, part 11: design and operation guidance. *ASRAE Transact* 1999, 105:1–10.

16. Centers for Disease Control and Prevention: Guidelines for preventing the transmission of Mycobacterium tuberculosis in health-care facilities. *MMWR* 1994, 43 (RR-13):1–132.

17. Centers for Disease Control and Prevention: Tuberculosis elimination revisited: obstacles, opportunities and a renewed commitment. *MMWR* 1999, 48(RR-9).

18. Centers for Disease Control and Prevention: Recommendation for prevention and control of tuberculosis among foreign-born persons: report of a working group on tuberculosis among foreign-born persons. *MMWR* 1998, 47(RR-16).

HIV/AIDS AND FUNGAL INFECTION

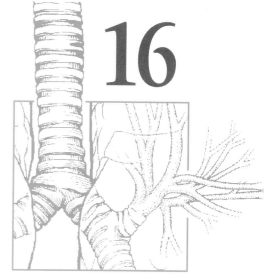

16

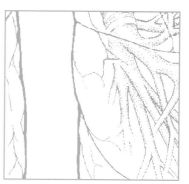

Robert W. Bradsher

Human immunodeficiency virus is the cause of AIDS, first described in the late 1980s. Initially, most of the cases were in men who had sex with men and those with injection drug use. Over the past 5 years, an increasing number of women have been diagnosed with AIDS after infection with HIV from heterosexual contact. Rather than the virus remaining in a latent state for a prolonged period, the virus is associated with a substantial amount of replication at a set point that sets the duration of the infection. This is determined by measuring the quantitative amount of virus in the bloodstream in an assay of polymerase chain reaction detection of viral RNA. The object of highly active antiretroviral therapy (HAART) is to reduce the viral load and thereby reduce the destruction of lymphocytes associated with clearance of HIV on a daily basis.

The major loss of the immune system in HIV/AIDS is related to cell-mediated immunity. This arm of immunity is directed by T-lymphocytes and controls the progression of many infectious pathogens, such as parasites, certain bacteria, and fungi. Depending on the geographical location, fungal organisms are among the leading cause of opportunistic infections in patients with AIDS. These include histoplasmosis, coccidioidomycosis, cryptococcal infection, candidiasis, and penicilliosis. To a lesser degree, aspergillosis, sporotrichosis, and blastomycosis may be diagnosed in patients with HIV infection. Amphotericin B or one of the azole agents, itraconazole or fluconazole, have been useful in controlling progressive infection or preventing relapse of infection in patients with AIDS.

The two modes of the epidemiology of fungal infections are opportunistic and endemic. The opportunistic fungi include *Aspergillus*, *Candida*, *Fusarium*, and *Rhizopus* species; some of the fungi more traditionally characterized as endemic fungi, including *Histoplasma*, *Blastomyces*, *Cryptococcus*, *Sporothrix*, and *Coccidioidomyces*, may also present as an opportunistic infection in the immunocompromised patient. However, the organisms considered as opportunistic fungi do not cause endemic or geographically localized diseases. *Aspergillus*, *Candida*, *Fusarium*, and *Rhizopus* species and the like are ubiquitous in nature and found throughout the world.

The endemic fungi are more likely to present from a community acquisition rather than nosocomial. These infections, other than sporotrichosis, originate by aerosol inhalation with the primary infection in the lung. This infection may never cause symptomatic disease and may resolve spontaneously or the organism may escape host defenses and cause progressive infection in the lung or at sites of hematogenous dissemination. Therefore, disease may range from the asymptomatic to life-threatening manifestations. Although there has been some evidence of development of resistance by *H. capsulatum* to fluconazole, antifungal resistance has not been a major factor in the endemic mycosis.

The opportunistic fungi are more likely to be nosocomial and to occur in specialized patient groups. These include those with HIV/AIDS, transplantation, and immunosuppressive chemotherapy, and those treated with corticosteroids. Resistance to antifungal chemotherapy, particularly with *Candida* and fluconazole, has been increasing.

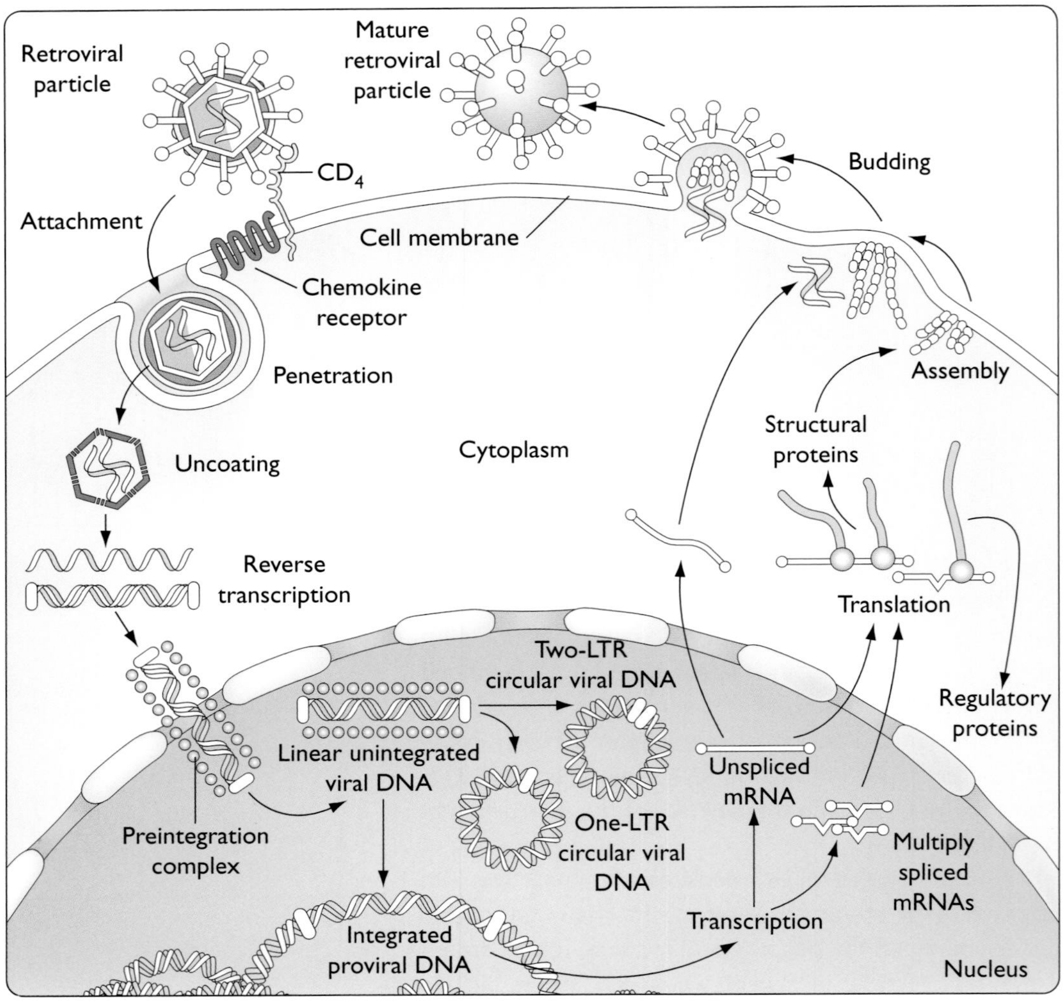

Figure 16-1.
The life cycle of HIV. (*Adapted from* [1].)

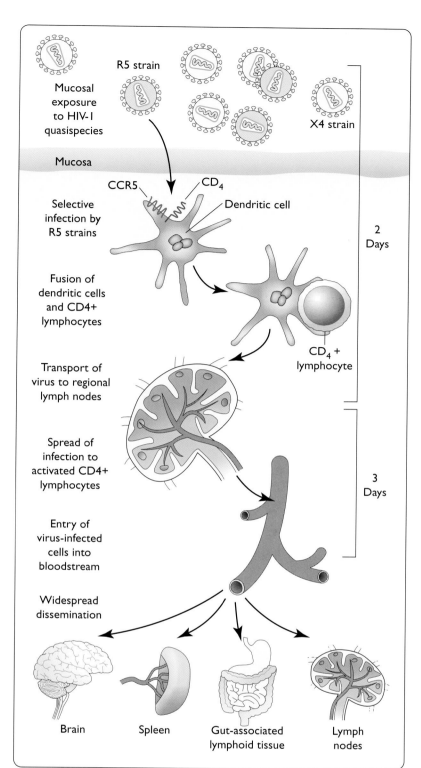

Figure 16-2.

HIV pathogenesis. This figure illustrates infection with the X4 (T trophic) and R5 (M trophic) strains. Note the dendritic (Langerhan's) cells, CD4 lymphocyte, and regional lymph nodes, as well as the systemic spread and bloodstream dissemination. The tissues involved include the tonsil, thymus, brain, gut-associated lymphoid tissue, and lymph nodes. The virus enters the bloodstream within 3 to 10 days of primary sexual infection. Progressive and persistent viral replication occurs with the removal of the virus by CD_4 lymphocyte over the prolonged period. AIDS is diagnosed when the pool of lymphocyte does not proliferate. (*Adapted from* Kahn and Walker[2].)

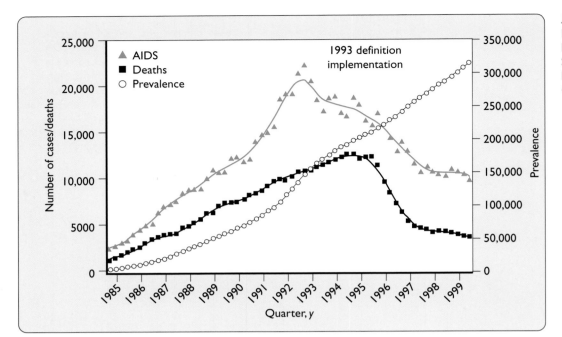

Figure 16-3.
Estimated incidence of AIDS, deaths, and prevalence by quarter year of diagnosis/death—United States, 1985–1999. The estimated incidence has been adjusted for reporting delays. (*Adapted from* CDC [3].)

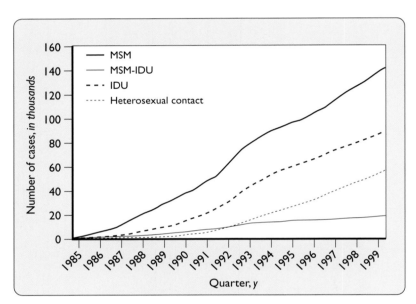

Figure 16-4.
Estimated AIDS prevalence among adults and adolescents by risk exposure—United States, 1985–1999. The estimated prevalence rates have been adjusted for reporting delays and unreported risk. IDU—injection drug used; MSM—men who have sex with men. (*Adapted from* CDC [3].)

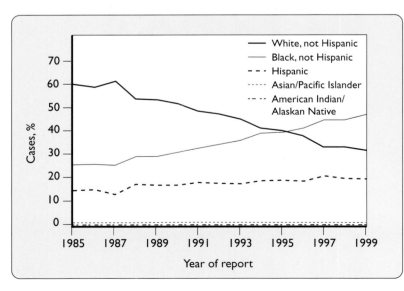

Figure 16-5.
Proportion of AIDS cases by race and ethnicity—United States, 1985–1999. The distribution of AIDS cases among racial and ethnic groups has shifted since the beginning of the epidemic. The proportion of cases among whites has decreased over time while increasing among blacks and Hispanics. As of 1996, a greater proportion of cases was reported among blacks than among whites. The proportion of cases reported among Asian/Pacific Islanders and American Indian/Native Alaskans has remained relatively constant, representing approximately 1% of all cases. In 1999, 32% of the reported AIDS cases were white, 47% black, 19% Hispanic, 1% Asian/Pacific Islander, and less than 1% American Indian/Native Alaskan. (*Adapted from* CDC [3].)

AIDS CASES IN ADULTS AND ADOLESCENTS BY EXPOSURE CATEGORY AND RACE/ETHNICITY

Exposure category	White Number, %	Black Number, %	Hispanic Number, %
Men who have sex with men (MSM)	216,564, 68	74,434, 28	45,867, 35
Injection drug use (IDU)	37,930, 12	97,550, 36	47,951, 36
MSM and IDU	23,880, 8	14,965, 6	7253, 6
Heterosexual contact	15,709, 5	40,840, 15	17,208, 13
Other/not identified*	22,752, 7	39,988, 15	13,419, 10
Total	316,835	267,777	131,698

*Includes patients with hemophilia- or transfusion-related exposures and those whose medical record review is pending; patients who died, were lost to follow-up, or declined interview, and those with other or undetermined reasons.

Figure 16-6.
AIDS cases in adults and adolescents by exposure category and race and ethnicity—United States, 1999. Most of the cases of AIDS reported among whites, Asian/Pacific Islanders, and American Indian/Native Alaskans have been among men who have sex with men (MSM). Among blacks and Hispanics, injection drug use (IDU) has been the primary mode of exposure to HIV (36%). In 1999, 74,406 cases of AIDS (with a known race/ethnicity) attributed to heterosexual contact were reported. Sixty-four percent of these was among women; more than half of these women (25,719) black. Since the beginning of the epidemic, there have been 5075 cases of AIDS among persons with hemophilia or coagulation disorders, and 8531 cases attributed to the receipt of blood transfusions, blood components, or tissue. These cases include persons of all racial and ethnic groups. (*Adapted from* CDC [3].)

HIV TESTING

HIV-RNA	CD4	% Alive at 10 years
<10,000	787	70
>10,000	781	30
	CD4 level	
	Viral load	
	RT-PCR	
	Branched DNA	

Figure 16-7.
HIV testing. The CD4 level is the best marker for the level of progression of the HIV disease. The viral load is the best marker for how rapidly the HIV disease is progressing.

HIV ANTIRETROVIRAL AGENTS

Nucleoside analogues
  Zidovudine (ZDV, AZT): Retrovir*
  Didanosine (ddI): Videx†
  Zalcitabine (ddC): Hivid‡
  Stavudine (d4T): Zerit†
  Lamivudine (3TC): Epivir*
  Abacavir (ABC): Ziagen*
  AZT, 3TC & ABC: Trizivir*
Non-nucleoside reverse transcriptase inhibitors (NNRTI)
  Nevirapine: Viramune
  Delaviridine: Rescriptor
  Efavirenz: Sustiva
  Adofovir (nucleotide): Prevenon (removed from market)
  Tenofovir (nucleotide): Investigational
Protease inhibitors (PI)
  Saquinavir: Fortovase, Invirase‡
  Ritonavir: Norvir
  Indinavir: Crixivan
  Nelfinavir: Viracept
  Amprenivir: Agenerase*
  Lopinavir (with ritonavir): Kaletra

Figure 16-8.
HIV antiretroviral agents.
*Glaxo Wellcome, Research Triangle Park, NC.
†Bristol Myers Squibb, Princeton, NJ.
‡Roche, Nutley, NJ

INDICATIONS TO TREAT

Acute HIV syndrome
Symptomatic patient
Asymptomatic patient with:
  CD4 < 500
  Viral load >10,000/mL

Figure 16-9.
Indications to treat. In asymptomatic patients, the treatment is dictated by patient acceptance and proof of adherence to the regimen.

A. METHOD OF GOODWIN AND DES PREZ

Normal host	Abnormal host
Mild exposure	Opportunistic
Usual Asx primary	Chronic pulmonary
Occ symptomatic	Structural
Asx symptomatic	Progressive disseminated
Heavy exposure	Immunologic
Acute pulmonary	Excess fibrosis
Primary	Histoplasmoma
Reinfection	Mediastinal fibrosis

Figure 16-10.
Classification of histoplasmosis. **A**, Method of Goodwin and Des Prez. **B**, Buckshot calcification as a result of prior pulmonary histoplasmosis. **C**, A schema showing correlations between degree of parasitization of the monocyte phagocytic system and pathologic and clinical manifestations of disease in disseminated histoplasmosis. The contrast between disease in infants and adults can be seen here. (*Adapted from* Goodwin and Des Prez [7].)

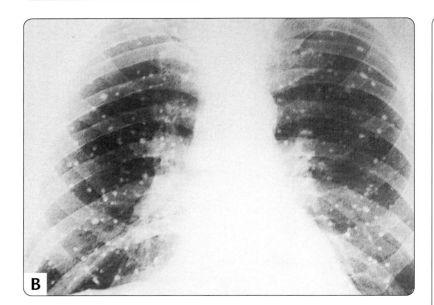

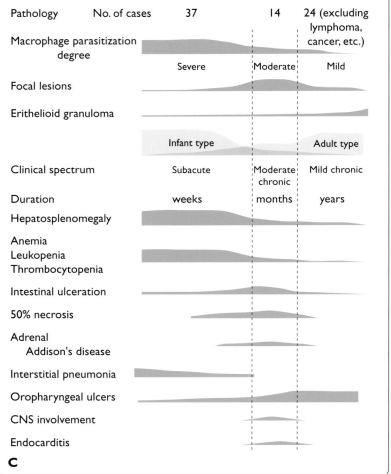

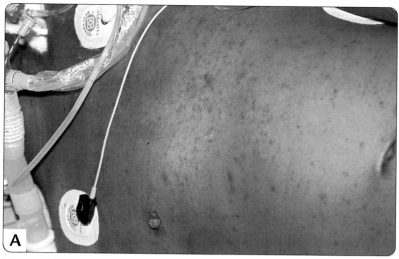

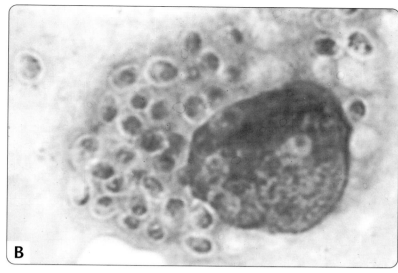

Figure 16-11.
Progressive disseminated histoplasmosis [7]. In Southeast Asia, patients infected with HIV have an illness caused by *Penicillium marnefeii*, which resembles histoplasmosis. Itraconazole is effective in this condition as it is in histoplasmosis. **A,** Patient with HIV and cutaneous manifestations of progressive disseminated histoplasmosis. (*See* color plate.) **B,** Organisms of *Histoplasma capsulatum* inside human macrophage. (*See* color plate.)

GUIDELINES FOR MANAGEMENT OF PATIENTS WITH HISTOPLASMOSIS, 2000

	Severe	Moderate
Acute pulmonary	AmB, steroids, then itra	None, itra if symptomatic 4 wk
Chronic pulmonary	AmB, then itra 12–24 mo	Itra 12–24 mo
Disseminated non-HIV	AmB, then itra 6–8 mo	Itra 6–18 mo
Disseminated AIDS	AmB, then itra life	Itra life
Meningitis	AmB 3 mo, then flucon 1 y	Same, because of poor prognosis
Granulomatous mediastinitis	AmB, then itra 6–12 mo	Itra 6–12 mo
Fibrosing mediastinitis	Itra 3 mo	Itra 3 mo
Pericarditis	Steroids	NSAID
Rheumatologic	NSAID	NSAID

Figure 16-12.
Guidelines for management of patients with histoplasmosis, 2000. AmB—amphotericin B; Flucon—fluconazole; Itra—itraconazole; NSAID—nonsteroidal anti-inflammatory drug. (*Adapted from* Wheat et al. [8].)

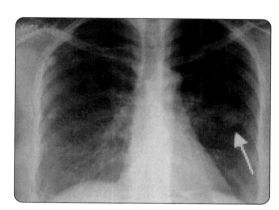

Figure 16-13.
Blastomycosis. Case report of a 42-year-old patient with AIDS and schizophrenia who lives in New Hampshire. He was on HAART, T/S, weekly azithromycin. He had 2 weeks of cough and sputum and a remote history of outdoor exposure, including eating beaver meat. The organism is *Blastomyces dermatitidis*. It is found in south central and southeastern United States. The lung is the primary site of infection with subsequent dissemination to skin, soft tissue, or other organ. (*Adapted from* Bradsher [9] and Pappas *et al.* [10].)

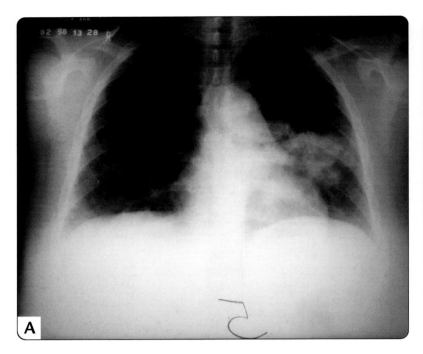

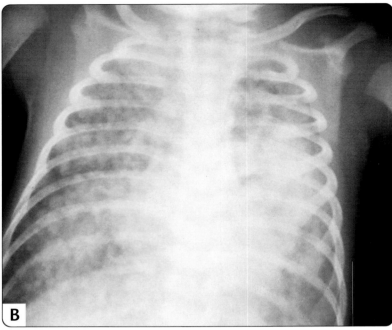

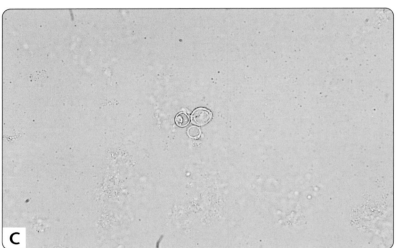

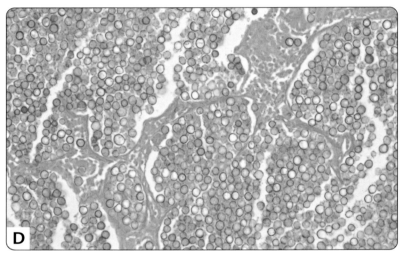

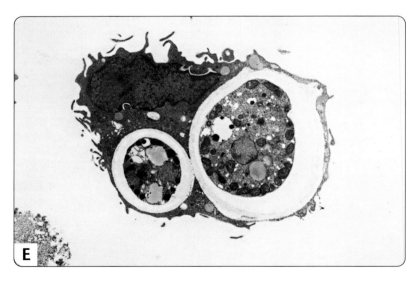

Figure 16-14.
A and **B**, Pneumonia caused by *Blastomyces dermatitidis* may present with an acute process, like bacterial pneumonia or ARDS, as in these two examples, or in a more chronic process resembling tuberculosis or malignancy. **C**, Sputum smear positive for organism by KOH preparation. (*See* color plate.) **D**, Lung biopsy positive for organisms by Methenamine silver stain. (*See* color plate.) **E**, Organisms are phagocytized by alveolar macrophages or peripheral macrophages. (*See* color plate.)

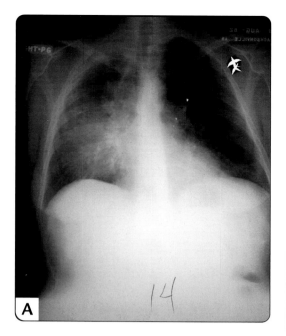

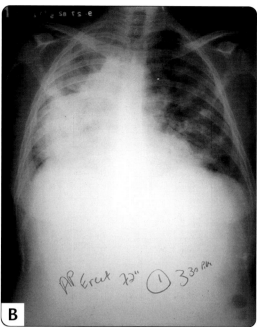

Figure 16-15.
Pneumonia with blastomycosis can progress, as in this patient, over a 3-week period. She previously had tuberculosis and apical pleural thickening. The right lung infiltrate spread from an alveolar process to widespread and bilateral pneumonia because she was noncompliant with therapy.

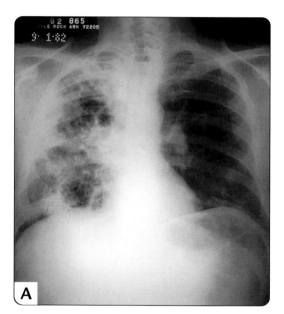

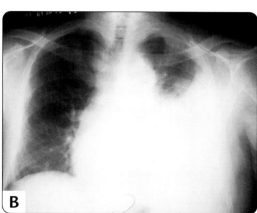

Figure 16-16.
Chronic pneumonia with blastomycosis may mimic cavitary tuberculosis or lung cancer with a mass-like lesion with effusion.

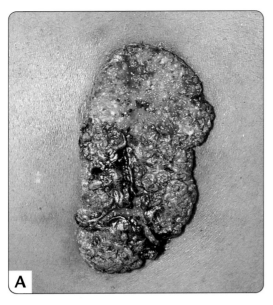

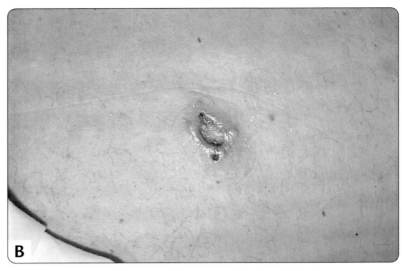

Figure 16-17.
Cutaneous blastomycosis: verrucous ulcerative. **A** and **B**, the most common extrapulmonary site of blastomycosis is the skin. Lesions may have a verrucous appearance or the roof of the lesion may slough to leave an ulcerative lesion. Microscopy of scrapings from the fungating lesion or the base of the ulcer will show the thick-walled, budding yeast cell after destruction of human tissue of KOH. (*See* color plates.)

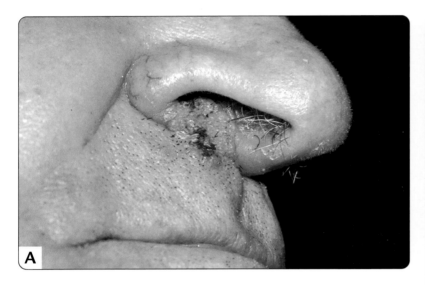

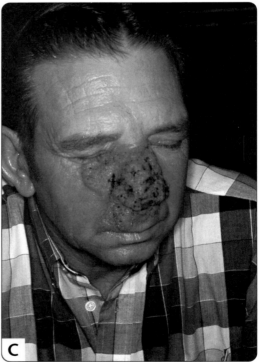

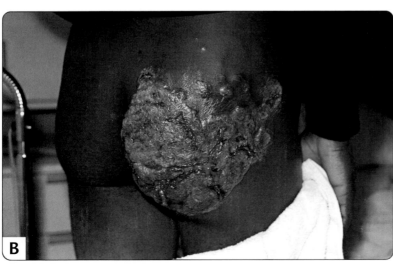

Figure 16-18.
Blastomycosis may present with a range: hardly noticeable lesions *(panel A)* to destructive and disfiguring sites of infection (panels B and C). (*See* color plates.)

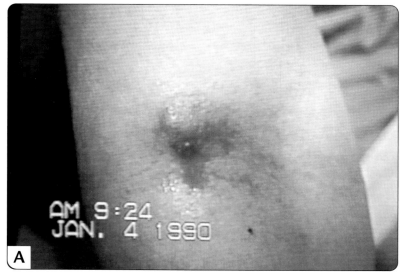

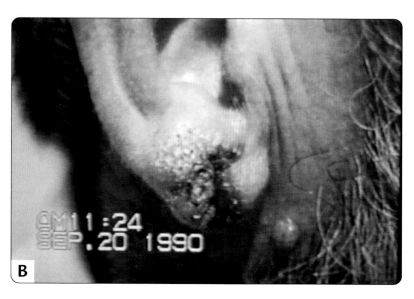

Figure 16-19.
Blastomycosis (disseminated). **A**, Patient who had improvement of his pulmonary blastomycosis with fluconazole therapy but developed this cutaneous lesion on his ear lobe. (*See* color plate.) **B**, Patient with multiple cutaneous lesions of blastomycosis who developed a site of dissemination at a venipuncture from the antecubital fossae 1 week prior. (*See* color plate.)

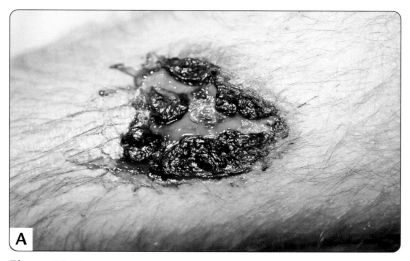

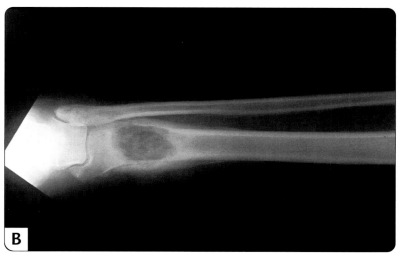

Figure 16-20.
A and **B**, Ulcers caused by blastomycosis may have a marked degree of exudate in the base or a relative lack of inflammatory cells. (*See* color plates.)

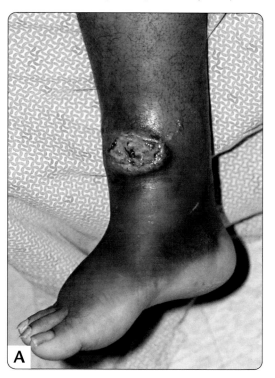

Figure 16-21.
A and **B**, Extrapulmonary blastomycosis can present in any organ in addition to the skin. (*See* color plate.) The next common involvement is bone followed by the genitourinary system and then by the central nervous system.

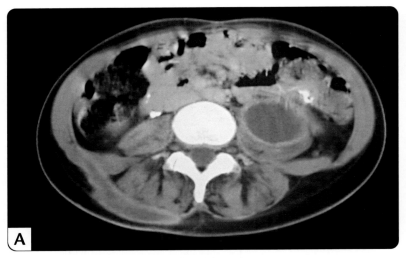

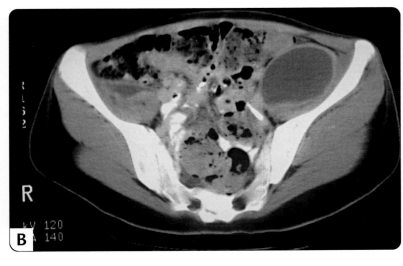

Figure 16-22.
Computed tomographic (CT) scan of woman with psoas abscess. This woman had a psoas abscess caused by *Blastomyces dermatitidis* that extended from her lumbar area down into her thigh. With CT-guided drainage and oral itraconazole, her infection was cured.

Figure 16-23.
Guidelines for management of patients with blastomycosis, 2000. AmB—amphotericin B; Flucon—fluconazole; Itra—itraconazole; ketocon—ketoconazole. (*Adapted from* Chapman et al. [11].)

GUIDELINES FOR MANAGEMENT OF PATIENTS WITH BLASTOMYCOSIS, 2000

Pulmonary	First-line	Alternate
Life threatening	AmB 1.5–2.5 g	AmB; itra when stable
Mild/moderate	Itra 200–400 mg/d	Flucon/ketocon
Disseminated		
CNS	AmB >2 g	?Flucon if intolerant
Non-CNS, severe	AmB 1.5–2.5 g	AmB; itra when stable
Non-CNS, mild/moderate	Itra 200–400 mg/d	Flucon/ketocon
Immunocompromised	AmB 1.5–2.5 g	Suppressive itra or flucon
Special circumstances		
Pregnancy	AmB	None
Pediatric	AmB or itra	?Flucon

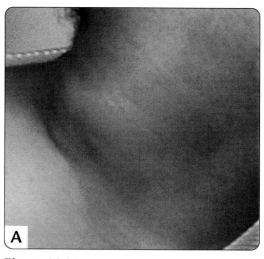

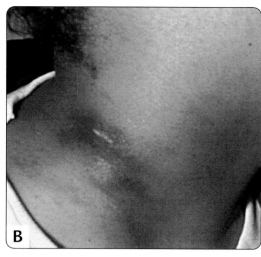

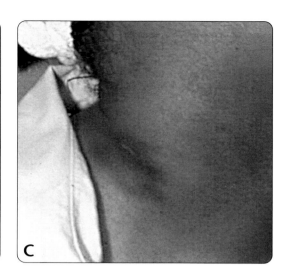

Figure 16-24.

Extrapulmonary blastomycosis treated with itraconazole [12]. This figure shows the rapid resolution of blastomycosis with oral itraconazole over 1 month. **A**, February 4, 1999. **B**, February 18, 1999. **C**, March 4, 1999. (See color plates.)

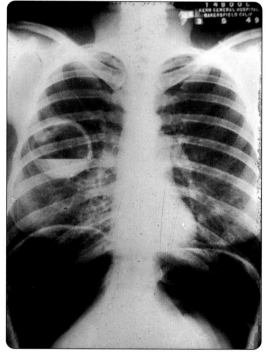

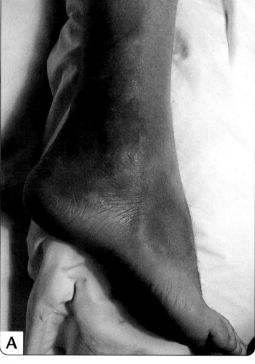

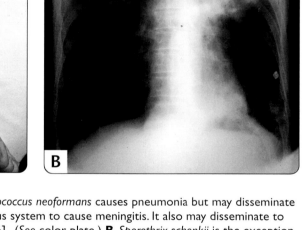

Figure 16-25.

Coccidioidomycosis is an endemic fungus that occurs in the Lower Sonoran Life Zone in areas that have alkaline soil with hot summers and mild winters and little rainfall [13–15]. Pulmonary involvement may be nodular or cavitary, typically with a thin cavitary wall, as in this radiograph from the CDC teaching files. Note the location of Bakersfield for the location of the patient.

Figure 16-26.

Cryptococcosis and sporotrichosis. **A**, *Cryptococcus neoformans* causes pneumonia but may disseminate to other sites, particularly the central nervous system to cause meningitis. It also may disseminate to the skin as in this renal transplant patient [16]. (See color plate.) **B**, *Sporothrix schenkii* is the exception to the other endemic fungi in that cutaneous inoculation is the primary means of infection. Pulmonary involvement with cavitary disease may be found after dissemination, particularly in patients with chronic lung disease [17].

Aspergillosis

Allergic bronchopulmonary

Invasive pulmonary

Aspergilloma (fungus ball)

Ulcerative tracheobronchitis

Semi-invasive

Disseminated: rhinocerebral, CNS, cutaneous, major organ

Treatment: amphotericin B, itraconazole

Hyalohyphomycosis

Nonpigmented septate hyphae

Fusarium, scedosporium, pseudallescheria

Clinical manifestations of fusariosis

Foreign body: contact lens, CAPD catheter

Localized: skin, nail, bone, brain

Disseminated: nodular skin, blood (60%)

Therapy: ?response to ampho B, surgery

Mucormycosis (phycomycosis)

Rhizopus, Mucor, Absidia, Cunninghamella

Risk factors of diabetes, neutropenia

Clinical manifestations

Sinus-rhinocerebral, necrotic, progressive

Lung-cavity, hemoptysis, ulcerative

Skin/wound trauma, burns, necrotic

Disseminated CNS, heart, kidney, gastrointestinal

Mycology: broad, nonseptate hyphae

Treatment: surgery, amphotericin B

Phaeohyphomycosis

Darkly pigmented septate hyphae

Curvularia, bipolaris, exoserhilum, alternaria, exophialia, drechslera, others

Clinical manifestations of Curvularia infection

Allergic: sinusitis (surgery)

Localized: skin, nail, lung, CAPD

Disseminated: heart, lung, CNS, deep abscess

Therapy: ampho B, surgery, itraconazole

Figure 16-27.

Aspergillosis, mucomycosis (phycomycosis), hyalohyphomycosis, and phaeohyphomycosis.

PENICILLIUM MARNEFEII

Immunosuppression: HIV, lymphoma

Southeast and East Asia

Clinical presentation similar to histoplasmosis

Skin, nodes, bone, joints, liver, spleen

Oval yeast with cross wall septation

Dimorphic at room/body temperatures

Therapy with amphotericin B or itraconazole

Figure 16-28.

Penicillium marnefeii [19–22].

REFERENCES

1. Manohar RF, Callaway DS, Phair JP, et al.: Persistence of HIV-1 transcription in peripheral-blood mononuclear cells in patients receiving potent antiretroviral therapy. N Engl J Med 1999, 340:1614–1622.

2. Kahn JO, Walker BD: Current concepts: acute human immunodeficiency virus type 1 infections. N Engl J Med 1998, 339:33–39.

3. Centers for Disease Control and Prevention: AIDS surveillance—trends. National Center for HIV, STD and TB Prevention: Divisions of HIV/AIDS Prevention Web site. http://www.cdc.gov/hiv/graphics/trends.htm. Accessed February 15, 2001.

4. Fauci AS: The AIDS epidemic—considerations for the 21st Century. N Engl J Med 1999, 341:1046–1050.

5. Kovacs JA, Masur H: Drug therapy: prophylaxis against opportunistic infections in patients with human immunodeficiency virus infection. N Engl J Med 2000, 342:1416–1429.

6. Goodwin RA Jr, Des Prez RM: Histoplasmosis. Am Rev Respir Dis 1978, 117:929–956.

7. Bradsher RW: Histoplasmosis and blastomycosis. Clin Infect Dis 1996, 22 (suppl 2):S102–S111.

8. Wheat J, Sarosi G, McKinsey D, et al.: Practice guidelines for the management of patients with histoplasmosis. Infectious Diseases Society of America. Clin Infect Dis 2000, 30:688–695.

9. Bradsher RW: Blastomycosis. Infect Dis Clin North Am 1988, 2:877–898.

10. Pappas PG, Pottage JC, Powderly WG, et al.: Blastomycosis in patients with the acquired immunodeficiency syndrome. Ann Intern Med 1992, 116:847–853.

11. Chapman SW, Bradsher RW, Campbell GD, Pappas PG, Kauffman CA: Practice guidelines for the management of patients with blastomycosis. Infectious Diseases Society of America. Clin Infect Dis 2000, 30:679–683.

12. Minamoto GY, Rosenberg AS: Fungal infections in patients with acquired immunodeficiency syndrome. Med Clin North Am 1997, 81:381–409.

13. Drutz DJ, Catanzaro A: Coccidioidomycosis. Am Rev Respir Dis 1978, 117:559–585, 727–771.

14. Stevens DA: Coccidioidomycosis. N Engl J Med 1995, 332:1077–1082.

15. Galgiani JN: Coccidioidomycosis: a regional disease of national importance. Ann Intern Med 1999, 130:293–300.

16. Kwon-Chung JK, Bennett JE: Cryptococcosis: P 397. In Medical Mycology. Philadelphia: Lea & Febiger; 1992.

17. Kaufman CA: Sporotrichosis. Clin Infect Dis 1999, 29:231–237.

18. Manns BJ, Baylis BW, Urbanski SJ, Gibb AP, Rabin HR: Paracoccidiomycosis: case report and review. Clin Infect Dis 1996, 23:1026–1032.

19. Duong RA: Infection due to Penicillium marneffei, an emerging pathogen: review of 155 reported cases. Clin Infect Dis 1996, 23:125–130.

20. Supparatpinyo K, Khamwan C, Baosoang V, Nelson KE, Sirisanthana T: Disseminated Penicillium marneffei infection in Southeast Asia. Lancet 1994, 344:110–113.

21. Chariyalertsak S, Sirisanthana T, Supparatpinyo K, et al.: Case-control study of the risk factors for Penicillium marneffei infection in human immunodeficiency virus-infected patients in northern Thailand. Clin Infect Dis 1997, 24:1080–1086.

22. Supparatpinyo K, Perrieus J, Nelson KE, Sirisanthana T: A controlled trial of itraconazole to prevent relapse of Penicillium marneffei infection in patients infected with the human immunodeficiency virus. N Engl J Med 1998, 339:1739–1743.

SARCOIDOSIS

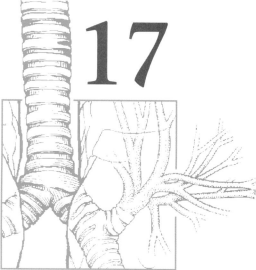

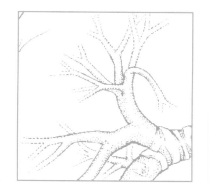

Robert P. Baughman

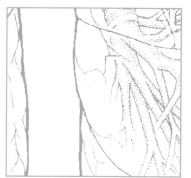

Sarcoidosis is a multisystem disease with a worldwide distribution. The hallmark of the disease is the presence of noncaseating granulomas [1]. The cause of sarcoidosis remains unclear, but several potential etiologies have been proposed. The disease seems to be caused by an environmental agent (infectious or noninfectious) that affects only certain individuals. The susceptibility and manifestation of the disease may be determined genetically.

The disease occurs most commonly in people 20 to 50 years of age, although at least one study suggests a second peak incidence in people older than age 60 [2]. It affects certain populations more frequently than others. These differences are based on more than investigator interest. A report from a clinic in London indicated a marked difference in the prevalence of the disease among racial groups [3]. The relative frequency of the disease appears to be lower in the United States than in Europe, although that may reflect incomplete reporting of the disease. In the United States, it appears more frequently in blacks than whites [4].

Genetic background appears to affect the disease manifestation. For example, erythema nodosum is more common among the Irish or Scandinavians than among blacks [3]. Other manifestations, such as lupus pernio and hypergammaglobulinemia, are more common among blacks and persons of West Indian descent than among whites [5]. Hypercalcemia and renal stones are more common among whites [6,7]. Cardiac disease appears far more frequently in Japan than elsewhere [8,9]. This does not mean that the disease always has a specific pattern in each group, but suggests that genetic disposition is important.

The diagnosis of sarcoidosis is one of exclusion. The initial evaluation should include a focused history and physical examination. Because the chest is involved in 90% of the patients, a chest radiograph is part of the initial evaluation. The findings of a chest radiograph can have several patterns. Scadding [10] proposed a staging system for the chest plain radiograph. It has proved useful for characterizing disease and for making a prognosis. Chest computed tomographic (CT) scans provide more detailed information. In most cases, CT patterns characteristic of sarcoidosis include perivascular thickening and adenopathy [11]. However, the increased cost does not warrant routine use of the CT scan in known cases of sarcoidosis.

Several clues indicating sarcoidosis may be available to the physician during a patient examination, including skin disease (especially lupus pernio), eye symptoms, a history of seventh nerve palsy, and a chest radiograph with findings that seem out of proportion with the patient's symptoms. Overall, sarcoidosis is a systemic disease. Consequently, the clinician is advised to consider the whole patient during evaluation.

The treatment of sarcoidosis remains controversial [12], especially because many patients with sarcoidosis never need therapy. Some manifestations of the disease clearly require treatment, including neurologic disease, cardiac disease, uveitis, and hypercalcemia. In these cases, therapy may be organ-sparing and sometimes life-saving. Treatment options for pulmonary disease are less clear cut [13,14]. Because some patients die as a result of pulmonary disease [15], lifetime therapy may be necessary for patients with severe pulmonary disease [16].

Given the toxicity of corticosteroids, steroid-sparing agents have been sought for some time [17]. Several have shown some benefit for patients with the disease. A recently proposed strategy for distinguishing acute versus chronic disease has been useful in directing therapy. Sarcoidosis is considered acute if it has been present for less than 2 years. There have been several predictors of chronic disease [7,18].

17

Steroid-sparing alternatives are most effective for patients with chronic disease. We have developed much experience with the use of methotrexate [19]. It has been used successfully with more than one third of the patients treated at our institution. A similar rate of response has been seen with azathioprine. Hydroxychloroquine has been associated with a lower response rate [20]; however, given the low toxicity of hydroxychloroquine and other antimalarials, these drugs should be considered for some patients with chronic disease. This is true especially for patients with easily measurable associated effects, such as hypercalcemia and skin lesions [21,22].

Thus, sarcoidosis is the most common disease of unknown etiology causing symptomatic interstitial lung disease. The clinician should consider it as part of the differential diagnosis of any pulmonary case that presents with evidence of infiltrates or adenopathy of unclear etiology. Looking for systemic disease will often yield evidence in support of the diagnosis. Although many patients do not require treatment, therapy should always be considered for the symptomatic patient. By following some simple rules, the clinician can minimize treatment-associated toxicity.

EPIDEMIOLOGY

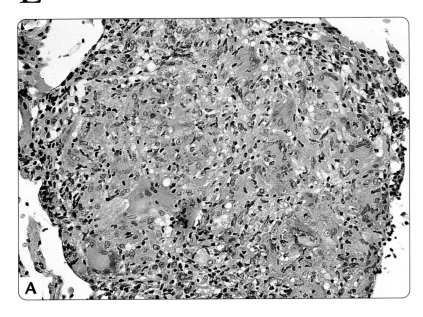

A

B. HOW SPECIFIC IS NONCASEATING GRANULOMA FOR SARCOIDOSIS?

In liver, granulomas are almost always noncaseating

In skin, noncaseating granulomas can represent a nonspecific reaction to foreign body (*eg*, splinter)

Not all granulomas are caused by sarcoidosis:
  Histoplasmosis
  Tuberculosis
  Cancer
  Lymphoma (especially Hodgkin's)

Figure 17-1.
Noncaseating granuloma as a sign of sarcoidosis. Sarcoidosis is characterized by noncaseating granulomas. **A**, Transbronchial biopsy specimen shows noncaseating granuloma. (*See* Color Plate.) **B**, Not all granulomas are caused by sarcoidosis [1].

SARCOIDOSIS IS A WORLDWIDE DISEASE

Country	Prevelance per 100,000
Sweden	500–1000
Ireland	300
Great Britain	
Irish immigrant	300
Londoner	10
West Indian	100
United States	
White	5
Black	80

Figure 17-2.
Relative incidence of sarcoidosis in Europe and United States.

RATE OF ORGAN INVOLVEMENT IN SARCOIDOSIS

Organ	Rate, %	Symptomatic, %
Lungs	90	60
Liver	50	10
Skin	30	20
Eyes	20	20
Heart	10	10
Central nervous system	15	10

Figure 17-3.
Rate of organ involvement by sarcoidosis. In some cases, patients may have organ involvement without symptoms.

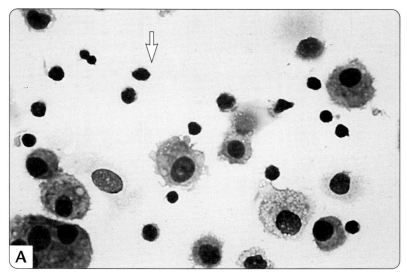

B. LYMPHOCYTES IN BRONCHOALVEOLAR LAVAGE

	Prednisone	Methotrexate
Lymphocytes		
Pretherapy	30+3.5%*	37+3.4%
Posttherapy	16+2.7%[†]	13+2.9%[†]
Change with therapy	12±3.2%	24±3.2%
CD4:CD8 ratio		
Pretherapy	7.3±1.52	7.4±2.69
Posttherapy	3.3±0.67	4.0±1.90

*Mean + SEM.
[†]Differs from pretherapy, P<0.001.

Figure 17-4.
Pathophysiology of sarcoidosis. Sarcoidosis is characterized by an increased number and level of activation of T-helper (CD4) lymphocytes in the area of disease activity [23,24]. This has been demonstrated most frequently by bronchoalveolar lavage (BAL). **A,** A cytocentrifuge-prepared BAL specimen from a patient with active sarcoidosis is shown. Normally, the lymphocyte (*arrow*) represents less than 10% of cells retrieved; in sarcoidosis, it can represent more than 50% of the recovered cells. (*See Color Plate.*) **B,** The figure indicates the percentage of lymphocytes and the CD4:CD8 ratio before and after 6 months of therapy with prednisone or methotrexate. Both drugs reduced the number of lymphocytes and relative percentage of helper T (CD4) cells [25].

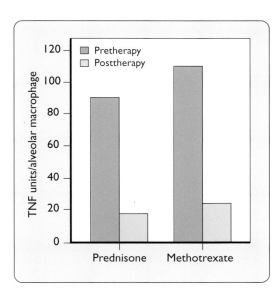

Figure 17-5.
Role of the immune system in sarcoidosis. Sarcoidosis results in activation of the alveolar macrophage [26]. Activation is indicated by the release of tumor necrosis factor (TNF) by macrophages retrieved by bronchoalveolar lavage in patients with active sarcoidosis. Alveolar macrophages from normal subjects do not usually release TNF [27]. TNF release levels decrease after therapy [25]. Both groups differ in pre- and posttherapy (*P* < 0.05).

A. MANIFESTATIONS OF SARCOIDOSIS

Manifestation	Examples
Minimal disease	Erythema nodosum
Mild single-organ involvement	Anterior uveitis
	Cough with normal pulmonary function tests
Generalized disease	Posterior uveitis
	Hypercalcemia
Chronic mild-moderate disease	Lupus pernio
	Chronic uveitis
Chronic severe disease	Pulmonary fibrosis
	Cardiac signs
	Neurologic signs
Refractory disease	Cor pulmonale
	Neurologic signs

Figure 17-6.

Manifestations of sarcoidosis. **A**, Certain complications are associated with specific degrees of severity of disease. The organ most commonly affected by sarcoidosis is the lung. **B**, A staging system has proved useful for describing patients with the disease and predicting its rate of resolution [10]. Also shown is the rate of resolution, *ie*, percentage of patients who develop a normal radiograph within 3 years of diagnosis. Finally, a differential diagnosis for each radiographic pattern is provided.

B. CHEST RADIOGRAPHIC STAGING SYSTEM

Stage	Description	Rate of resolution, %	Differential diagnosis
0	Normal	—	—
1	Hilar adenopathy	80	Fungal infection, tuberculosis, lymphoma
2	Nodes plus infiltrate	50	Tuberculosis, IPF, cancer, pneumoconiosis, PIE
3	Infiltrate alone	30	Same as stage 2 plus berylliosis, scleroderma, alveolar proteinosis
4	Fibrosis	0	Same as stage 3

IPF—idiopathic pulmonary fibrosis; PIE—pulmonary infiltrates with eosinophilia.

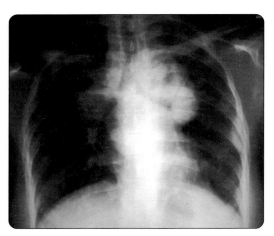

Figure 17-7.
Chest radiograph of a patient with stage 1 sarcoidosis with severe adenopathy.

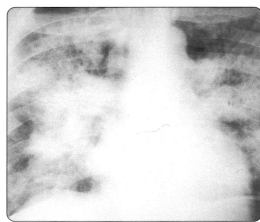

Figure 17-8.
Chest radiograph of a patient with stage 2 sarcoidosis with adenopathy and diffuse infiltrates.

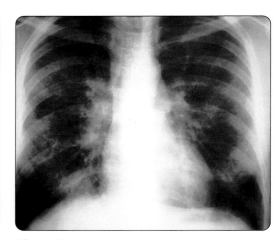

Figure 17-9.
Chest radiograph of a patient with stage 3 sarcoidosis.

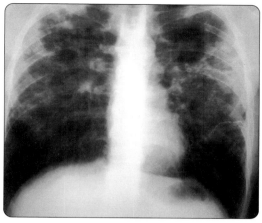

Figure 17-10.
Chest radiograph of a patient with stage 4 sarcoidosis with fibrosis. Sarcoidosis tends to cause upper-lobe fibrosis. Despite extensive fibrosis, this patient had no symptoms.

SARCOIDOSIS RESOLUTION WITHIN 2 YEARS OF DIAGNOSIS*		
Sarcoidosis involvement	Number[†]	Resolution, %
Erythema nodosum	210/251	84
Acute arthritis	148/178	83
Hilar adenopathy	334/458	73
Nodes plus infiltrate	77/150	51
Ocular	105/224	47
Heart	3/9	33
Central nervous system	19/77	25
Lupus pernio	5/33	15
SURT	3/21	14
Cor pulmonale	0/18	0

*n = 818 patients.
[†]Number resolving/number with condition.
SURT—sarcoidosis of upper respiratory tract.

Figure 17-11.
The manifestations of sarcoidosis. The rates of resolution of some symptoms of the disease within 2 years of diagnosis are shown [18]. Disease that is present longer than 2 years is considered chronic; patients with chronic disease may require long-term therapy.

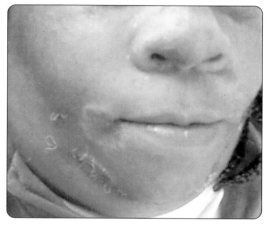

Figure 17-12.
Lupus pernio. The macular lesions also occur on the eyelids and spread across the bridge of the nose. This form of the disease is usually chronic. (*See* Color Plate.)

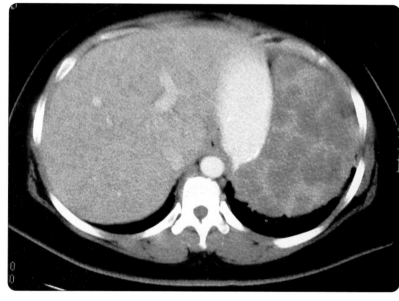

Figure 17-13.
Computed tomographic scan of the spleen of a patient with sarcoidosis. Liver and spleen abnormalities are often found in sarcoidosis. Increased liver function tests usually include increased alkaline phosphatase levels, but almost any abnormality can be seen [19,28]. The computed tomographic scan demonstrates the multiple defects in the spleen, which can be seen in sarcoidosis [29].

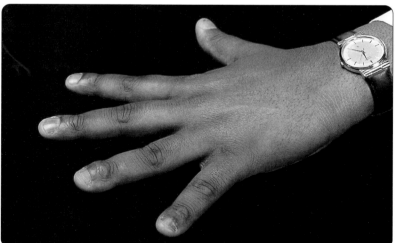

Figure 17-14.
Finger clubbing in a patient with sarcoidosis. Sarcoidosis can cause cystic changes in the distal phalanxes of the hands [30]. This is usually associated with chronic disease. In this patient, clubbing is most prominent on the fourth digit.

NEUROLOGIC MANIFESTATIONS OF SARCOIDOSIS

Manifestation*	Patients affected, n (%)†
Cranial nerves	
VII	24 (34)
VII plus other	15 (21)
I	1 (1)
II	7 (10)
III, IV, and/or VI	8 (11)
VIII	2 (3)
Diabetes insipidus	6 (8)
Seizure	5 (7)
Peripheral neuropathy	3 (4)
Dural invasion	2 (3)
Psychosis	2 (3)
Cavernous sinus thrombosis	1 (1)

*Patients may have more than one neurologic involvement.
†Number = percent positive of 71 patients with neurosarcoidosis (n = 71).

Figure 17-15.
Neurologic manifestations of sarcoidosis. Neurologic complications are significant for patients with sarcoidosis. Common manifestations of neurologic sarcoidosis seen with 71 patients at our institution are shown [31]. Other investigators have also found that the seventh cranial nerve is the most commonly affected nerve in patients with sarcoidosis [32,33].

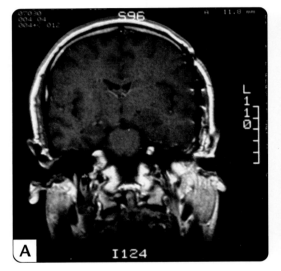

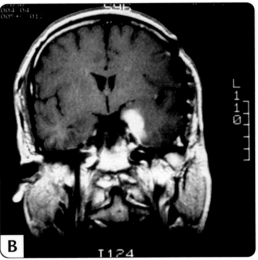

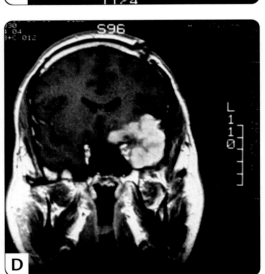

HEMATOLOGIC MANIFESTATIONS OF UNTREATED SARCOIDOSIS

Hematologic abnormality	Patients affected, n (%)
Anemia	21 (26)
Lymphopenia	41 (55)
Leukopenia	31 (41)
Eosinophilia	12 (16)
Monocytosis	9 (12)

Number of patients in study = 76.

Figure 17-17.
Hematologic manifestations of untreated sarcoidosis. Sarcoidosis causes many hematologic manifestations, as shown [35]. They occur through the replacement of bone marrow with granulomatous tissue [36]. Lymphopenia can occur through local sequestration of cells in the area of disease activity, such as the lung [24]. (From Lower et al. [35].)

Figure 17-16.
A–D, Magnetic resonance imaging scans of brain, demonstrating gadolinium uptake in a sarcoidosis mass. Magnetic resonance imaging with contrast has become the procedure of choice to demonstrate neurosarcoidosis [34]. The scan is positive for approximately 80% of patients [31,34]. The most diagnostic pattern is leptomeningeal uptake or hypothalamic disease.

DIFFERENTIAL DIAGNOSIS

COMPARISON OF SARCOIDOSIS, TUBERCULOSIS, AND HODGKIN'S LYMPHOMA

Sign/predisposing condition	Sarcoidosis	Tuberculosis	Hodgkin's lymphoma
Erythema nodosum	Common	Rare	Rare
Uveitis	Common	Rare	Unknown
Skin lesions	Common	Rare	Rare
Parotid enlargement	Present	Rare	Rare
Pleural disease	Rare	Common	Common
Hilar adenopathy	Common	Rare*	Common
Bone disease	Cysts in hands	Paget's of spine	Sclerotic changes
Elevated ACE	60%–80%	5%–10%	<1%
Corticosteroid therapy	Helpful	Harmful alone	May induce temporary remission

*In patients with HIV, bilateral adenopathy seen in tuberculosis.
ACE—angiotensin-converting enzyme.

Figure 17-18.
Comparison of sarcoidosis, tuberculosis, and Hodgkin's lymphoma. Patients with chest radiographs such as that shown in Fig. 16-7 present a common diagnostic dilemma. They can cause the clinician to consider several different diseases, including infectious granulomatous diseases (eg, tuberculosis) and malignancy (eg, Hodgkin's lymphoma). A method designed to help the clinician distinguish among the three groups is shown, although tissue for pathology and culture is the preferred method of diagnosis.

TREATMENT

THERAPIES PROPOSED FOR SARCOIDOSIS

None
Systemic steroids
Inhaled steroids
Methotrexate
Azathioprine
Hydroxychloroquine
Etanercept

Radiation
Thalidomide
Pentifylline
Chlorambucil
Cyclophosphamide
Cyclosporine
Infliximab

Figure 17-19.
Proposed therapies for patients with sarcoidosis. No therapy remains the best therapy for some patients with sarcoidosis. However, symptoms may lead the clinician to select one of the therapeutic regimens shown. Certain manifestations of sarcoidosis are considered definitive reasons for therapy; they include neurologic disease (other than facial nerve palsy), cardiac disease, posterior uveitis, and hypercalcemia.

TRIALS OF CORTICOSTEROIDS FOR PULMONARY SARCOIDOSIS

Study	Study design	Patients, n	Duration of therapy, mo	Duration of observation, y	Outcome
Israel et al. [37]	Randomized, double-blind	90	3	5.2	No difference
Selroos and Sellergren [38]	Randomized	39	7	4	Steroids helped only during treatment
Zaki et al. [39]	Randomized block, blind	183	24	3	No difference
Harkleroad et al. [40]	Randomized, double-blind	25	6	2, 15	No difference
Gibson et al. [41]	Randomized, double-blind	58	18	5	Steroids helpful
Emirgil et al. [42]	Nonrandomized	38	24	12	Corticosteroids helpful
Johns et al. [43]	Single-arm	153	>9	10	Steroids helpful
Stone and Schwartz [44]	Single-arm	37	3–9	6	No benefit from steroids
Sharma et al. [45]	Nonrandomized	43	12–36	6	No difference

Figure 17-20.
Effects of corticosteroids in patients with pulmonary sarcoidosis. The use of corticosteroids remains controversial in patients with sarcoidosis. A summary of several trials comparing steroids to placebo is shown. With the exception of one study [41], the double-blind randomized trials did not demonstrate a difference between the placebo and steroid treatment. Many open-label studies did find benefits for treated patients. (*Adapted from* Baughman et al. [12].)

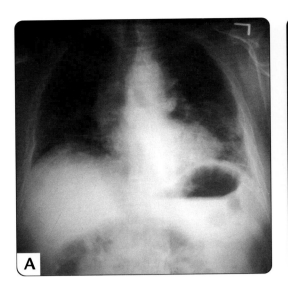

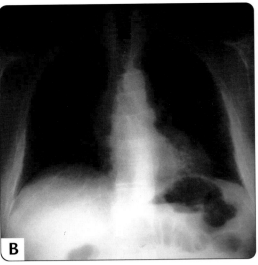

Figure 17-21.
A and **B**, Chest radiographs of a patient with sarcoidosis taken before (*panel A*) and after (*panel B*) corticosteroid therapy.

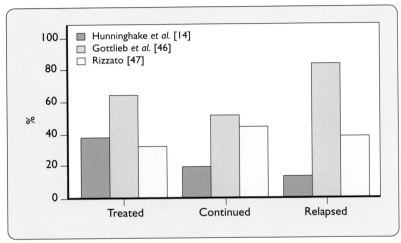

Figure 17-22.
The results of withdrawal of corticosteroid therapy in sarcoidosis. The results of corticosteroid therapy have been summarized recently by three groups reporting on all the patients treated at their centers. The figure summarizes the percentage of patients treated with corticosteroids (*treated*), the percentage who were continued on corticosteroids (*continued*), and the percentage who relapsed when therapy was stopped (*relapsed*). Although there was variation among the three groups, all of them found a significant number of patients who could not have corticosteroid therapy stopped or who relapsed when it was discontinued. (*Adapted from Rizzato [47].*)

RULES FOR TREATING SARCOIDOSIS

One is always giving too much or too little prednisone

Treat topically if possible

Once systemic steroids are started, they should be administered for at least 1 y (tapering the dose)

The dose to induce remission of symptoms is higher than the dose to maintain remission

Figure 17-23.
Rules for treating patients with sarcoidosis. The rules presented for treating sarcoidosis remain helpful guides to therapy.

SARCOIDOSIS TREATMENT BASED ON MANIFESTATION

Manifestation	Usual therapy	Alternative therapy
Minimal disease	None	NSAIDs
		Prednisone
Mild single-organ involvement	Topical steroids	Prednisone
		Hydroxychloroquine
		Pentoxifylline
Generalized disease	Prednisone	Methotrexate
		Hydroxychloroquine
		Azathioprine
Chronic mild-moderate disease	Prednisone	Methotrexate
		Azathioprine
		Hydroxychloroquine
Chronic severe disease	Prednisone	Methotrexate
		Azathioprine
		Chlorambucil
		Thalidomide
Refractory disease	Prednisone	Methotrexate
		Azathioprine
		Cyclophosphamide
		Cyclosporine
		Etanercept
		Infliximab

NSAIDs—nonsteroidal anti-inflammatory drugs.

Figure 17-24.
The proposed therapy for sarcoidosis based on manifestation of the disease. Some of the examples presented consist of well-established drugs, such as hydroxychloroquine and methotrexate. Others involve more controversial therapy, such as thalidomide, which has been reported in only a few cases.

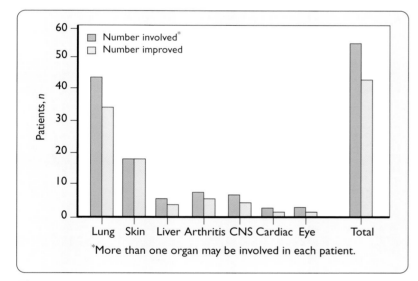

Figure 17-25.
Response to methotrexate therapy. We have used methotrexate extensively as a steroid-sparing agent in sarcoidosis. A summary of the response rate in 54 patients treated for at least 2 years with methotrexate is shown [19]. CNS—central nervous system.

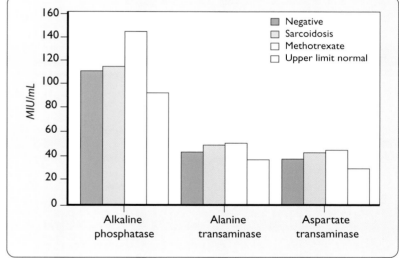

Figure 17-26.
Liver function abnormalities associated with methotrexate therapy. Liver biopsy specimens were obtained from 41 patients after 2 or more years of methotrexate therapy. Of these, 19 biopsy results showed normal tissue, 16 showed evidence of sarcoidosis, and six showed evidence of methotrexate toxicity. A summary of these liver function tests is shown [19]. The mean highest value for liver function tests was not significantly different for the three patient groups.

TOXICITY OF THERAPEUTIC ALTERNATIVES

Therapy	Nausea	Mucositis	Hematologic	Teratogenic	Carcinogenic
Methotrexate	Minimal	Occasional	Minimal	Occasional	None
Azathioprine	Occasional	Minimal	Occasional	Significant	Minimal
Cyclophosphamide	Significant	Minimal	Significant	Significant	Significant
Hydroxychloroquine	Minimal	None	None	None	None
Cyclosporine	Minimal	Minimal	Minimal	Occasional	Occasional
Thalidomide	None	None	None	Significant	None

Figure 17-27.
Summary of the usual toxicity in steroid alternative therapies. Methotrexate is also associated with hypersensitivity pneumonitis and hepatotoxicity. Hydroxychloroquine can also cause eye disease; routine eye examinations are recommended when using the drug. Cyclosporine is associated with significant toxicity; it was not useful in routine cases of sarcoidosis [48], but it has been reported as useful in some cases of neurosarcoidosis [49].

REFERENCES

1. Sheffield EA, Jones WW: Pathology. In *Sarcoidosis and Other Granulomatous Disease.* Edited by James DG. New York: Marcel Dekker; 1994:45–67.

2. Hillerdal G, Nou E, Osterman K, Schmekel B: Sarcoidosis: epidemiology and prognosis: a 15-year European study. *Am Rev Respir Dis* 1984, 130:29–32.

3. Honeybourne D: Ethnic differences in the clinical features of sarcoidosis in South-East London. *Br J Dis Chest* 1980, 74:63–69.

4. Keller AZ: Hospital, age, racial, occupational, geographical, clinical and survivorship characteristics in the epidemiology of sarcoidosis. *Am J Epidemiol* 1971, 94:222–230.

5. Goldstein RA, Israel HL: An assessment of serum protein electrophoresis in sarcoidosis. *Am J Med Sci* 1968, 256:306–313.

6. Goldstein RA, Israel HL, Becker KL, Moore CF: The infrequency of hypercalcemia in sarcoidosis. *Am J Med* 1971, 51:21–30.

7. Rizzato G, Fraioli P, Montemurro L: Nephrolithiasis as a presenting feature of chronic sarcoidosis. *Thorax* 1995, 50:555–559.

8. Hirose Y, Ishida Y, Hayashida K, et al.: Myocardial involvement in patients with sarcoidosis: an analysis of 75 patients. *Clin Nucl Med* 1994, 19:522–526.

9. Iwai K, Sekiguti M, Hosoda Y, et al.: Racial difference in cardiac sarcoidosis incidence observed at autopsy. *Sarcoidosis* 1994, 11:26–31.

10. Scadding JG: Prognosis of intrathoracic sarcoidosis in England. *Br Med J* 1961, 4:1165–1172.

11. Brauner MW, Grenier P, Mompoint D, et al.: Pulmonary sarcoidosis: evaluation with high-resolution CT. *Radiology* 1989, 172:467–471.

12. Baughman RP, Lower EE, Lynch JP: Treatment modalities for sarcoidosis. *Clin Pulm Med* 1994, 1:223–231.

13. DeRemee RA: The present status of therapy of pulmonary sarcoidosis: a house divided. *Chest* 1977, 71:388–393.

14. Hunninghake GW, Gilbert S, Pueringer R, et al.: Outcome of the treatment for sarcoidosis. *Am J Respir Crit Care Med* 1994, 149:893–898.

15. Baughman RP, Winget DB, Bowen EH, Lower EE: Predicting respiratory failure in sarcoidosis patients. *Sarcoidosis* 1997, 14:154–158.

16. Johns CJ, Zachary JB, MacGregor MI, et al.: The longitudinal study of chronic sarcoidosis. *Trans Am Clin Climatol Assoc* 1982, 94:173–181.

17. Baughman RP, Lower EE: Steroid-sparing alternative treatments for sarcoidosis. *Clin Chest Med* 1997, 18:853–864.

18. Neville E, Walker AN, James DG: Prognostic factors predicting the outcome of sarcoidosis: an analysis of 818 patients. *Q J Med* 1983, 208:525–533.

19. Lower EE, Baughman RP: Prolonged use of methotrexate for sarcoidosis. *Arch Intern Med* 1995, 155:846–851.

20. Baughman RP, Lower EE: Alternatives to corticosteroids in the treatment of sarcoidosis. *Sarcoidosis* 1997, 14:121–130.

21. Jones E, Cagen JP: Hydroxychloroquine is effective therapy for control of cutaneous sarcoidal granulomas. *Am Acad Dermatol* 1990, 23:487–490.

22. Adams JS, Diz MM, Sharma OP: Effective reduction in the serum 1,25-dihydroxyvitamin D and calcium concentration in sarcoidosis-associated hypercalcemia with short-course chloroquine therapy. *Ann Intern Med* 1989, 111:437–438.

23. Hunninghake GW, Crystal RG: Pulmonary sarcoidosis: a disorder mediated by excess helper T-lymphocyte activity at sites of disease activity. *N Engl J Med* 1981, 305:429–432.

24. Thomas PD, Hunninghake GW: Current concepts of the pathogenesis of sarcoidosis. *Am Rev Respir Dis* 1987, 135:747–760.

25. Baughman RP, Lower EE: The effect of corticosteroid or methotrexate therapy on lung lymphocytes and macrophages in sarcoidosis. *Am Rev Respir Dis* 1990, 142:1268–1271.

26. Pueringer RJ, Schwartz DA, Dayton CS, et al.: The relationship between alveolar macrophage TNF, IL-1, and PGE$_2$ release, alveolitis, and disease severity in sarcoidosis. *Chest* 1993, 103:832–838.

27. Baughman RP, Strohofer SA, Buchsbaum J, Lower EE: Release of tumor necrosis factor by alveolar macrophages of patients with sarcoidosis. *J Lab Clin Med* 1990, 115:36–42.

28. Maddrey WC, Johns CJ, Boitnott JK, Iber FL: Sarcoidosis and chronic hepatic disease: a clinical and pathologic study of 20 patients. *Medicine* 1970, 49:375–395.

29. Warshauer DM, Molina PL, Hamman SM, et al.: Nodular sarcoidosis of the liver and spleen: analysis of 32 cases. *Radiology* 1995, 195:757–762.

30. Rohatgi PK: Osseous sarcoidosis. *Semin Resp Med* 1992, 13:468–488.

31. Lower EE, Broderick JP, Brott TG, Baughman RP: Diagnosis and management of neurologic sarcoidosis. *Arch Intern Med* 1997, 157:1864–1868.

32. Sharma OP: Neurosarcoidosis: a personal perspective based on the study of 37 patients. *Chest* 1997, 112:220–228.

33. James DG: Differential diagnosis of facial nerve palsy. *Sarcoidosis* 1997, 14:115–120.

34. Miller DH, Kendall BE, Barter S, et al.: Magnetic resonance imaging in central nervous system sarcoidosis. *Neurology* 1988, 38:378–383.

35. Lower EE, Smith JT, Martelo OJ, Baughman RP: The anemia of sarcoidosis. *Sarcoidosis* 1988, 5:51–55.

36. Browne PM, Sharma OP, Salkin D: Bone marrow sarcoidosis. *JAMA* 1978, 240:43–50.

37. Israel HL, Fouts DW, Beggs RA: A controlled trial of prednisone treatment of sarcoidosis. *Am Rev Respir Dis* 1973, 107:609–614.

38. Selroos O, Sellergren TL: Corticosteroid therapy of pulmonary sarcoidosis. *Scand J Resp Dis* 1979, 60:212–215.

39. Zaki MH, Lyons HA, Leilop L, Huang CT: Corticosteroid therapy in sarcoidosis: a five year controlled follow-up. *NY State J Med* 1987, 87:496–499.

40. Harkelroad LE, Young RL, Savage PJ, et al.: Pulmonary sarcoidosis: long-term follow-up of the effects of steroid therapy. *Chest* 1982, 82:84–87.

41. Gibson GJ, Prescott RJ, Muers MF, et al.: British Thoracic Society Sarcoidosis study: effects of long term corticosteroid treatment. *Thorax* 1996, 51:238–247.

42. Emirgil C, Sobol BJ, Williams MHJ: Long-term study of pulmonary sarcoidosis: the effect of steroid therapy as evaluated by pulmonary function studies. *J Chronic Dis* 1969, 22:69–86.

43. Johns CJ, Zachary JB, Ball WC: A ten year study of corticosteroid treatment of pulmonary sarcoidosis. *Johns Hopkins Med* 1974, 134:271–283.

44. Stone DJ, Schwartz A: A long-term study of sarcoid and its modification by steroid therapy: lung function and other factors in prognosis. *Am J Med* 1966, 41:528–540.

45. Sharma OP, Colp C, Williams MHJ: Course of pulmonary sarcoidosis with and without corticosteroid therapy as determined by pulmonary function studies. *Am J Med* 1966, 41:541–551.

46. Gottlieb JE, Israel HL, Steiner RM, et al.: Outcome in sarcoidosis: the relationship of relapse to corticosteroid therapy. *Chest* 1997, 111:623–631.

47. Rizzato G: Long-term outcome of patients treated for sarcoidosis. *Sarcoidosis Vasc Diffuse Lung Dis* 1998, in press.

48. Wyser CP, van Schalkwyk EM, Alheit B, et al.: Treatment of progressive pulmonary sarcoidosis with cyclosporin A: a randomized controlled trial. *Am J Respir Crit Care Med* 1997, 156:1571–1576.

49. Agbogu BN, Stern BJ, Sewell C, Yang G: Therapeutic considerations in patients with refractory neurosarcoidosis. *Arch Neurol* 1995, 52:875–879.

INTERSTITIAL LUNG DISEASES

Joseph P. Lynch III &
Jeffrey L. Myers

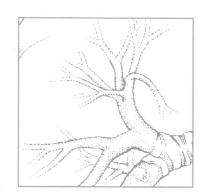
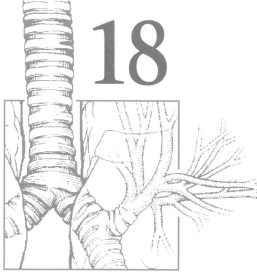
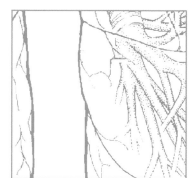

Interstitial lung disease (ILD) is a heterogeneous group of diseases characterized by a spectrum of inflammatory and fibrotic changes affecting alveolar walls and airspaces [1–13]. Clinical manifestations are protean, but progressive cough, dyspnea, parenchymal infiltrates on chest radiographs, loss of pulmonary function, and histopathologic features of inflammation and fibrosis in the lung parenchyma are characteristic [1,3,7,8].

Chest radiographs are often the first clue to the presence of ILD. Parenchymal infiltrates, cystic radiolucencies, nodules, or reduced lung volumes are present in most patients with ILDs. The distribution and pattern of radiographic lesions may suggest specific ILDs. Although chest radiographs are nonspecific, serial chest radiographs are invaluable in assessing chronicity or evolution of ILDs. In this context, review of old films is critical, even in patients with newly diagnosed ILD.

High-resolution computed tomographic scanning, using 1- to 2-mm thin sections of the lung parenchyma, more clearly demarcates honeycombing, cystic changes, alveolar opacities, and interstitial disease compared with standard chest radiographs [4,6]. There is no doubt that this imaging modality is far superior to conventional chest radiographs in depicting fine parenchymal details, identifying the nature and extent of the pulmonary disease, and discriminating end-stage fibrosis (*eg*, honeycombing) from potentially reversible disease.

More than 150 causes of ILD have been identified and include disorders in which specific agents or antigens are known (*eg*, pneumoconioses, asbestosis, silicosis, berylliosis, granulomatous infections, hypersensitivity pneumonia) and disorders in which the etiologic factors (or inciting stimuli) are unknown [8]. A discussion of these myriad disorders is beyond the scope of this chapter. A few ILDs, such as sarcoidosis, connective tissue disorders, pulmonary vasculitis, and bronchiolitis obliterans organizing pneumonia, are discussed elsewhere in this book. This chapter limits the discussion to a few rare ILDs, each of which has distinctive characteristics but shares overlapping clinical, radiographic, and physiologic features with other ILDs.

ETIOLOGY OF INTERSTITIAL LUNG DISORDERS

Known causes

Granulomatous infections
 (*eg*, tuberculosis, fungal infections)
Hypersensitivity pneumonitis
 (*eg*, farmer's lung, bird fancier's disease)
Malignant neoplasms
 (*eg*, lymphangitic carcinomatosis, lymphoproliferative
 neoplasms, bronchio-alveolar cell carcinomas)
Pneumoconiosis
 (*eg*, asbestosis, silicosis, berylliosis, hard metal
 pneumoconiosis)
Respiratory bronchiolitis (caused by cigarette smoking)
Toxic pneumonitis
 (*eg*, drugs, fumes, chemicals, radiation therapy)

Inherited causes

Hermanszky-Pudlak syndrome
Neurofibromatosis
Metabolic storage disorders
Hypocalciuric hypercalcemia
Tuberous sclerosis
Familial
 (*eg*, subsets of IPF, sarcoidosis)

Unknown causes

Bronchiolitis obliterans organizing pneumonia
IPF
Collagen vascular disease–associated
 pulmonary fibrosis
Eosinophilic granuloma
Eosinophilic pneumonia (chronic or acute)
Lymphangioleiomyomatosis
Pulmonary alveolar proteinosis
 (alveolar phospholipidosis)
Pulmonary vasculitis
 (*eg*, Wegener's granulomatosis, alveolar
 hemorrhage syndromes)
Sarcoidosis

IPF—idiopathic pulmonary fibrosis.

Figure 18-1.
Etiology of interstitial lung disorders.

DIAGNOSTIC EVALUATION OF INTERSTITIAL LUNG DISEASE

Careful occupational, exposure, drug, and family histories, and risk factors
Conventional chest radiographs (compare with old films)
Pulmonary function tests
 Spirometry, flow-volume loop, lung volumes, DLCO, oximetry (rest, exercise)
 Formal cardiopulmonary exercise tests (arterial cannulation) for selected patients
Serologies for selected patients (*eg*, collagen vascular disease profile, complement fixation
 for fungi, serum angiotensin-converting enzyme, hypersensitivity pneumonitis screen)
High-resolution thin-section computed tomographic scan
Lung biopsy for selected patients
 Fiberoptic bronchoscopy with transbronchial lung biopsies and bronchoalveolar lavage
 Video-assisted thoracoscopic lung biopsy (when fiberoptic bronchoscopy is
 nondiagnostic and no contraindications to surgical biopsy exist)

DLCO—diffusing capacity of lung for carbon monoxide.

Figure 18-2.
Diagnostic evaluation of interstitial lung disease. Idiopathic pulmonary fibrosis, a chronic lung disorder primarily affecting older adults, is characterized by cough, dyspnea, end-inspiratory velcro rales, diffuse parenchymal infiltrates on chest radiographs, hypoxemia, and a restrictive ventilatory defect on pulmonary function tests [11,14–16]. The need for lung biopsy depends on extent, severity, chronicity, and nature of the disease. The risks and benefits of biopsy and the therapeutic options available must be assessed carefully. In most patients, transbronchial lung biopsies and bronchoalveolar lavage are performed before considering video-assisted thoracoscopic surgery because a specific diagnosis can sometimes be made by transbronchial biopsies (eg, sarcoidosis, pulmonary alveolar proteinosis, malignancy, granulomatous infections), averting the need for surgical biopsies.

IDIOPATHIC PULMONARY FIBROSIS

HIGH-RESOLUTION COMPUTED TOMOGRAPHIC FEATURES OF IDIOPATHIC PULMONARY FIBROSIS

Typical findings

Predilection for the basilar and subpleural regions
Patchy involvement, with areas of intervening normal lung
Honeycomb cysts (4–20 mm in diameter)
Coarse reticular (linear) opacities; thick septal lines
Patchy ground glass opacities
Possible coexisting zones of emphysema in smokers

Late findings

Anatomic distortion, severe
 volume loss
Traction bronchiectasis or
 bronchiolectasis
Dilated pulmonary arteries

Figure 18-3.
High-resolution computed tomographic (HRCT) features of idiopathic pulmonary fibrosis. HRCT scans are superior to conventional chest radiographs in depicting the salient parenchymal aberrations (eg, honeycomb cysts, alveolar or reticular opacities, distortion) and demarcating the extent and distribution of the disease [4–6,9,17,18]. Salient HRCT features of idiopathic pulmonary fibrosis (usual interstitial pneumonia variant) are outlined here.

PROGNOSTIC VALUE OF HRCT PATTERN IN IDIOPATHIC PULMONARY FIBROSIS

Pattern of HRCT scans

Ground glass (alveolar) opacities

Usually associated with alveolitis and a favorable response to therapy

In some cases, ground glass opacities represent irreversible fibrosis involving intralobular and alveolar septae

Reticular pattern (intersecting fine or coarse lines)

May reflect fibrosis or inflammation

The prognosis of reticular or mixed ground glass/reticular patterns is less favorable than predominant ground glass patterns

Regression occurs with therapy in some patients

Honeycomb cysts

Indicates end-stage, irreversible fibrosis

Traction bronchiectasis, bronchiolectasis, and distortion also indicate irreversible fibrosis.

Extent of abnormality of HRCT scans

Quantitative scoring systems assessing the *extent* and *pattern* of HRCT have prognostic value

HRCT—high-resolution computed tomography.

Figure 18-4.
Prognostic value of high-resolution computed tomographic (HRCT) patterns in idiopathic pulmonary fibrosis. The extent of disease on HRCT correlates roughly with severity of functional impairment [15,18]. Specific HRCT patterns may discriminate early alveolar inflammation (alveolitis) from fibrosis and have prognostic value [15,17–19].

HISTOLOGIC PATTERNS OR VARIANTS IN IDIOPATHIC PULMONARY FIBROSIS

Usual interstitial pneumonia

Patchy, heterogeneous involvement; lack of uniformity

Minimal intra-alveolar component

Prominent interstitial inflammatory infiltrate

Destruction of alveolar walls

Fibrosis, honeycombing, destruction of the alveolar architecture

Desquamative interstitial pneumonia

Uniform process throughout all fields

Filling of the alveolar spaces with alveolar macrophages

Interstitial infiltration (less striking than usual interstitial pneumonia)

Prominent type II pneumocytes

Intact alveolar walls

Preservation of alveolar architecture

Mild or absent fibrosis or honeycombing

Nonspecific interstitial pneumonia/fibrosis

Foci of fibrosis and inflammation (intra-alveolar and interstitial)

Temporally uniform

Features overlap with usual interstitial pneumonia and desquamative interstitial pneumonia

Foci of bronchiolitis obliterans organizing pneumonia

± Collections of intra-alveolar macrophages

± Loosely formed granulomas

Acute interstitial pneumonia

Acute and organizing alveolar damage

Hyaline membranes

Fibrinous exudates

Epithelial cell necrosis

Interstitial and intra-alveolar edema

Figure 18-5.
Histologic patterns or variants in idiopathic pulmonary fibrosis (IPF). The histologic features of IPF include varying degrees of inflammation and fibrosis of alveolar walls and spaces, excessive collagen and extracellular matrix within the alveolar walls, fibroblastic foci, patchy involvement and temporal heterogeneity, areas of relatively uninvolved lung parenchyma, distortion or destruction of the alveolar architecture, reduced airspace volume, and honeycomb lung [20–22]. The term *usual interstitial pneumonia* [20] describes the typical histopathologic features seen in IPF. Other histopathologic variants have been described including desquamative interstitial pneumonia [19,20,23], nonspecific interstitial pneumonia/fibrosis [20,21,24–26], and acute interstitial pneumonia [27]. Whether these represent variants of IPF or distinct disorders is controversial. The extent of honeycombing or alveolar inflammation (cellularity) and specific histologic features or subtypes have prognostic value [20,24–26].

USUAL INTERSTITIAL PNEUMONIA

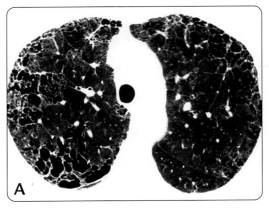

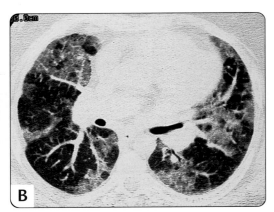

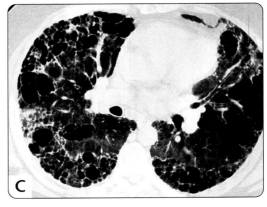

Figure 18-6.
High-resolution computed tomographic scans showing usual interstitial pneumonia. **A,** Thin section cuts from mid portions of lower lobes show focal honeycomb cysts distributed in a peripheral (subpleural) distribution. **B,** Thin section cuts from extreme bases of lower lobes of another patient show evidence of foci of alveolar opacification (ground glass) in a patchy distribution. No definite honeycomb cysts are evident. **C,** Thin section cuts from lower lobes of a third patient reveal extensive honeycomb cysts. Note the predominantly peripheral (subpleural) distribution.

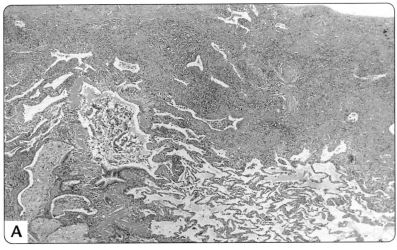

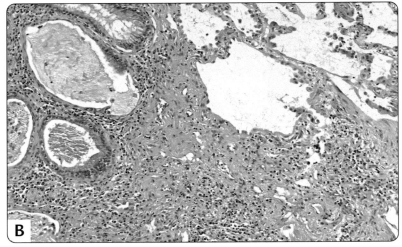

Figure 18-7.
Open-lung biopsy specimens showing usual interstitial pneumonia. **A,** Low-magnification photomicrograph shows patchy irregular interstitial thickening as a result of inflammation and fibrosis. The changes are accentuated in peripheral subpleural parenchyma and include areas of early honeycomb change. (*See Color Plate*). **B,** Higher magnification shows inflammation and fibrosis. The fibrosis includes dense eosinophilic collagen deposition and foci of fibroblast proliferation. An area of honeycomb change is present on the left and comprises cystically dilated fibrotic air spaces lined by bronchiolar-type epithelium.

DESQUAMATIVE INTERSTITIAL PNEUMONIA

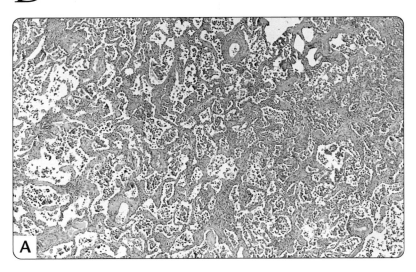

Figure 18-8.
Open-lung biopsy specimens showing desquamative interstitial pneumonia. **A,** Low-magnification photomicrograph shows uniform alveolar septal thickening, which is associated with prominent clusters of lightly pigmented alveolar histiocytes. (*See Color Plate.*)

(*Continued on next page*)

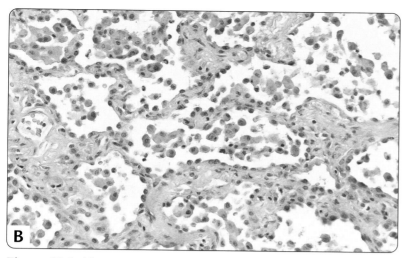

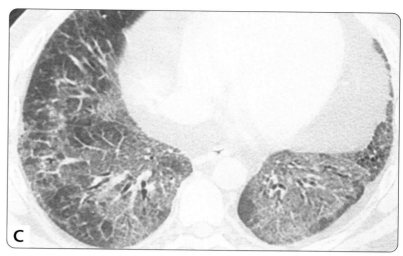

Figure 18-8. (*Continued*)
B, Higher magnification depicts relatively uniform alveolar septal thickening caused by mild inflammatory infiltrate, fibrosis, and hyperplasia of alveolar lining cells. Alveolar spaces contain lightly pigmented "smoker's"

macrophages. **C**, High-resolution computed tomographic scan shows desquamative interstitial pneumonia. Bilateral ground glass opacities are associated with minimal architectural distortion. (Panel C *courtesy of* Jeff Myers, MD.)

NONSPECIFIC INTERSTITIAL PNEUMONIA

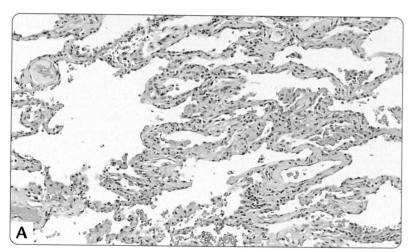

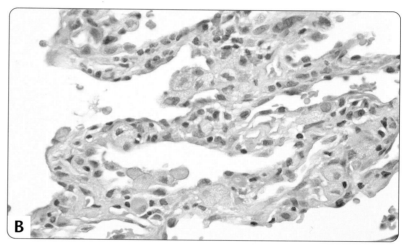

Figure 18-9.
Open-lung biopsy specimens showing nonspecific interstitial pneumonia. **A**, Low-magnification photomicrograph illustrates temporally uniform interstitial thickening. The pattern contrasts sharply with the more heterogeneous, variegated pattern seen in classic usual interstitial

pneumonia (*see* Fig. 18-7A). (*See* Color Plate.) **B**, Higher magnification shows uniform expansion of alveolar septa by a combination of inflammation and fibrosis in nonspecific interstitial pneumonia.

LYMPHOCYTIC INTERSTITIAL PNEUMONIA

ASSOCIATED DISORDERS OF LYMPHOID INTERSTITIAL PNEUMONIA

HIV infection (particularly infants and children)
Miscellaneous immunodeficiency or immunologic disorders
    Sjögren's syndrome
    Dysproteinemias (*eg*, hypogammaglobulinemia, monoclonal gammopathies)
    Allogeneic bone marrow transplant recipients
    Systemic lupus erythematosus
    Myasthenia gravis
    Common variable immunodeficiency syndrome
    Primary biliary cirrhosis

Figure 18-10.
Associated disorders of lymphoid interstitial pneumonia (LIP). LIP is a rare disorder characterized by dense infiltration of alveolar septa by small lymphocytes and plasma cells with relative sparing of airways [28–31]. LIP usually occurs in patients infected with HIV (particularly children) [28,30,31–33] and occurs less commonly in HIV-negative patients with diverse underlying immunologic disorders [28,29,32]. In HIV-negative patients, LIP affects adults older than 40 years of age and rarely affects children; women are affected twice as often as men [28,29].

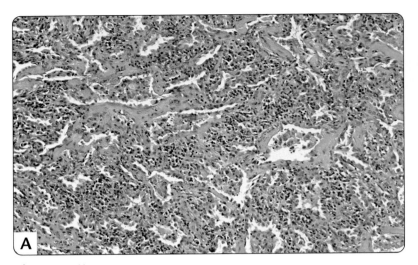

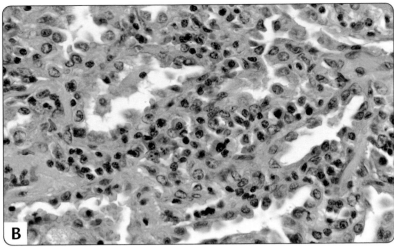

Figure 18-11.
Open-lung biopsy specimens showing lymphocytic interstitial pneumonia. **A,** Low-magnification photomicrograph presents an interstitium that is expanded markedly by a dense infiltrate of lymphocytes and plasma cells.

(*See Color Plate.*) **B,** Higher magnification shows dense alveolar septal infiltrate of lymphocytes and plasma cells.

HYPERSENSITIVITY PNEUMONIA

SELECTED CAUSES OF HYPERSENSITIVITY PNEUMONITIS

Disease syndrome	Source	Offending antigen
	Plant products	
Farmer's lung	Moldy hay or corn	Thermophilic actinomycetes
Ventilator lung	Air conditioner, humidifier	Thermophilic actinomycetes
Bagassosis	Moldy sugar cane	Thermophilic actinomycetes
Mushroom worker's lung	Moldy compost	Thermophilic actinomycetes
Hot tub lung	Mold on ceiling	*Cladosporium* spp
Suberosis	Moldy cork	*Penicillium* spp
Maple bark stripper's disease	Contaminated maple	*Cryptostroma corticale*
Malt worker's lung	Contaminated barley	*Aspergillus clavatus*
Tobacco worker's lung	Mold on tobacco	*Aspergillus* spp
Wine grower's disease	Mold on grapes	*Aspergillus* spp
Wood pulp worker's disease	Wood pulp	*Alternaria* spp
Japanese summer house hypersensitivity pneumonia	House dust	*Trichosporon cutaneum*
	Animal products	
Pigeon breeder's disease	Excreta or feathers	Avian antigens
Laboratory worker's lung	Rat fur	Rat urine protein
Pituitary snuff	Pituitary powder	Vasopressin
Miller's lung	Grain weevils in wheat flour	*Sitophilius granarius* proteins
	Reactive chemicals	
Toluene diisocyanate hypersensitivity pneumonia	Toluene diisocyanate	Altered proteins
Trimellitic anhydride hypersensitivity pneumonia	Trimellitic anhydride	Altered proteins

Figure 18-12.
Selected causes of hypersensitivity pneumonitis. Hypersensitivity pneumonia (also termed *extrinsic allergic alveolitis*) is a cell-mediated response to a variety of inhaled organic dusts or inorganic chemicals [34–38]. Exposure in the workplace environs (*eg,* agricultural or textile occupations), hobbies (*eg,* raising birds), or home (*eg,* humidifiers) may elicit the syndrome. The prototype of hypersensitivity pneumonia is "farmer's lung," caused by inhalation of thermophilic *Actinomycetes* spores from moldy hay, which occurs in 1% to 8% of exposed farmers [35,39,40]. Other syndromes elicited by thermophilic actinomycetes in occupational settings include air conditioner (humidifier) lung, mushroom worker's lung, and bagassosis [35]. In Mexico, domestic exposure to pigeon antigens (pigeon breeder's lung) is the most common cause of hypersensitivity pneumonia [41]. This occurs in 6% to 15% of pigeon breeders [35,41]. More than 50 different occupational and environmental sources of antigen associated with hypersensitivity pneumonia have been described [36,37]. (*Adapted from* Curtis and Schuyler [13].)

DISCRIMINATING CHRONIC HYPERSENSITIVITY PNEUMONIA FROM IPF USING HRCT

HRCT feature	Chronic hypersensitivity pneumonia, n (%) (n=19)	IPF, n (%) (n=32)
Honeycombing	3 (16)	29 (88)
Micronodules	8 (42)	2 (6)
Extensive ground glass opacities	6 (32)	4 (12)
Lower lobe predominance	8 (42)	27 (81)
Peripheral predominance	10 (53)	30 (91)

HRCT—high-resolution computed tomography; IPF—idiopathic pulmonary fibrosis.

Figure 18-13.
Discriminating chronic hypersensitivity pneumonia from idiopathic pulmonary fibrosis using high-resolution computed tomography. Although chronic hypersensitivity pneumonia overlaps with idiopathic pulmonary fibrosis in clinical, physiologic, and radiographic features, high-resolution computed tomography may assist in differentiating these conditions. (*Adapted from* Lynch et al. [34].)

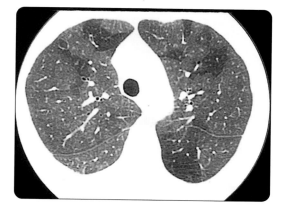

Figure 18-14.
High-resolution computed tomographic scan showing hypersensitivity pneumonitis. A mosaic pattern of attenuation is accompanied by small centrilobular nodules. Salient high-resolution computed tomographic features in hypersensitivity pneumonitis include micronodules, ground glass opacities, a peribronchiolar distribution, a predilection for mid or upper lung zones, and variable areas of attenuation [40,42]. Bronchial obstruction may cause patchy areas of hyperlucency in a lobular distribution [40,42]. With end-stage disease, fibrosis and areas of emphysema may be observed [34,39,40].

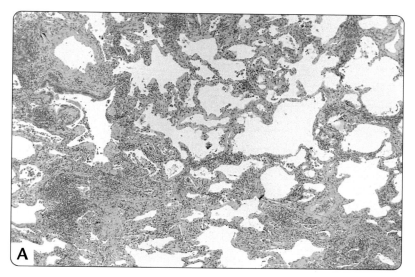

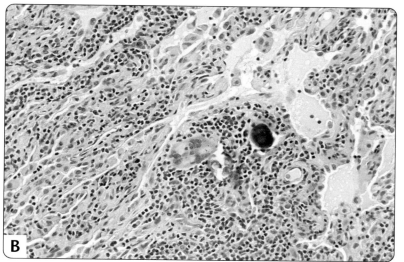

Figure 18-15.
Open-lung biopsy specimens showing hypersensitivity pneumonia (extrinsic allergic alveolitis). **A,** Low-magnification photomicrograph shows a patchy, cellular interstitial pneumonia accentuated around bronchioles. (*See Color Plate.*) **B,** Higher magnification shows a combination of lymphocytes and isolated multinucleated giant cells in hypersensitivity pneumonia. The giant cells contain a variety of nonspecific calcified and noncalcified cytoplasmic inclusions.

CHRONIC EOSINOPHILIC PNEUMONIA

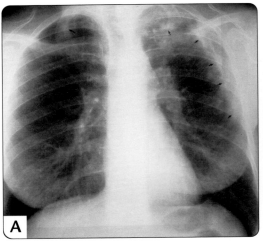

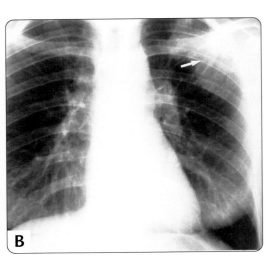

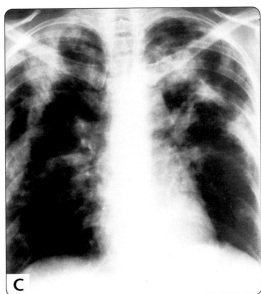

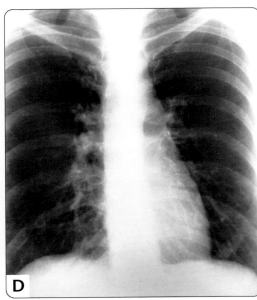

Figure 18-16.
Chronic eosinophilic pneumonia [43–46].
A, Postero-anterior chest radiograph from a 37-year-old woman demonstrates focal peripheral alveolar infiltrates (*arrows*). Transbronchial lung biopsies showed aggregates of eosinophils and scattered multinucleated giant cells. Symptoms and chest radiographs normalized with corticosteroid therapy. **B,** Posteroanterior chest radiograph from the same patient 5 years later demonstrates a peripheral alveolar infiltrate in the apical region of the left upper lobe (*arrow*). Symptoms of cough, malaise, and wheezing improved promptly, and chest radiographs normalized with intensification of corticosteroid therapy. **C,** Postero-anterior chest radiograph from a 33-year-old woman with dyspnea, wheezing, and blood eosinophilia demonstrates focal alveolar infiltrates. Fiberoptic bronchoscopy with bronchoalveolar lavage (BAL) revealed intense BAL eosinophilia (>30%). Prednisone 60 mg/d was initiated. **D,** Posteroanterior chest radiograph from the same patient 5 days later demonstrates nearly complete resolution of infiltrates. (Panel B *from* Lynch and Flint [46]; with permission.)

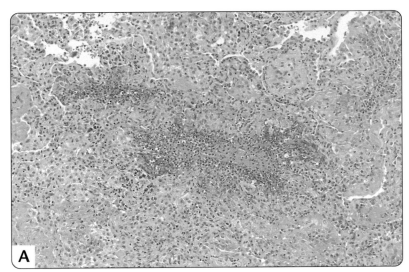

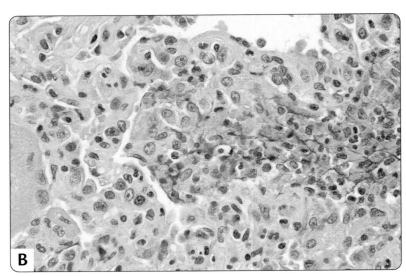

Figure 18-17.
Open-lung biopsy specimens showing chronic eosinophilic pneumonia. **A,** Low-magnification photomicrograph depicts a partially necrotic air space exudate. The necrotic zones represent eosinophilic abscesses, a finding characteristic of chronic eosinophilic pneumonia. (*See Color Plate.*) **B,** Higher magnification photomicrograph shows an air space exudate of eosinophils and histiocytes.

PULMONARY ALVEOLAR PROTEINOSIS

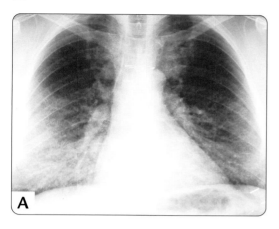

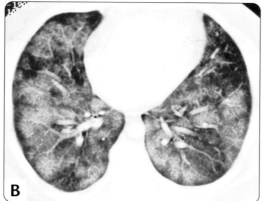

Figure 18-18.
Pulmonary alveolar proteinosis [47]. **A,** Postero-anterior chest radiograph demonstrates bilateral, predominantly basilar, alveolar infiltrates in a 50-year-old man with progressive exertional dyspnea. **B,** Computed tomographic scan from the same patient shows multiple foci of ground glass opacification throughout the lung parenchyma. Open-lung biopsy demonstrated classic features of pulmonary alveolar proteinosis. (*From* Lynch and Raghu [3]; with permission.)

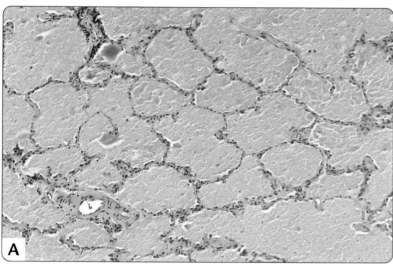

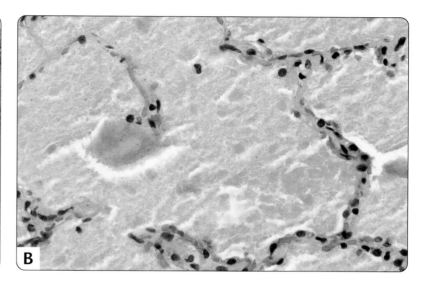

Figure 18-19.
Open-lung biopsy specimens showing pulmonary alveolar proteinosis. **A,** Photomicrograph demonstrates complete filling of alveolar spaces with a dense proteinaceous exudate. The alveolar architecture is preserved.

(*See* Color Plate.) **B,** Higher magnification photomicrograph shows characteristic air space exudate and relatively normal alveolar septa.

EOSINOPHILIC GRANULOMA

DIFFERENTIAL DIAGNOSIS OF CYSTIC LESIONS ON HIGH-RESOLUTION COMPUTED TOMOGRAPHY

	Pulmonary eosinophilic granuloma	Lymphangioleiomyomatosis	Usual interstitial pneumonia/ idiopathic pulmonary fibrosis
Cysts	Thin-walled; often regular in size	Thin-walled; often regular in size; may coalesce	Less-defined walls; variable size
Location	Upper, midlung zones; peribronchiolar; subpleural; spare costophrenic angles	Uniform; all lobes	Peripheral (subpleural); bibasilar; patchy, heterogeneous
Associated findings	Peribronchiolar nodules	Lack nodules	Reticular or alveolar opacities; distortion; traction bronchiolectasis

Figure 18-20.
Differential diagnosis of cystic lesions on high-resolution computed tomography. Cysts are highly characteristic of pulmonary eosinophilic granuloma, lymphangioleiomyomatosis, and usual interstitial pneumonia but may be seen in any chronic lung disorder that destroys alveolar walls and distorts the alveolar architecture. Honeycomb cysts may be observed in advanced cases of pulmonary sarcoidosis, chronic hypersensitivity pneumonitis, granulomatous infections, and so forth. In some cases, associated features may depict the underlying nature of the disorder. For example, upper lobe predominance, a predilection for central bronchovascular bundles and lymphatics, concomitant nodules, alveolar opacities, distortion, or hilar or mediastinal lymphadenopathy may be clues to the diagnosis of sarcoidosis. In chronic obstructive pulmonary disease caused by cigarette smoking, emphysematous "cysts" are more irregular in size, lack well-formed walls, and are more extensive in the upper lobes.

HISTOLOGIC FEATURES OF PULMONARY EOSINOPHILIC GRANULOMA

Combination of cystic, nodular, and fibrotic lesions

Bronchocentric distribution

Intervening zones of normal lung parenchyma

Stellate pattern of fibrosis (low-power magnification)

Cellular granulomatous lesions (high-power magnification)

Proliferation of atypical histiocytes (Langerhans' cells)

    Moderately large, ovoid histiocytes

    Pale eosinophilic cytoplasm

    Indented (grooved nuclei), inconspicuous nucleoli

    Positive staining for S100 protein or common thymocyte antigen (OKT6)

    Intracytoplasmic rod- or racquet-shape inclusions 42–45 nm in thickness (electron microscopy)

Destruction of bronchioles and alveolar parenchyma

Blebs, subpleural cysts, honeycomb lung (late features)

Figure 18-21.
Histologic features of pulmonary eosinophilic granuloma. Histologically, pulmonary eosinophilic granuloma is characterized by inflammatory, cystic, nodular, and fibrotic lesions distributed in a bronchocentric fashion [48,49]. Langerhans' cells (also termed *histiocytosis X cells*), are the cornerstone of the diagnosis. Langerhans' cells can usually be identified by hematoxylin-eosin stains. In equivocal cases, immunohistochemical stains (eg, S100 protein or common thymocyte antigen [OKT6]) may substantiate the identity of Langerhans' cells.

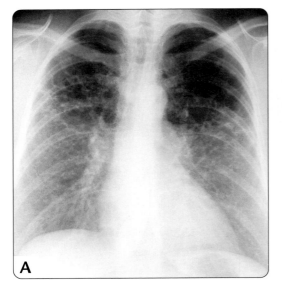
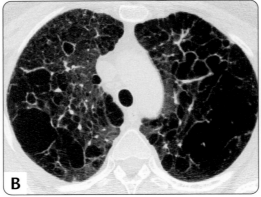
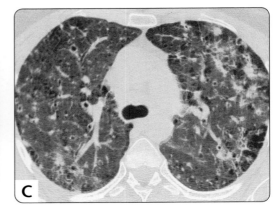

Figure 18-22.
Eosinophilic granuloma. **A,** Posteroanterior chest radiograph demonstrates diffuse reticular and cystic changes. Note the upper lobes are hyperlucent, reflecting extensive cystic destruction of the lung parenchyma. **B,** High-resolution computed tomographic scan from the same patient illustrates cuts from the upper lobes, which demonstrate multiple cystic spaces, with coalescence, reflecting destruction of alveolar walls. A nodular component is not obvious. **C,** High-resolution computed tomographic scan from the same patient (lower lobes) reveals multiple well-defined cystic spaces. In addition, peribronchiolar infiltrates and a slight nodular component is evident.

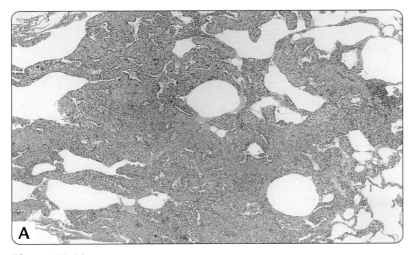
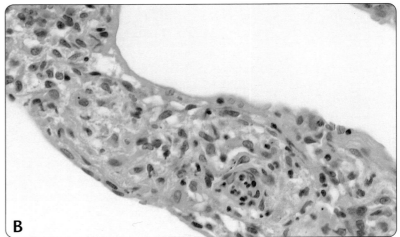

Figure 18-23.
Open-lung biopsy specimens showing eosinophilic granuloma. **A,** Low-magnification photomicrograph shows stellate bronchiolocentric nodule. There is associated paracictricial airspace enlargement ("scar emphysema"), which accounts for the frequent finding of cystic change. (*See Color Plate.*)

B, Higher magnification photomicrograph shows a polymorphic inflammatory infiltrate in eosinophilic granuloma, which includes diagnostic Langerhans' cells with highly convoluted nuclear contours. (*See Color Plate.*)

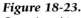

LYMPHANGIOLEIOMYOMATOSIS

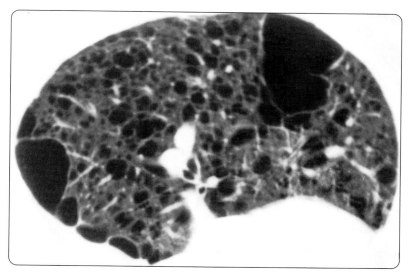

Figure 18-24.
High-resolution computed tomographic scan in a 44-year-old woman with lymphangioleiomyomatosis demonstrating multiple, thin-walled cystic radiolucencies bilaterally [50–52]. Note the two large lesions, representing confluent cysts. (*From* Lynch and Raghu [3]; with permission.)

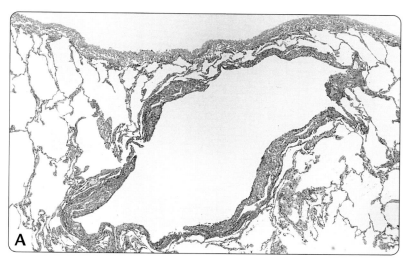

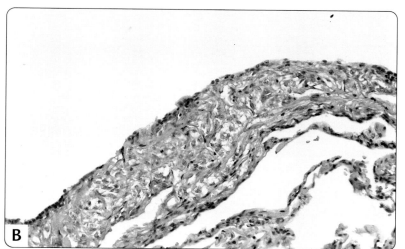

Figure 18-25.
Open-lung biopsy specimens showing lymphangioleiomyomatosis. **A**, Low-magnification photomicrograph illustrates characteristic cyst in lymphangioleiomyomatosis. (*See* Color Plate.) **B**, Higher magnification photomicrograph shows characteristic smooth muscle cells in lymphangioleiomyomatosis. (*See* Color Plate.)

REFERENCES

1. Crystal RG, Bitterman PB, Rennard LI, *et al.*: Interstitial lung diseases of unknown cause: disorders characterized by chronic inflammation of the lower respiratory tract. *N Engl J Med* 1984, 310:154–166, 235–244.

2. Corrin B: Pathology of interstitial lung disease. *Semin Respir Crit Care Med* 1994, 15:61–76.

3. Lynch JP III, Raghu G: Major disease syndromes of unknown etiology. In *Textbook of Pulmonary Diseases,* edn 6. Edited by Baum GA. Boston: Little, Brown Publishers; 1998:431–476.

4. Colby TV, Swensen SJ: Anatomic distribution and histopathologic patterns in diffuse lung disease: correlation with HRCT. *J Thorac Imaging* 1996, 11:1–26.

5. Grenier P, Chevret S, Beigelman C, *et al.*: Chronic diffuse infiltrative lung disease: determination of the diagnostic value of clinical data, chest radiography, and CT with Bayesian analysis. *Radiology* 1994, 191:383–390.

6. Raghu G: Interstitial lung disease, a diagnostic approach: Are CT scan and lung biopsy indicated in every patient? *Am J Respir Crit Care Med* 1995, 151:909–914.

7. Coultas DB, Zumwalt RE, Black WC, Sobonya RE: The epidemiology of interstitial lung diseases. *Am J Respir Crit Care Med* 1994, 150:967–972.

8. Mapel DW, Coultas DB: The environmental epidemiology of idiopathic interstitial lung disease including sarcoidosis. *Semin Respir Crit Care Med* 1999, 20:521–529.

9. Johkoh T, Muller NL, Cartier Y, *et al.*: Idiopathic interstitial pneumonias: diagnostic accuracy of thin-section CT in 129 patients. *Radiology* 1999, 211:555–560.

10. Beckett WS: Occupational respiratory diseases. *N Engl J Med* 2000, 342:406–413.

11. American Thoracic Society and European Respiratory Society: Idiopathic pulmonary fibrosis: diagnosis and treatment. International Consensus Statement. *Am J Respir Crit Care Med* 2000,161:646–664.

12. British Thoracic Society and Standrads of Care Committee: The diagnosis, assessment, and treatment of diffuse parenchymal lung disease in adults. Thorax 1999, 54(suppl 1):S1–S30.

13. Curtis JL, Schuyler M: Immmunologically mediated lung diseases. In *Textbook of Pulmonary Diseases.* Edited by Baum G, Crapo J, Celli B, Karlinsky J. Philadelphia: Lippincott-Raven; 1998, 1:367–406.

14. Lynch JP III, Toews GB: Idiopathic pulmonary fibrosis. In *Textbook of Pulmonary Diseases and Disorders,* edn 3. Edited by Fishman A. New York: McGraw Hill; 1997:1193–1210.

15. Wells AU: Clinical usefulness of high resolution computed tomography in cryptogenic fibrosing alveolitis. Thorax 1998, 53:1080–1087.

16. Douglas WW, Rhy JH, Schroeder DR: Idiopathic pulmonary fibrosis: impact of oxygen and colchicine, prednisone, or no therapy on survival. *Am J Respir Crit Care Med* 2000, 161:1172–1178.

17. Gay SE, Kazerooni EA, Toews GB, Lynch JP III, *et al.*: Idiopathic pulmonary fibrosis: predicting response to therapy and survival. *Am J Respir Crit Care Med* 1998, 157:1063–1072.

18. Wells AU, King AD, Rubens MB, Cramer D, du Bois RM, Hansell DM: Lone cryptogenic fibrosing alveolitis: a functional-morphologic correlation based on extent of disease on thin section computed tomography. *Am J Respir Crit Care Med* 1997, 155:1367–1375.

19. Hartman TE, Primack SL, Swensen SJ, Hansell D: Desquamative interstitial pneumonia: thin-section CT findings in 22 patients. *Radiology* 1993, 187:787–790.

20. Katzenstein AL, Myers J: Idiopathic pulmonary fibrosis: clinical relevance of pathological classification. *Am J Respir Crit Care Med* 1998, 157:1301–1315.

21. Nicholson AG, Colby TV, duBois RM, Hansell DM, Wells AU: The prognostic significance of the histologic pattern of interstitial pneumonia in patients presenting with the clinical entity of cryptogenic fibrosing alveolitis. *Am J Respir Crit Care Med* 2000, 162:2213–2217.

22. Travis WD, Matsui K, Moss J, et al.: Idiopathic nonspecific interstitial pneumonia: prognostic significance of cellular and fibrosing patterns: survival comparison with usual interstitial pneumonia and desquamative interstitial pneumonia. *Am J Surg Pathol* 2000, 24:19–33.

23. Moon J, du Bois RM, Colby TV, et al.: Clinical significance of respiratory bronchiolitis on open lung biopsy and its relationship to smoking-related interstitial lung disease. *Thorax* 1999, 54:1009–1114.

24. Bjoraker JA, Ryu JH, Edwin MK, et al.: Prognostic significance of histopathological subsets in idiopathic pulmonary fibrosis. *Am J Respir Crit Care Med* 1998, 157:199–203.

25. Nagai S, Kitaichi M, Itoh H, et al.: Idiopathic nonspecific interstitial pneumonia/fibrosis: comparison with idiopathic pulmonary fibrosis and BOOP. *Eur Respir J* 1998, 12:1010–1019.

26. Daniil ZD, Gilchrist FC, Nicholson AG, et al.: A histological pattern of nonspecific interstitial pneumonia is associated with a better prognosis than usual interstitial pneumonia in patients with cryptogenic fibrosing alveolitis. *Am J Respir Crit Care Med* 1999, 160:899–905.

27. Vourlekis JS, Brown KK, Cool CD, et al.: Acute interstitial pneumonitis: Case series and review of the literature. *Medicine* 2000, 79:369.

28. Schneider RF: Lymphocytic interstitial pneumonitis and nonspecific interstitial pneumonitis. *Clin Chest Med* 1996, 17:763–766.

29. Koss MN, Hochholzer L, Langloss JM, Wehung WD, Lazarus AA: Lymphoid interstitial pneumonia: clinicopathological and immunopathological findings in 18 cases. *Pathology* 1987, 19:178–185.

30. Griffiths MH, Miller RF, Semple SJ: Interstitial pneumonitis in patients infected with human immunodeficiency virus. *Thorax* 1995, 50:1141–1146.

31. McGuinness G, Schloes JV, Jagirdar JS, Lubat E: Unusual lymphoproliferative disorders in nine adults with HIV or AIDS: CT and pathological findings. *Radiology* 1995, 197:59–66.

32. Fishback N, Koss M: Update on lymphoid interstitial pneumonitis. *Curr Opin Pulm Med* 1996, 2:429–433.

33. Travis WD, Fox CH, Devaney KO: Lymphoid interstitial pneumonitis in 50 adult patients infected with the human immunodeficiency virus: lymphocytic interstitial pneumonitis versus nonspecific interstitial pneumonia. *Hum Pathol* 1992, 23:529–541.

34. Lynch DA, Newell JD, Logan PM, King TE Jr, Muller NL: Can CT distinguish hypersensitivity pneumonitis from idiopathic pulmonary fibrosis? *AJR* 1995, 165:807–811.

35. Sharma OP, Fujimura N: Hypersensitivity pneumonitis: a noninfectious granulomatosis. *Semin Respir Infect* 1995: 10:96–106.

36. Selman M: Hypersensitivity pneumonitis. In *Interstitial Lung Disease*. Edited by Schwartz M, King TE. Hamilton, Canada: Decker Inc; 1998, 393–422.

37. Schuyler M, Cormier Y: The diagnosis of hypersensitivity pneumonitis. *Chest* 1997, 111:534–536.

38. Miyagawa T, Hamagami S, Tanigawa N: *Cryptococcus albidus*-induced summer-type hypersensitivity pneumonitis. *Am J Respir Crit Care Med* 2000, 161:961–966.

39. Lalancette M, Carrier G, Laviolette M, Ferland S: Farmer's lung. Long-term outcome and lack of predictive value of bronchoalveolar lavage fibrosing factors. *Am Rev Respir Dis* 1993, 148:216–221.

40. Erkinjutti-Pekkanen R, Rytkonen H, Kokkarinene JI, et al.: Long-term risk of emphysema in patients with farmer's lung and matched control farmers. *Am J Respir Crit Care Med* 1998, 158:662–665.

41. Perez-Padilla R, Salas J, Chapela R, Sanchez M, Carillo G, Perez R: Mortality in Mexican patients with chronic pigeon breeders lung compared with those with usual interstitial pneumonia. *Am Rev Respir Dis* 1993, 148:49–53.

42. Adler BD, Padley SP, Muller NL, Remy-Jardin M, Remy J: Chronic hypersensitivity pneumonitis: high-resolution CT and radiographic features in 16 patients. *Radiology* 1992, 185:91–95.

43. Allen JN, Davis WB: Eosinophilic lung diseases. *Am J Respir Crit Care Med* 1994, 150:1423–1438.

44. Shannon J, Lynch JP III: Eosinophilic pulmonary syndromes. *Clin Pulm Med* 1995, 2:19–38.

45. Naughton M, Fahy J, Fitzgerald MX: Chronic eosinophilic pneumonia: a long-term follow-up of 12 patients. *Chest* 1993, 103:162–165.

46. Lynch JP III, Flint A: Sorting out the pulmonary eosinophilic syndromes. *J Respir Dis* 1984, 5:61–78.

47. Shah PL, Hansell D, Lawson PR, Reid KBM, Morgan C: Pulmonary alveolar proteinosis: clinical aspects and current concepts on pathogenesis. *Thorax* 2000, 55:67–77.

48. Tazi A, Soler P, Hance AJ: Adult pulmonary Langerhans' cell histiocytosis. *Thorax* 2000, 55:405–416.

49. Vassallo R, Rhu JH, Colby TV, Hartman T, Limper AH: Pulmonary Langerhans' cell histiocytosis. *N Engl J Med* 2000, 342:1969–1978.

50. Johnson SR: Lymphangioleiomyomatosis: clinical features, management and basic mechanisms. *Thorax* 1999, 54:254–264.

51. Urban T, Lazor R, Lacronique M, et al.: Pulmonary lymphangioleiomyomatosis: a study of 69 cases. *Medicine* 1999, 78:321–337.

52. Chu SC, Horiba K, Usuki J, et al.: Comprehensive evaluation of 35 patients with lymphangioleiomyomatosis. *Chest* 1999, 115:1041–1052.

CONNECTIVE TISSUE DISEASE

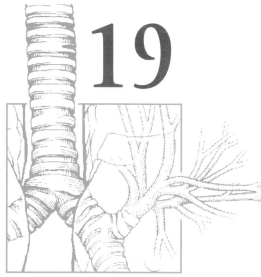

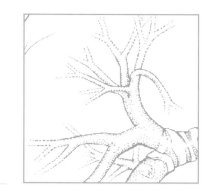

Seth Mark Berney & Maureen Heldmann

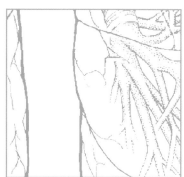

Many autoimmune connective tissue diseases involve the lung directly or as a complication of treatment. Rheumatoid arthritis, systemic lupus erythematosus, scleroderma, polymyositis and dermatomyositis, ankylosing spondylitis, and Sjögren's syndrome are all systemic autoimmune disorders of unknown etiology that cause pulmonary pathology. This chapter highlights the pulmonary manifestations of the most common of the disorders (*see* Chapter 20 for a discussion of necrotizing vasculitides).

Rheumatoid arthritis affects 1% to 2% of the world's population. The peak age of onset is 25 to 55 years with a female-to-male ratio of 2.5:1 [1,2]. Rheumatoid arthritis is characterized by symmetric polyarthritis, circulating autoantibodies (rheumatoid factor), inflammatory laboratory abnormalities (*eg*, elevated erythrocyte sedimentation rate, "anemia of chronic disease," thrombocytosis, and increased inflammatory cytokines), and extra-articular manifestations. Genetics appears to play a role in development or severity of disease; HLA-DR4 (DRB10401) and -DR1 (DRB10101) frequently occur in patients with more severe disease [3]. Extra-articular manifestations typically occur in patients with severe joint disease and high-titer rheumatoid factor and include subcutaneous or pulmonary nodules, vasculitis, pleuropericarditis, pneumonitis, bronchiolitis, episcleritis, or scleritis. Rheumatologists treat patients aggressively with slow-acting antirheumatic drugs, which include hydroxychloroquine, methotrexate, gold, sulfasalazine, and D-penicillamine. Cytotoxic therapy (azathioprine, cyclophosphamide, and chlorambucil) and immunomodulators (cyclosporine and FK-506) are reserved for resistant synovitis or potentially life-threatening extra-articular manifestations. In addition, because of the multitude of adverse side effects, systemic steroids (administered orally, intramuscularly, or intravenously) are reserved for potentially life-threatening extra-articular manifestations.

Systemic lupus erythematosus affects approximately one in 2000 individuals. The peak age of onset is 15 to 40 years with a female-to-male ratio of 5:1 [4]. Lupus is characterized by immune complex deposition, circulating autoantibodies, rash, cytopenias, arthritis, cerebritis, and nephritis. Genetics plays an important role in the development of the disease as evidenced by the increased frequency of HLA-DR2 and -DR3 in white patients with systemic lupus erythematosus [5]. However, other undetermined genetic or environmental factors are also important. Therapy depends on the severity of the disease, with systemic steroids and cytotoxic agents reserved for potentially life-threatening or major organ manifestations.

Progressive systemic sclerosis (diffuse scleroderma) and limited scleroderma (formerly known as CREST syndrome) affect approximately one in 5000 to 20,000 individuals. The peak age of onset is 40 to 60 years, with women being affected more commonly [6,7]. Scleroderma manifests with circulating autoantibodies and fibrosis of the skin, vasculature, lungs, kidneys, heart, and gastrointestinal tract. Treatment is restricted to aggressive angiotensin-converting enzyme inhibitor therapy, which decreases renal crises and subsequent renal failure, vasodilators for Raynaud's syndrome, and systemic steroids and cytotoxics for inflammatory organ involvement.

Polymyositis and dermatomyositis are inflammatory myopathies, which affect one in 100,000 to 200,000 individuals per year with a female predominance [8]. Although the cause is also unknown, dermatomyositis affecting older individuals (older than 50 to 60 years of age) may be paraneoplastic. Up to 10% of these older patients are diagnosed with a malignancy within 1 year of the onset of their myositis symptoms [9]. Polymyositis and dermatomyositis cause lymphocyte infiltration of proximal skeletal muscle, manifesting as weakness but sparing sensation and facial/distal extremity muscles. The disease also affects the lungs, heart, skin, esophagus, joints, and vasculature. The mainstay of therapy is systemic steroids. If the disease is steroid resistant or involves vital organs, methotrexate or cytotoxics are often effective.

Ankylosing spondylitis is a systemic inflammatory arthropathy, which primarily affects the axial skeleton. This disease is strongly associated with HLA-B27 and is three times more common in men. Onset usually occurs before 40 years of age [10]. Ankylosing spondylitis manifests as sacroiliitis and spondylitis resulting in fused sacroiliac joints and the classic bamboo spine. Uncommon extra-axial manifestations include peripheral arthritis, anterior uveitis, aortic root dilation, apical lung fibrosis, and cauda equina syndrome. Patient treatment includes physical therapy, nonsteroidal anti-inflammatory drugs, sulfasalazine,

and if necessary, ophthalmic immunosuppressants and orthopedic, cardiothoracic, or spinal surgery.

Sjögren's syndrome is a systemic autoimmune disease of the exocrine glands. Primary Sjögren's syndrome affects one in 1250 individuals (middle-aged women are at greatest risk) but can also complicate rheumatoid arthritis, systemic lupus erythematosus, progressive systemic sclerosis, and myositis (considered secondary Sjögren's) [11]. Sjögren's syndrome manifests as autoantibody formation, keratoconjunctivitis sicca (dry eyes), and xerostomia (dry mouth), which result from lymphocytic infiltration of lacrimal and salivary glands. Other organs affected include musculoskeletal, renal, skin, pulmonary, gastrointestinal, pancreatic, hematologic peripheral, and central nervous systems, with subsequent organ failure. Treatment includes replenishment of deficient hormones (thyroid, insulin, artificial tears, and artificial saliva) and immunosuppression if life-threatening or major organ involvement occurs.

A. PULMONARY MANIFESTATIONS OF CONNECTIVE TISSUE DISEASES

Disease	Manifestation					
	Parenchymal	Serosal	Vascular	Neuromuscular	Airway	Other
Systemic lupus erythematosus	Infectious pneumonia Pneumonitis Diffuse alveolar hemorrhage Acute reversible hypoxemia syndrome	Pleurocarditis Pericarditis	Pulmonary hypertension Thrombosis Thromboembolism	Shrinking lung syndrome	—	—
Rheumatoid arthritis	Interstitial pneumonitis Interstitial fibrosis Nodulosis	Pleuritis	Arteritis	—	Bronchiolitis obliterans and organizing pneumonia	—
Progressive systemic sclerosis	Interstitial pneumonitis Interstitial fibrosis	Pleurocarditis Pericarditis	Pulmonary hypertension	—	—	Respiratory restriction secondary to skin tightness Dilated esophagus
Polymyositis/ dermatomyositis	Interstitial pneumonitis Interstitial fibrosis	—	Pulmonary hypertension	Respiratory muscle weakness Pharyngeal muscle weakness with recurrent aspiration	—	—
Ankylosing spondylitis	Apical fibrosis	—	—	—	—	Respiratory restriction secondary to loss of thoracic expansion Bamboo spine Aortic root dilation
Sjögren's syndrome	Interstitial pneumonitis	—	—	—	—	—

Figure 19-1.
A, Pulmonary manifestations of connective tissue diseases.

(Continued on next page)

B. PULMONARY SIDE EFFECTS OF COMMONLY USED ANTIRHEUMATIC MEDICATION

Methotrexate
    Interstitial pneumonitis
    Alveolar pneumonitis
    Interstitial fibrosis
Gold
    Interstitial pneumonitis
    Alveolar pneumonitis
Cyclophosphamide
    Interstitial fibrosis
Sulfasalazine
    Interstitial pneumonitis

Figure 19-1. (*Continued*)
B, Pulmonary side effects of commonly used antirheumatic medication.

SYSTEMIC LUPUS ERYTHEMATOSUS

CLASSIFICATION CRITERIA FOR SYSTEMIC LUPUS ERYTHEMATOSUS

S	Serositis	Pleuritis or pericarditis
O	Oral ulcers	Oral or nasopharyngeal ulcerations (usually painless)
A	Arthritis	Nonerosive arthritis involving two or more peripheral joints with synovitis
P	Photosensitivity	Skin rash from sun
B	Blood dyscrasias	Hemolytic anemia with reticulocytosis *or*
		Leukopenia <4000/mm^3 leukocytes on two or more occasions *or*
		Lymphopenia <1500/mm^3 on two occasions *or*
		Thrombocytopenia <100 000/mm^3
R	Renal disorder	Persistent proteinuria >0.5 g/d or cellular (erythrocytes or leukocytes) casts
A	Antinuclear antibody	
I	Immunologic disorder	Anti–double-stranded DNA (ds-DNA) antibody *or*
		Anti–Smith (Sm) antibody *or*
		Antiphospholipid antibody based on one of the following:
		Abnormal serum IgG or IgM anticardiolipin antibody *or*
		Positive lupus anticoagulant *or*
		False-positive rapid plasma reagin or Venereal Disease Research Laboratory tests known positive for ≥6 mo and confirmed by *Treponema pallidum* immobilization or fluorescent treponemal antibody absorption test
N	Neurologic disorder	Seizures or psychosis
M	Malar rash	Fixed erythema, flat or raised, over the malar eminences, sparing the nasolabial folds
D	Discoid rash	Erythematous raised patches with scaling and follicular plugging; atrophic scarring may occur in older lesions

Figure 19-2.
Systemic lupus erythematosus classification criteria. Four of the 11 manifestations listed in the figure are required for classification of systemic lupus erythematosus. The mnemonic is "SOAP BRAIN MD." (*Adapted from* Hochberg [12] and Tan *et al.* [13].)

Manifestation	Incidence	Comments
Pleuro- and pericarditis	50%–80% [14]	—
Infection	Unknown	Most common cause of infiltrate in systemic lupus erythematosus: typical (especially encapsulated organisms) and opportunistic (especially nocardia, fungal)
Interstitial lung disease	25% [15]	—
Pulmonary hypertension	9% [16]	—
Acute pneumonitis	1%–9% [17–19]	Patient is acutely ill with hypoxemia; chest radiograph has diffuse bibasilar infiltrates with or without effusions [17–19]
Diffuse alveolar hemorrhage	1%–2% [20,21]	—
Thrombosis and thromboembolism	Unknown	Hypercoagulability state secondary to nephrosis or antiphospholipid antibody syndrome
Shrinking lung syndrome	Unknown	Secondary to respiratory muscle dysfunction with atelectasis and diaphragm elevation
Acute reversible hypoxemia syndrome	Unknown	—

Figure 19-3.
The most common pulmonary manifestations of systemic lupus erythematosus.

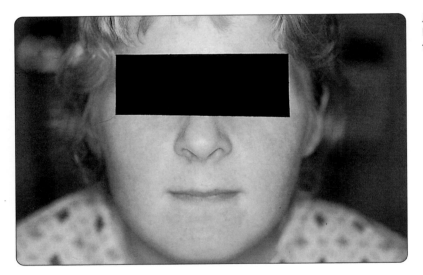

Figure 19-4.
Malar rash. The classic malar (butterfly) rash typically spares the nasolabial folds and is commonly precipitated by solar irradiation. (See Color Plate.)

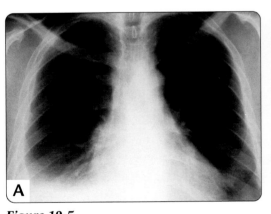
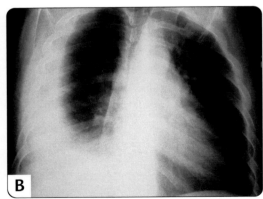
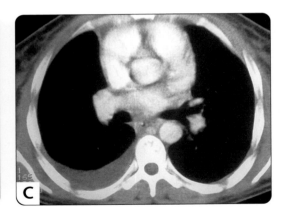

Figure 19-5.
A–C, Erect posteroanterior (*panel A*) and right lateral decubitus (*panel B*) radiographs and chest computed tomographic scan (*panel C*) revealing a free-flowing right pleural effusion. Lupus pleural fluid is exudative with a leukocyte count of less than 10,000 (monocytes/lymphocytes); the glucose level is normal and the pH is greater than 7.35. Pleural fluid lupus erythematosus cell is insensitive but specific for systemic lupus erythematosus. Pleural fluid antinuclear antibody and complement levels are not specific for systemic lupus erythematosus and have been found in patients with empyema and malignancy. Their presence has not been tested extensively in other autoimmune diseases, and as a result, routine measurements of antinuclear antibody or C3/C4 are unhelpful [22].

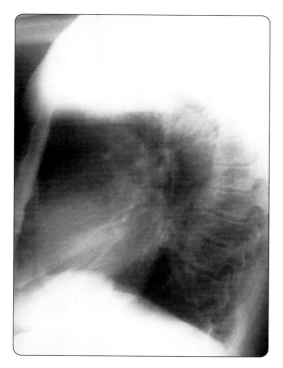

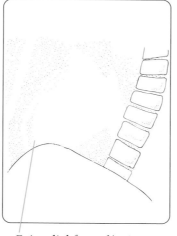

Epicardial fat pad/stripe

Figure 19-6.
The presence of pericardial effusion from systemic lupus erythematosus illustrated by lateral chest radiograph showing separation of the epicardial fat pad from the sternum. The heart is normally closely applied to the posterior sternum. This separation suggests the presence of some substance (usually fluid) between the epicardium and pericardium.

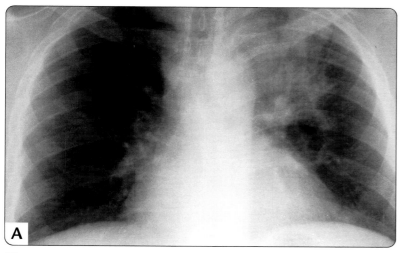

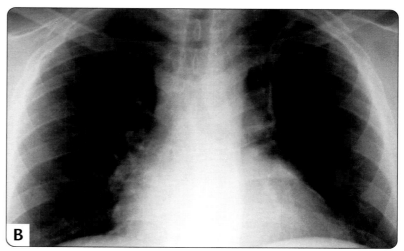

Figure 19-7.
A, Erect posteroanterior chest radiograph of a patient with lupus demonstrating left upper lobe consolidation with associated air bronchogram. During treatment for glomerulonephritis with cyclophosphamide and prednisone, this patient developed fever, dyspnea, and a slightly purulent cough. Sputum culture revealed blastomycosis, which responded to decreasing his immunosuppression and beginning itraconazole. **B,** Chest radiograph after therapy revealing a small scar.

RHEUMATOID ARTHRITIS

CLASSIFICATION CRITERIA FOR RHEUMATOID ARTHRITIS

Morning stiffness in and around joints lasting ≥1 h before maximal improvement

Soft-tissue swelling of three or more joint areas observed by a physician (PIP, MCP, wrist, elbow, knee, ankle, MTP)

Swelling of the PIP, MCP, or wrist joints

Symmetric joint swelling

Subcutaneous nodules over bony prominence or extensor surface or in juxta-articular regions

Positive test result for rheumatoid factor

Radiographic erosions or periarticular osteopenia in hand or wrist joints

---

MCP—metacarpophalangeal; MTP—metatarsophalangeal; PIP—proximal interphalangeal.

Figure 19-8.
Classification criteria for rheumatoid arthritis. Four of the seven manifestations listed must be present for classification as rheumatoid arthritis [23].

PULMONARY MANIFESTATIONS OF RHEUMATOID ARTHRITIS

Manifestation	Incidence	Comments
Pleural disease	20%–40% [24,25]	Pleurisy with or without effusion (very low glucose)
Interstitial pneumonitis	5%–10% [26]	Interstitial infiltrate with predilection for lung bases and periphery
Nodulosis	≤1% [27]	Solitary or multiple with or without pneumoconiosis (Caplan's syndrome); more common in men with high-titer rheumatoid factor, subcutaneous nodules, active rheumatoid arthritis; upper and midlung zone predominance
Interstitial fibrosis	Unknown	Basal predilection
Bronchiolitis obliterans and organizing pneumonia	Rare	—
Arteritis	Rare	Usually occurs in setting of diffuse alveolar hemorrhage

Figure 19-9.
The most common pulmonary manifestations of rheumatoid arthritis.

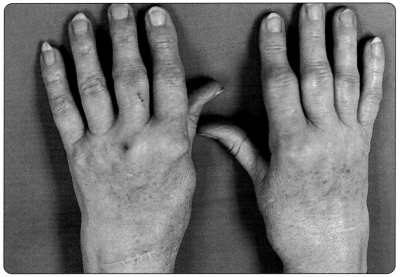

Figure 19-10.
Synovitis. This patient with rheumatoid arthritis has synovitis of both wrists and several metacarpophalangeal and proximal interphalangeal joints. This patient also had rupture of the left wrist extensor tendon, which was repaired (evidenced by left wrist scar).

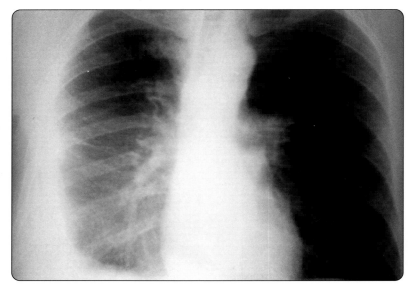

Figure 19-11.
Erect posteroanterior chest radiograph showing rheumatoid pleural disease with effusion. In this patient, the disease is represented by a moderate-sized right pleural-based density. Rheumatoid pleural fluid is exudative with a pH of less than 7.2, a glucose level of 30 mg/dL or less, and a leukocyte count of 15,000 or less. Because pleural rheumatoid factor is found in tuberculosis, malignancy, and other infections, this test is unhelpful [26].

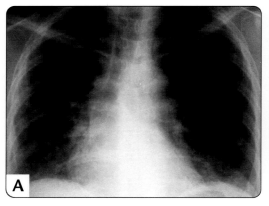
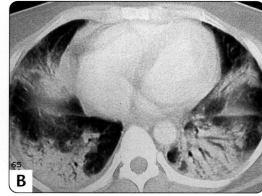
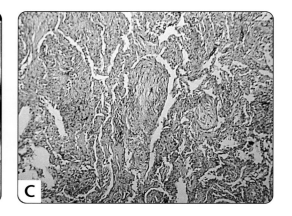

Figure 19-12.
A and **B,** Erect posteroanterior chest radiograph (*panel A*) and lung window chest computed tomographic scan (*panel B*) demonstrating patchy bibasilar areas of consolidation. These areas are notably peribronchiolar in distribution and are associated with mild bronchiolar dilation in affected areas, which are common findings in bronchiolitis obliterans organizing pneumonia (BOOP). **C,** Lung biopsy specimen from the same patient containing balls of fibroblasts within a respiratory bronchiole and surrounding air spaces consistent with BOOP. (Panel C *courtesy of* W.D. Grafton, MD.)

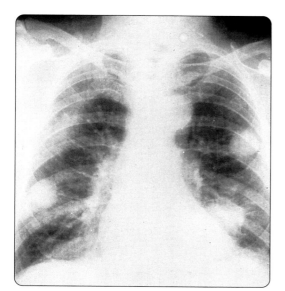

Figure 19-13.
Chest radiograph demonstrating bilateral pulmonary nodules in a patient with rheumatoid arthritis. These nodules are discrete and similar to metastatic malignant nodules; however, they are histologically identical to subcutaneous rheumatoid nodules. Excisional biopsy is usually needed to differentiate rheumatoid nodules from malignancy-related nodules. (*From* the Visual Aids Subcommittee of the Professional Education Committee of the Arthritis Foundation [28]; with permission.)

PROGRESSIVE SYSTEMIC SCLEROSIS

CLASSIFICATION CRITERIA FOR PROGRESSIVE SYSTEMIC SCLEROSIS

Major criterion

Proximal scleroderma

  Symmetric thickening, tightening, and induration of the skin of the fingers and the skin proximal to the metacarpophalangeal or metatarsophalangeal joints

  The changes may affect the entire extremity, face, neck, and trunk

Minor criteria

Sclerodactyly

  Skin changes listed under major criterion limited to the fingers

Digital pitting scars or loss of substance from the finger pad

  Depressed areas at tips of fingers or loss of digital pad tissue as a result of ischemia

Bibasilar pulmonary fibrosis

  Bilateral reticular or reticular pattern or reticulonodular densities most pronounced in basilar portions of the lungs on standard chest radiograph; may assume appearance of diffuse mottling or "honeycomb lung"; these changes should not be attributable to primary lung disease

Figure 19-14.
Classification criteria for progressive systemic sclerosis (scleroderma). One major or two minor criteria are needed for classification [29].

PULMONARY MANIFESTATIONS OF PROGRESSIVE SYSTEMIC SCLEROSIS

	Incidence	
	Diffuse, %	Limited, %
Interstitial pneumonitis—alveolar effusions (ground glass appearance)	30–90	30–90
Interstitial fibrosis	35	35
Pulmonary hypertension	≤ 1	10
Dilated esophagus	75	75
Pleuro- and pericarditis	40	?
Respiratory restriction secondary to chest wall skin tightness	?	0

Figure 19-15.
Pulmonary manifestations of diffuse and limited scleroderma [30].

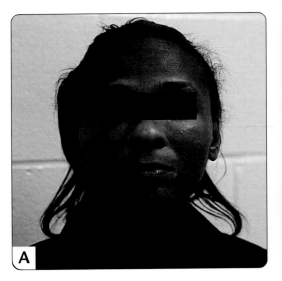

A

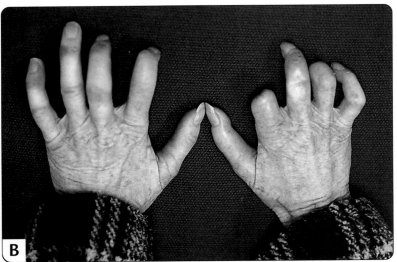

B

Figure 19-16.
Sclerodactyly in a patient with scleroderma. **A,** This patient with scleroderma has tight skin (*ie,* lack of wrinkles), which has caused a decreased oral aperture. (*See* Color Plate.) **B,** This patient with Raynaud's phenomenon of the fingers has autoamputation of right index and ring fingers and areas of blanching and cyanosis. (*See* Color Plate.)

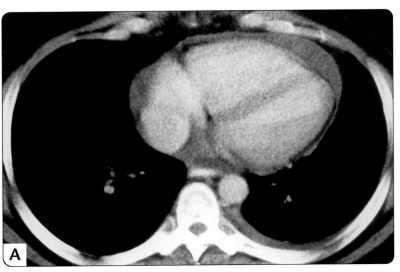

A

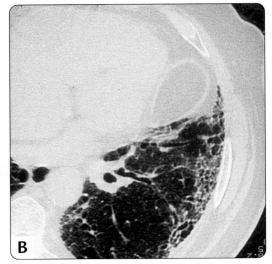

B

Figure 19-17.
A, Computed tomographic scan showing small left pleural and pericardial effusions in a patient with scleroderma. **B,** High-resolution computed tomographic scan of a different patient demonstrates typical subpleural honeycombing with lower zonal posterior predominance of pulmonary fibrosis.

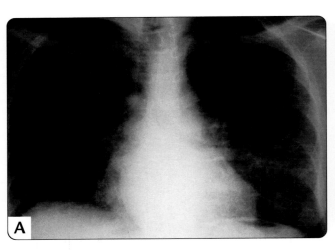

A

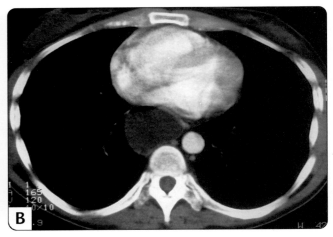

B

Figure 19-18.
A, Erect posteroanterior chest radiograph showing lower and midzonal coarse reticular interstitial disease in a patient with scleroderma. Note the double density of the right cardiac border. **B,** Chest computed tomographic scan displays the same density as in *panel A,* which represents a dilated, fluid-filled esophagus.

(*Continued on next page*)

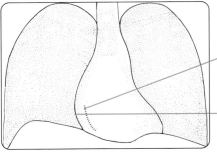

Dilated
esophageal border

Right cardiac border
(Right atrium)

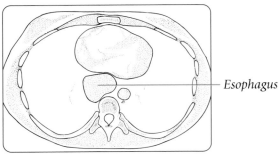

Esophagus

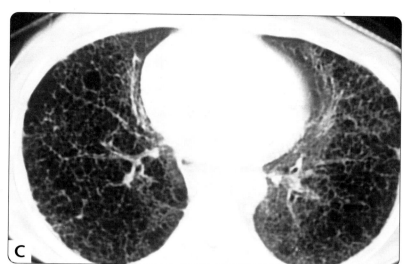

Figure 19-18. *(Continued)*
C, Lung window computed tomographic scan of the same patient illustrates honeycomb, end-stage lung disease.

POLYMYOSITIS AND DERMATOMYOSITIS

CLASSIFICATION CRITERIA FOR POLYMYOSITIS AND DERMATOMYOSITIS

Symmetric proximal muscle weakness (limb girdle and anterior neck muscles) ± tenderness

Elevated serum muscle enzymes (creatine phosphokinase, lactate dehydrogenase, aldolase, aspirate aminotransferase, alanine aminotransferase)

Myopathic changes on electromyography manifested as the triad of:

  Short, small polyphasic motor units

  Fibrillations, positive waves, and insertional irritability

  Bizarre high-frequency discharges

Muscle biopsy specimen demonstrating inflammation (muscle fiber necrosis/ regeneration/atrophy in a perifascicular distribution with an inflammatory exudate)

Skin rash

  Heliotrope (lilac-colored) discoloration of eyelids with periorbital edema

  Scaly, erythematous dermatitis over the dorsa of the hands (especially over the metacarpophalangeal and proximal interphalangeal joints [Gottron's sign]) and involvement of the knees, elbows, medial malleoli, face, neck, and upper torso

Figure 19-19.
Classification criteria for polymyositis and dermatomyositis. (*Adapted from* Wortmann [31] and Bohan and Peter [32].)

POLYMYOSITIS AND DERMATOMYOSITIS ANTISYNTHETASE ANTIBODY SYNDROME

Polymyositis/dermatomyositis with the following:

  Relatively acute onset

  Interstitial lung disease

  Fever

  Arthritis

  Raynaud's phenomenon

  "Mechanic's hands" (darkened or dirty-appearing cracking and fissuring of the lateral and palmar aspects of the fingers)

Presence of the myositis-specific antisynthetase antibodies to:

  Histidyl-tRNA synthetase (Jo-1)

  Threonyl-tRNA synthetase (PL-7)

  Alanyl-tRNA synthetase (PL-12)

  Glycyl-tRNA synthetase (EJ)

  Isoleucyl-tRNA synthetase (OJ)

Figure 19-20.
Polymyositis and dermatomyositis antisynthetase antibody syndrome. (*Adapted from* Wortmann [31].)

PULMONARY MANIFESTATIONS OF POLYMYOSITIS AND DERMATOMYOSITIS

Manifestation	Incidence, %
Interstitial lung disease (but increased in patients with antisynthetase antibody)	5–30 [33,34]
Interstitial fibrosis (but increased in patients with antisynthetase antibody)	5–10 [35]
Diaphragm/respiratory muscle weakness	≤5 [36]
Pharyngeal muscle weakness with recurrent aspiration	>50 [37]
Pulmonary hypertension	Unknown

Figure 19-21.
Pulmonary manifestations of polymyositis and dermatomyositis.

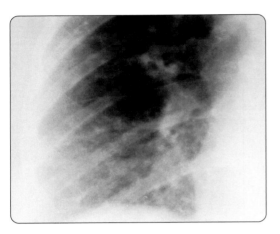

Figure 19-22.
Magnification of the lower zone of a posteroanterior chest radiograph showing fine reticular lower zonal interstitial lung disease in a patient with polymyositis.

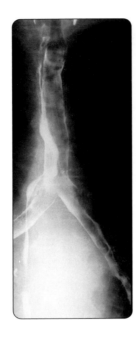

Figure 19-23.
Upper gastrointestinal examination of a patient with dermatomyositis. Pharyngeal dysmotility predisposes to aspiration, as seen by contrast material coating the trachea and proximal bronchi. Barium pools in the pyriform sinuses, with only a small amount traversing the esophagus.

ANKYLOSING SPONDYLITIS

THORACIC AND PULMONARY MANIFESTATIONS OF ANKYLOSING SPONDYLITIS

Manifestation	Incidence
Bamboo spine and chest wall fixation	Develops in many patients
Apical fibrosis (which may cavitate and become infected with *Aspergillus* spp or mycobacteria)	<2% [38]
Aortic root dilation and aortic valve regurgitation	3.5% in ankylosing spondylitis >15 y [39]

Figure 19-24.
Thoracic and pulmonary manifestations of ankylosing spondylitis.

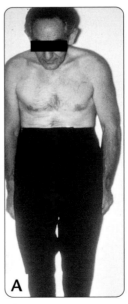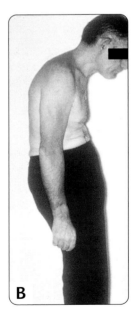

A   **B**

Figure 19-25.
A and **B,** Frontal (*panel A*) and side (*panel B*) views of a patient with advanced ankylosing spondylitis. The patient maintains fixed forward protrusion of the head, thoracic kyphosis, and loss of normal lumbar lordosis. (*From* the Visual Aids Subcommittee of the Professional Education Committee of the Arthritis Foundation [28]; with permission.)

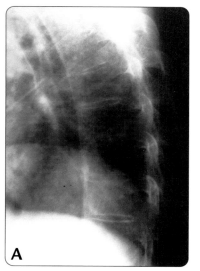 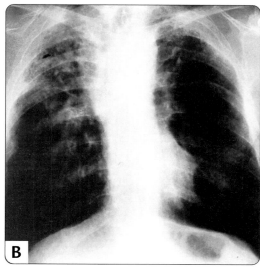

Figure 19-26.
A, Lateral thoracic spine radiograph revealing flowing ossification of the paraspinal soft tissues producing the classic "bamboo spine" of ankylosing spondylitis. **B,** Chest radiograph of patient with ankylosing spondylitis and bilateral upper-zone fibro-nodular infiltrates. (Panel B *from* Schwarz [26]; with permission.)

A. DRUG TOXICITY

Drug	Indications	Description	Treatment
Methotrexate	Alveolar/interstitial infiltrate	Frequently acute onset with fever, dyspnea 1%–11% incidence in rheumatoid arthritis May be a hypersensitive reaction and may result in fibrosis	Drug withdrawal or in severe cases prednisone (1 mg/kg) [40,41]
Gold	Alveolar/interstitial infiltrate with upper lung predominance	Dyspnea, cough, fever, peripheral eosinophilia	Drug withdrawal or in severe cases prednisone (1 mg/kg)
Cyclophosphamide	Interstitial pulmonary fibrosis	—	—
Sulfasalazine	Diffuse interstitial infiltrate	Hypersensitivity lung disease with cough, fever, and dyspnea	Drug withdrawal or in severe cases prednisone (1 mg/kg)

B. RHEUMATOLOGIC DRUGS THAT MAY PREDISPOSE TO INFECTION

Glucocorticoids (prednisone, solumedrol)
Cyclophosphamide (cytoxan)
Azathioprine (imuran)
Cyclosporin A
Methotrexate
Etanercept (Enbrel; Boehringer Ingelheim, Ridgefield, CT)
Infliximab (Remicade; Centocor, Malvern, PA)

Figure 19-27.
A, Toxicity of common antirheumatic medications. **B,** Rheumatologic drugs that may predispose to infection.

AUTOANTIBODIES AND THEIR INCIDENCES IN CONNECTIVE TISSUE DISEASE

Autoantibody	Rheumatoid arthritis	Systemic lupus erythematosus	Sjögren's syndrome	PSS (scleroderma)	Polymyositis/ dermatomyositis	Ankylosing spondylitis
Rheumatoid factor	Common*	Common	Common	Common	Rare†	Undetectable
Antinuclear antibody	Common	Common	Common	Common	Rare	Undetectable
Double-stranded DNA (ds-DNA)	Undetectable	Diagnostic	Undetectable	Undetectable	Undetectable	Undetectable
Smith (Sm) antibody	Undetectable	Diagnostic	Undetectable	Undetectable	Undetectable	Undetectable
Ro(SSA)/La(SSB) ("Sjögren's antibodies")	Uncommon‡ (associated with Sjögren's)	Uncommon (associated with Sjögren's)	Common	Uncommon	Rare	Undetectable
Centromere	Undetectable	Undetectable	Rare	Common in limited PSS	Rare	Undetectable
SCL-70 (topoisomerase 1)	Undetectable	Undetectable	Rare	Common in diffuse PSS	Rare	Undetectable
Jo-1 (synthetase)	Undetectable	Undetectable	Undetectable	Rare	Common in patients with interstitial lung disease	Undetectable
Antineutrophil cytoplasmic antibody (ANCA)	Rare	Rare	Uncommon	Undetectable	Uncommon	Undetectable

*>25% of patients; †<5% of patients; ‡5%–25% of patients; PSS—progressive systemic sclerosis.

Figure 19-28.
Autoantibodies and their incidence in connective tissue disease. (*Adapted from* Froelich et al. [42] and Gross [43].)

REFERENCES

1. Kellgren JH: Epidemiology of rheumatoid arthritis. *Arthritis Rheum* 1966, 9:658–674.

2. Chan KA, Felson DT, Yood RA, Walker AM: Incidence of rheumatoid arthritis in central Massachusetts. *Arthritis Rheum* 1993, 36:1691–1696.

3. Weyand CM, Hicok KC, Conn DL, et al.: The influence of *HLA-DRB1* genes on disease severity in rheumatoid arthritis. *Ann Intern Med* 1992, 118:801–806.

4. Fessel WJ: Systemic lupus erythematosus in the community: incidence, prevalence, outcome and first symptoms; the high prevalence in black women. *Arch Intern Med* 1974, 134:1027–1035.

5. Howard PF, Hochberg MC, Bias WB, et al.: Relationship between C4 null genes, HLA-D region antigens, and genetic susceptibility to systemic lupus erythematosus in Caucasian and Black Americans. *Am J Med* 1986, 81:187–193.

6. Tamaki T, Mori S, Takehara K: Epidemiological study of patients with systemic sclerosis in Tokyo. *Arch Dermatol Res* 1991, 283:366–371.

7. Maricq HR, Weinrich MC, Keil JE, et al.: Prevalence of scleroderma spectrum disorders in the general population of South Carolina. *Arthritis Rheum* 1989, 32:998–1006.

8. Oddis CV, Conte CG, Steen VD, et al.: Incidence of polymyositis-dermatomyositis: a 20-year study of hospital diagnosed cases in Allegheny County, PA 1963–1982. *J Rheumatol* 1990, 17:1329–1334.

9. Sigurgeirsson B, Lindelof B, Edhag O, et al.: Risk of cancer in patients with dermatomyositis or polymyositis: a population-based study. *N Engl J Med* 1992, 326:363–367.

10. Khan MA, van der Linden SM: Ankylosing spondylitis and associated diseases. *Rheum Dis Clin North Am* 1990, 16:551–579.

11. Youinou P, Moutsopoulos HM, Pennec YL: Clinical features of Sjögren's syndrome. *Curr Opin Rheumatol* 1990, 2:687–693.

12. Hochberg MD: Updating the American College of Rheumatology revised criteria for the classification of systemic lupus erythematosus. *Arthritis Rheum* 1997, 40:1725.

13. Tan EM, et al.: The 1982 revised criteria for the classification of systemic lupus erythematosus. *Arthritis Rheum* 1982, 25:1271–1277.

14. Gross M, Esterley R, Earle RH: Pulmonary alterations in systemic lupus erythematosus. *Am Rev Respir Dis* 1972, 105:572–577.

15. Boulware DW, Hedgpeth MT: Lupus pneumonitis and anti-SSA(Ro) antibodies. *J Rheumatol* 1989, 16:479–481.

16. Badui E, Garcia-Rubi D, Robles E, et al.: Cardiovascular manifestations in systemic erythematosus: prospective study of 100 patients. *Angiology* 1985, 36:431–440.

17. Estes D, Christian CL: The natural history of systemic lupus erythematosus by prospective analysis. *Medicine* 1971, 50:85–95.

18. Bulgrin JG, Dubois EL, Jacobson G: Chest roentgenographic changes in systemic lupus erythematosus. *Radiology* 1960, 74:42–49.

19. Matthay RA, Schwartz MI, Petty TL, et al.: Pulmonary manifestations of systemic lupus erythematosus: review of twelve cases of acute lupus pneumonitis. *Medicine* 1975, 54:397–409.

20. Abud-Mendoza C, Diaz-Jouanen E, Alarcon-Segovia D: Fetal pulmonary hemorrhage in systemic lupus erythematosus: occurrence without hemoptysis. *J Rheumatol* 1985, 12:558–561.

21. Marino CT, Pertschuk LP: Pulmonary hemorrhage in systemic lupus erythematosus. *Arch Intern Med* 1981, 141:201–203.

22. Khare V, Baethge B, Lang S, et al.: Antinuclear antibodies in pleural fluid. *Chest* 1994, 106:866–871.

23. Arnett FC, Edworthy SM, Bloch DA, et al.: The American Rheumatism Association 1987 revised criteria for the classification of rheumatoid arthritis. *Arthritis Rheum* 1988, 31:315–324.

24. Jurik AG, Graudal H: Pleurisy in rheumatoid arthritis. *Scand J Rheumatol* 1983, 12:75–80.

25. Jurik AG, Davidsen D, Graudal H: Prevalence of pulmonary involvement in rheumatoid arthritis and its relationship to some characteristics of the patients: a radiological and clinical study. *Scand J Rheumatol* 1982, 11:217–224.

26. Schwarz MI: Pulmonary manifestations of the collagen vascular diseases. In *Fishman's Pulmonary Diseases and Disorders*, edn 3. Edited by Fishman AP, Elias JA, Fishman JA, *et al.* New York: McGraw-Hill; 1998:1115–1132.

27. Walker WC, Wright V: Pulmonary lesions and rheumatoid arthritis. *Medicine* 1968, 47:501–520.

28. The Visual Aids Subcommittee of the Professional Education Committee of the Arthritis Foundation: *Clinical Slide Collection of the Rheumatic Diseases.* New York: The Arthritis Foundation;1995.

29. Masi AT, Rodnan GP, Medsger TA Jr, *et al.*: Preliminary criteria for the classification of systemic sclerosis (scleroderma). *Arthritis Rheum* 1980, 23:581–590.

30. Medsger TA, Steen V: Systemic sclerosis and related syndromes: clinical features and treatment. In *Primer on the Rheumatic Diseases*, edn 10. Edited by Schumacher HR Jr, Klippel JH, Koopman WJ. Atlanta: Arthritis Foundation; 1993:120–127.

31. Wortmann RL: Inflammatory diseases of muscle. In *Textbook of Rheumatology* edn 5. Edited by Kelley WN, Harris ED Jr, Ruddy S, Sledge CB. Philadelphia: WB Saunders; 1997:1177.

32. Bohan A, Peter JB: Polymyositis and dermatomyositis (first of two parts). *N Engl J Med* 1975, 292:344.

33. Bernstein RM, Morgan SH, Chapman J, *et al.*: Anti-Jo-1 antibody: a marker for myositis with interstitial lung disease. *Br Med J* 1984, 289:151–152.

34. Schwarz MI, Matthay RA, Sahn SA, *et al.*: Interstitial lung disease in polymyositis-dermatomyositis: analysis of 6 cases and review of the literature. *Medicine* 1976, 55:89–104.

35. Tazelaar HD, Viggiano RW, Pickergill J, Colby TV: Interstitial lung disease in polymyositis and dermatomyositis: clinical features and prognosis as correlated with histologic findings. *Am Rev Respir Dis* 1990, 14:272.

36. Schwarz MI: Pulmonary and cardiac manifestations of polymyositis-dermatomyositis. *J Thorac Imaging* 1992, 7:46–54.

37. Dickey BF, Myers AR: Pulmonary disease in polymyositis-dermatomyositis. *Semin Arthritis Rheum* 1984, 14:60–76.

38. Boushea DK, Sundstrom WR: The pleuropulmonary manifestations of ankylosing spondylitis. *Semin Arthritis Rheum* 1989, 18:277–281.

39. Carette S, Graham DC, Little HA, *et al.*: The natural disease course of ankylosing spondylitis. *Arthritis Rheum* 1983, 26:186–190.

40. Carroll GJ, Thomas R, Phatouros CC, *et al.*: Incidence, prevalence, and possible risk factors for pneumonitis in patients with rheumatoid arthritis receiving methotrexate. *J Rheumatol* 1994, 21:51–54.

41. Hargreaves MR, Mowat AG, Benson MK: Acute pneumonitis associated with low dose methotrexate treatment for rheumatoid arthritis: report of five cases and review of published reports. *Thorax* 1992, 47:628–633.

42. Froelich CJ, Wallman J, Skosey JL, Teodorescu M: Clinical value of an integrated ELISA system for the detection of 6 autoantibodies (ssDNA, dsDNA, Sm, RNP/Sm, SSA, and SSB). *J Rheumatol* 1990, 17:192–200.

43. Gross WL: Antineutrophil cytoplasmic autoantibody testing in vasculitides. In *Rheumatic Disease Clinics of North America—Vasculitis*, vol 21. Edited by Hunder GG. Philadelphia: WB Saunders; 1995:997.

NECROTIZING VASCULITIS

Seth Mark Berney,
Steven N. Berney, &
Maureen Heldmann

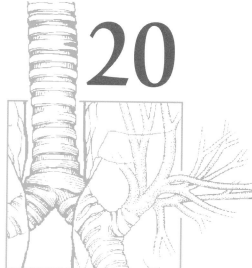

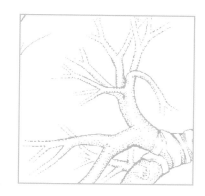

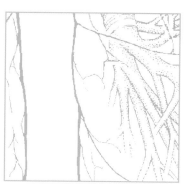

Vasculitis is a heterogeneous group of conditions characterized by inflammation and necrosis of blood vessel walls. Arteries and veins of various sizes and locations may be involved, resulting in a diversity of signs and symptoms. Significant bewilderment has existed regarding the nomenclature, identification, and diagnosis of vasculitis, which prompted the American College of Rheumatology in 1990 to issue classification criteria for the more common vasculitides [1–6]. However, physicians still experience confusion as a result of several different nomenclature systems. Vasculitis can be grouped according to affected vessel size, presence or absence of the antineutrophil cytoplasmic antibody, pathogenesis (immune complex–associated, antibody-associated, endothelium/cell–mediated), or the disease spectrum shown below, which is based on the intensity of the inflammatory cell infiltrate of the artery wall (angiitis). At one end of the spectrum are polyarteritis nodosa (PAN), the prototypic angiitis; hypersensitivity vasculitis; and the PAN-like diseases, including microscopic polyangiitis (formerly known as microscopic PAN), and allergic angiitis and granulomatosis (Churg-Strauss syndrome), which have abundant cellular infiltration of the artery walls of symptomatic tissue. At the other end of the spectrum is Wegener's granulomatosis, characterized by a paucity of cells infiltrating the affected vessel wall.

PAN	Microscopic	Churg-Strauss	Rheumatoid	Temporal	Wegener's
	polyangiitis	syndrome	arthritis	arteritis	granulomatosis
Hypersensitivity					
vasculitis			Systemic lupus	Takayasu's	
			erythematosus	arteritis	
			Cryoglobulins		

Polyarteritis nodosa is a necrotizing vasculitis affecting small to medium-sized arteries. It has a mean age of onset of 48 years and affects men slightly more than women (1.5:1) [7]. PAN usually presents with constitutional symptoms and vasculitis causing abdominal, joint, muscle, and testicular pain. In addition, patients develop nephritis with hypertension, peripheral nervous system vasculitis (mononeuritis multiplex), central nervous system vasculitis, hepatitis, and cutaneous vasculitis with palpable purpura. However, PAN typically spares the lung and is not associated with wheezing, eosinophilia, or granuloma formation.

Hypersensitivity vasculitis (leukocytoclastic vasculitis) affects arterioles, venules, and capillaries and is related to exposure to allergens, medications, infections, or noxious chemicals. It has an explosive onset, with skin the most commonly affected organ, yet hypersensitivity vasculitis has the potential for involving most organs without granulomas.

Microscopic polyangiitis is similar to PAN. However, lung involvement, more significant renal involvement, and small vessel (capillaries, venules, and arterioles) involvement distinguish it from PAN. It affects men slightly more often than women (1.5:1) and has an age of onset of 40 to 60 years.

Allergic angiitis and granulomatosis (Churg-Strauss syndrome) affects small to medium-sized arteries, has an age of onset of 15 to 75 years (mean, 38), and afflicts men twice as often as women (2:1) [8]. This disease is characterized by three phases: 1) allergic rhinitis and/or asthma, 2) peripheral and tissue eosinophilia (infiltrative eosinophilia such as eosinophilic pneumonia or gastroenteritis), and 3) granulomatous vasculitis and angiitis. The patient's asthma often subsides as the vasculitis appears, and constitutional symptoms may herald the onset of systemic disease. Several recent published reports associate the development of Churg-Strauss syndrome with the use of the leukotriene receptor antagonists: zafirlukast, montelukast, and pranlukast. Patients with asthma treated with these medications developed a Churg-Strauss-like syndrome as their physician tapered their systemic corticosteroids [9].

Takayasu's arteritis and temporal arteritis are histologically identical granulomatous inflammatory diseases (with multinucleated giant cells) of large arteries. Both diseases cause symptoms of narrowing or occlusion of the aorta or its branches. The major differences are epidemiologic. Takayasu's arteritis (pulseless disease) primarily affects Asian (Japanese) children and women younger than 40 years of age and usually presents with constitutional symptoms and upper extremity vascular insufficiency symptoms (aortic arch syndrome). Patients may eventually develop secondary hypertension, aortic insufficiency, coronary arteritis, congestive heart failure, pulmonary artery inflammation, glomerulonephritis, and cutaneous vasculitis [10]. In contrast, temporal arteritis (cranial arteritis) affects older patients (older than 50 years of age), also with a female predominance (female-to-male ratio, 2:1). Up to 50% of patients

with temporal arteritis already suffer from polymyalgia rheumatica. Patients with temporal arteritis may present with a sudden-onset flu-like syndrome with fever and weight loss or may develop cachexia and failure to thrive. Eventually they manifest symptoms indicative of cranial vascular involvement. These patients may also experience aortic arch syndrome symptoms and peripheral neuropathy [11].

Wegener's granulomatosis is a necrotizing granulomatous vasculitis with an age of onset of 30 to 50 years and a tendency to afflict men more often than women [12]. This disease is characterized by a triad of involved tissue: upper respiratory tract, lower respiratory tract, and kidney. The presence of the triad is the classic presentation; however, incomplete forms occur involving only one or two of the tissues, making the diagnosis more difficult.

This chapter concentrates on the most common necrotizing vasculitides affecting the lungs: microscopic polyangiitis, Churg-Strauss syndrome, and Wegener's granulomatosis.

5-YEAR PATIENT SURVIVAL WITH TREATMENT

Polyarteritis nodosa	80%
Microscopic polyangiitis	65%
Churg-Strauss syndrome	75%
Takayasu's/temporal arteritis	>90%
Wegener's granulomatosis	>75%

Figure 20-1.
Five-year patient survival rates with treatment. The diagnosis of vasculitis is based on appropriate symptoms, physical findings, laboratory values, and abnormal angiographic findings or a characteristic tissue biopsy. The prognosis for patients diagnosed with vasculitis has dramatically improved since the advent of glucocorticoids, and the inclusion of cyclophosphamide has further improved patient survival [12–16]. In addition, in patients with non-immediately life-threatening Wegener's granulomatosis (defined as creatinine < 2.5, PO_2 > 70 mm Hg and carbon monoxide diffusing capacity > 70% arterial predicted), methotrexate and prednisone have been used successfully [17].

VASCULITIDES INVOLVING THE RESPIRATORY TRACT

Microscopic polyangiitis—angiitis
Churg-Strauss disease (allergic angiitis and granulomatosis)—angiitis and granuloma formation
Wegener's granulomatosis—granuloma formation
Giant cell arteritis (Takayasu's arteritis and temporal arteritis)—granuloma formation
Cryoglobulinemia—immune complex deposition
Serum sickness—immune complex deposition
Behçet's disease—pulmonary artery aneurysms and thrombosis
Goodpasture's syndrome—glomerular basement membrane antibody deposition
Rheumatoid arthritis
Systemic lupus erythematosus

Figure 20-2.
Vasculitides involving the respiratory tract.

MICROSCOPIC POLYANGIITIS

CLINICAL MANIFESTATIONS OF MICROSCOPIC POLYANGIITIS

System	Manifestation
Renal	90%–100% patients develop rapidly progressive glomerulonephritis
Musculoskeletal	70% of patients experience myalgias, arthralgias, and a nondeforming arthritis
Pulmonary	50% of patients develop pulmonary manifestations
Gastrointestinal	50% of patients develop vasculitis manifested as abdominal pain
Cutaneous	50% of patients manifest as palpable purpura
Nervous	30% of patients have involvement of the nervous system primarily as peripheral neuropathy
Cardiac	15% of patients develop pericarditis or coronary arteritis

Figure 20-3.
Clinical manifestations of microscopic polyangiitis. Most patients develop constitutional symptoms, including fatigue, weight loss, and low-grade fever. (*Adapted from* Lhote *et al.* [8]).

PULMONARY MANIFESTATIONS OF MICROSCOPIC POLYANGIITIS

Manifestation	Incidence
Diffuse alveolar hemorrhage	30% of patients develop hemorrhage manifesting as hemoptysis or rapid anemia
Pleurisy (with or without effusion)	15%
Parenchymal infiltrates	—
Interstitial fibrosis secondary to vasculitis	—

Figure 20-4.
Pulmonary manifestations of microscopic polyangiitis [14].

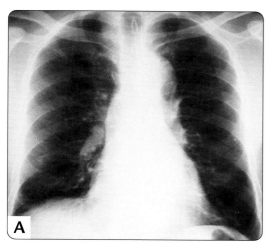
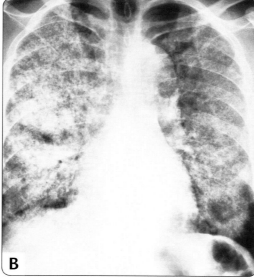

Figure 20-5.
Microscopic polyangiitis. **A**, Erect posteroanterior chest radiograph from a 62-year-old man. **B**, Erect posteroanterior radiograph from the same patient 1 month later. The patient developed diffuse pulmonary hemorrhage manifesting as airspace consolidation, sparing only the apices and costophrenic angles.

CHURG-STRAUSS SYNDROME

CLASSIFICATION CRITERIA FOR CHURG-STRAUSS SYNDROME

Asthma

Eosinophilia >10% leukocytes

Mononeuropathy or polyneuropathy

Transitory pulmonary infiltrates

Paranasal sinus abnormality

Biopsy specimen showing extravascular eosinophils

Figure 20-6.
Classification criteria for Churg-Strauss syndrome (allergic angiitis and granulomatosis). The patient must have four of the six criteria to meet the classification requirements [16].

CLINICAL MANIFESTATIONS OF CHURG-STRAUSS SYNDROME

System	Manifestation
Pulmonary	70% of patients
Nervous	70% of patients have peripheral nervous system manifestations (mononeuritis multiplex or polyneuropathy)
	Central nervous system involvement is uncommon
Cutaneous	60% of patients develop subcutaneous nodules, petechia, purpura, skin infarction
Cardiac	50% of patients develop coronary arteritis, congestive heart failure, peri-, myo-, endocarditis
Gastrointestinal	50% of patients develop vasculitis, which causes abdominal pain, distention, hematemesis, or melena
Musculoskeletal	50% of patients experience arthralgia or nondestructive arthritis
Renal	45% of patients develop glomerulonephritis; however, renal failure and nephrotic syndrome are infrequent
Prostate and lower genitourinary tract	Eosinophilic granulomatosis is unique to Churg-Strauss syndrome

Figure 20-7.
Clinical manifestations of Churg-Strauss syndrome. Most patients develop constitutional symptoms, including fatigue, weight loss, and low-grade fever. (*Adapted from* Jennette and Falk [18] and Lanham *et al.* [19].)

PULMONARY MANIFESTATIONS OF CHURG-STRAUSS SYNDROME

Upper airway
   Sinusitis
   Nasal inflammation/polyps
Lower airway—chest radiographs are abnormal in 50% of
   patients and show:
Patchy shifting infiltrates
Massive bilateral nodular infiltrates without cavitation
Diffuse interstitial disease (suggesting eosinophilic
   pneumonia) [5,20]
Pleural effusions [19]

Figure 20-8.
Pulmonary manifestations of Churg-Strauss syndrome.

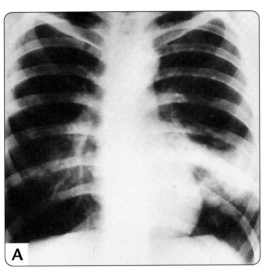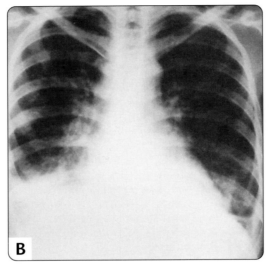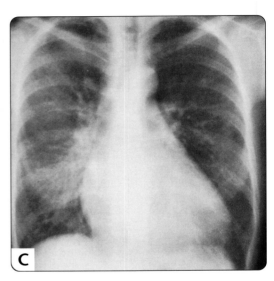

Figure 20-9.
Churg-Strauss syndrome. A 28-year-old woman with asthma had peripheral eosinophilia (10.3×10^9/L) and original right upper lung consolidation. **A**, Chest radiograph shows left lower lung zone consolidation. **B**, Chest radiograph 6 months later shows that the patient developed bilateral pleural effusions. **C**, Chest radiograph from the same patient 1 year later reveals the development of cardiomyopathy. (*From* Wilson [21]; with permission.)

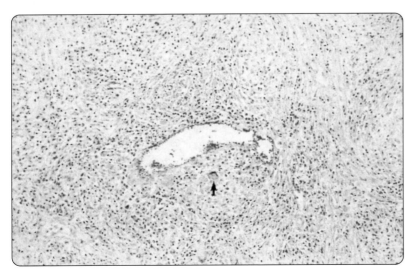

Figure 20-10.
Lung biopsy specimen from a patient with Churg-Strauss syndrome showing mixed inflammatory cell infiltrate with numerous eosinophils. A small pulmonary vessel is focally necrotic and is being destroyed by this process. Note the multinucleated giant cell in the wall of the vessel (*arrow*). (*From* Winterbauer [22]; with permission.)

WEGENER'S GRANULOMATOSIS

CLASSIFICATION CRITERIA FOR WEGENER'S GRANULOMATOSIS

Nasal or oral inflammation (oral ulcers or bloody nasal drainage)

Abnormal chest radiograph (nodules, fixed infiltrates, cavities)

Urinary sediment (>5 erythrocytes/high-power field or erythrocyte casts)

Granulomatous inflammation on biopsy specimen (in wall of artery or arteriole, perivascular or extravascular)

Figure 20-11.
Classification criteria for Wegener's granulomatosis. The patient must have two of the four criteria to meet the classification requirements [3].

CLINICAL MANIFESTATIONS OF WEGENER'S GRANULOMATOSIS

System	Manifestation
Pulmonary	90% of patients
Ear/nose/throat	90% of patients experience nasal ulcers, oropharyngeal pain/ulcers, sinusitis, or otitis media (which can injure facial nerve)
Renal	Glomerulonephritis is found in 20% of patients at presentation; however, 80% of patients eventually develop renal symptoms of proteinuria, hematuria, erythrocyte casts, renal insufficiency; hypertension is uncommon
Musculoskeletal	60% of patients experience arthralgias or mild nondestructive arthritis
Ocular	50% of patients; orbital involvement frequently occurs secondary to extension from sinusitis; proptosis, conjunctivitis, scleritis, episcleritis, uveitis, ophthalmoplegia
Nervous	50% of patients develop peripheral neuropathy with or without mononeuritis multiplex (30%), cranial neuropathy, seizures, cerebritis, cerebrovascular accident symptoms.
Gastrointestinal	50% of patients develop vasculitis, which causes abdominal pain, distention, hematemesis, or melena
Cutaneous	40% of patients develop subcutaneous nodules, purpura, skin infarction (lower >upper extremities)
Cardiac	Uncommon but dysrhythmias, pericarditis, and coronary arteritis have been observed

Figure 20-12.
Clinical manifestations of Wegener's granulomatosis. Most patients develop constitutional symptoms, including fatigue, weight loss, and low-grade fever. (*Adapted from* Jennette and Falk [18] and Hoffman *et al.* [12].)

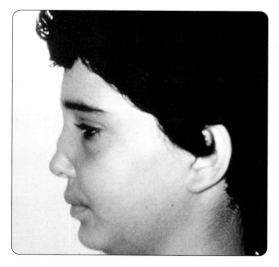

Figure 20-13.
Saddle nose deformity in a patient with Wegener's granulomatosis. Saddle nose deformity, which eroded nasal cartilage in this patient, can also occur in relapsing polychondritis, sarcoidosis, and congenital syphilis. (*From* the Visual Aids Subcommittee of the Professional Education Committee of the Arthritis Foundation [23]; with permission.)

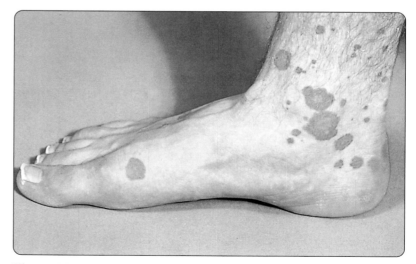

Figure 20-14.
Cutaneous vasculitis manifesting as palpable purpura. (*See* Color Plate.) (*Courtesy of* D. Hogan, MD.)

PULMONARY AND AIRWAY MANIFESTATIONS OF WEGENER'S GRANULOMATOSIS

Upper airway

    Tracheal/subglottic stenosis—15% of adults, 50% of children [24,25]

    Nasal/palatal ulcerations with or without destruction

    Destructive sinusitis

    Saddle nose deformity

Lower airway

    Unilateral or bilateral nodules with or without cavitation—60%

    Infiltrates—65%

    Pleuritis with or without effusions—28%

    Alveolar capillaritis resulting in diffuse alveolar hemorrhage (less fixed and more irregular infiltrates)—8% [12]

Figure 20-15.
Pulmonary and airway manifestations of Wegener's granulomatosis.

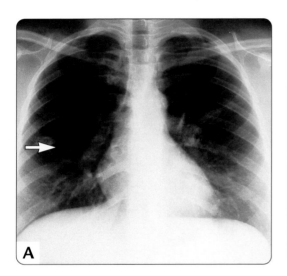

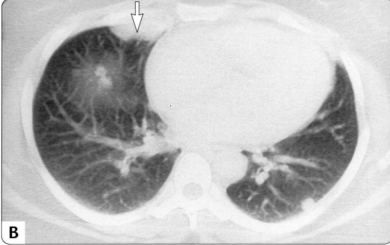

Figure 20-16.
Wegener's granulomatosis. **A,** Postero-anterior chest radiograph reveals a well-defined cavitary nodule in the right middle lobe (*arrow*). **B,** Lung window computed tomographic image shows multiple lesions, from defined nodules (some surrounded by edema and hemorrhage) to subpleural confluent opacity anteriorly (*arrow*).

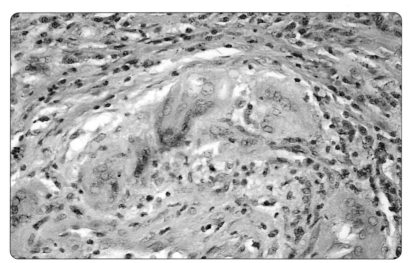

Figure 20-17.
Lung biopsy specimen from a patient with Wegener's granulomatosis demonstrating multiple granulomas with central necrosis and multinucleated giant cells. (*See* Color Plate.) (*Courtesy of* F. Abreo, MD.)

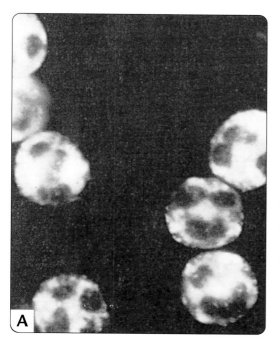
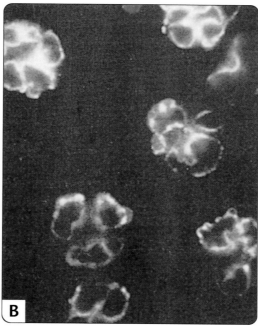

Figure 20-18.
Fluorescence patterns of antineutrophil cytoplasmic antibodies (ANCA). **A,** Cytoplasmic ANCA (cANCA) causes a cytoplasmic fluorescence. More than 90% of cANCA is directed against the neutrophil alpha granule enzyme proteinase 3. cANCA is associated strongly with Wegener's granulomatosis. **B,** Perinuclear ANCA (pANCA) causes a perinuclear fluorescence. More than 70% of pANCA is directed against the neutrophil alpha granule enzyme myeloperoxidase. Other pANCA antigens include cathepsin G, human leukocyte elastase, and lactoferrin. (*From* Gross [26]; with permission.)

HISTORY AND PHYSICAL CHARACTERISTICS OF VASCULITIS

DISTINGUISHING FEATURES OF NECROTIZING VASCULITIS

	Patients, %		
	Microscopic polyangiitis	Churg-Strauss syndrome	Wegener's granulomatosis
System			
Cutaneous	40	60	40
Renal	90	45	80
Pulmonary	50	70	90
Ear/nose/throat	35	50	90
Musculoskeletal	60	50	60
Neurologic	30	70	50
Gastrointestinal	50	50	50
ANCA	90*	70*	90†
Asthma and eosinophilia	—	Diagnostic	—
Granuloma formation	0	100	100

*Most patients have perinuclear ANCA antibody against myeloperoxidase.
†Most patients have cytoplasmic ANCA antibody against proteinase 3.
ANCA—antineutrophil cytoplasmic antibodies.

Figure 20-19.
Distinguishing features of necrotizing vasculitis. Treatment for microscopic polyangiitis includes glucocorticoid and cyclophosphamide. Churg-Strauss syndrome is treated with glucocorticoid alone. Wegener's granulomatosis is also treated with glucocorticoid and cyclophosphamide, as well as methotrexate for mild disease and possibly trimethoprim and sulfamethoxazole. (*Adapted from* Jennette and Falk [18].)

DIFFERENTIAL DIAGNOSIS OF VASCULITIS

Microscopic polyangiitis	Churg-Strauss syndrome	Wegener's granulomatosis
SLE	Wegener's granulomatosis	Fungal infection
Wegener's granulomatosis	PAN	Mycobacterial infection
Churg-Strauss syndrome	Acute sarcoidosis (Loffler's syndrome)	Lymphomatoid granulomatosis
Subacute bacterial endocarditis	Hypersensitivity vasculitis	Churg-Strauss syndrome
Atrial myxoma	Microscopic polyangiitis	PAN
Fibromuscular dysplasia	SLE	Cholesterol emboli
Cholesterol emboli	RA vasculitis	Goodpasture's syndrome
PAN		Microscopic polyangiitis
Goodpasture's syndrome		
RA vasculitis		

PAN—polyarteritis nodosa; RA—rheumatoid arthritis; SLE—systemic lupus erythematosus.

Figure 20-20.
Differential diagnosis of vasculitis.

RED FLAGS OF VASCULITIS

Fever of unknown origin
Unexplained multisystem disease
Unexplained inflammatory arthritis
Unexplained myositis
Unexplained glomerulonephritis
Unexplained cardiac/gastrointestinal/ central nervous system ischemia
Mononeuritis multiplex
Suspicious rash:
    Palpable purpura
    Maculopapular
    Nodules
    Ulcers
    Livedo reticularis

Figure 20-21.
Red flags of vasculitis. (*Adapted from* Calabrese [27].)

REFERENCES

1. Lightfoot BA Jr, Michel DA, Bloch GG, et al.: The American College of Rheumatology 1990 criteria for the classification of polyarteritis nodosa. *Arthritis Rheum* 1990, 33:1088–1093.

2. Calabrese LH, Michel BA, Bloch DA, et al.: The American College of Rheumatology 1990 criteria for the classification of hypersensitivity vasculitis. *Arthritis Rheum* 1990, 33:1108–1113.

3. Leavitt RY, Fauci AS, Bloch DA, et al.: The American College of Rheumatology 1990 criteria for the classification of Wegener's granulomatosis. *Arthritis Rheum* 1990, 33:1101–1107.

4. Hunder GG, Bloch DA, Michel BA, et al.: The American College of Rheumatology 1990 criteria for the classification of giant cell arteritis. *Arthritis Rheum* 1990, 33:1122–1128.

5. Masi AT, Hunder GG, Lie JT, et al.: The American College of Rheumatology 1990 criteria for the classification of Churg-Strauss syndrome (allergic granulomatosis and angiitis). *Arthritis Rheum* 1990, 33:1094–1100.

6. Arend WP, Michel BA, Bloch DA, et al.: The American College of Rheumatology 1990 criteria for the classification of Takayasu arteritis. *Arthritis Rheum* 1990, 33:1129–1136.

7. Cupps TR: Vasculitis epidemiology, pathology and pathogenesis. In *Primer on the Rheumatic Diseases*, edn 10. Edited by Schumacher HR Jr, Klippel JH, Koopman WJ. Atlanta: Arthritis Foundation; 1993:136–140.

8. Lhote F, Guillevin L: Polyarteritis nodosa, microscopic polyangiitis, and Churg-Strauss syndrome. In *Rheumatic Disease Clinics of North America—Vasculitis*, vol 21. Edited by Hunder GG. Philadelphia: WB Saunders; 1995:911–947.

9. Wechsler ME, Pauwels R, Drazen JM: Leukotriene modifiers and Churg-Strauss syndrome: adverse effect or response to corticosteroid withdrawal? *Drug Safety* 1999, 21:241–251.

10. Kerr GS: Takayasu's arteritis. In *Rheumatic Disease Clinics of North America—Vasculitis*, vol 21. Edited by Hunder GG. Philadelphia: WB Saunders; 1995:1041–1058.

11. Nordborg E, Nordborg C, Malmvall B, et al.: Giant cell arteritis. In *Rheumatic Disease Clinics of North America—Vasculitis*, vol 21. Edited by Hunder GG. Philadelphia: WB Saunders; 1995:1013–1026.

12. Hoffman GS, Kerr GS, Leavitt RY, et al.: Wegener granulomatosis: an analysis of 158 patients. *Ann Intern Med* 1992, 116:488–498.

13. Fauci AS, Katz P, Haynes BF, et al.: Cyclophosphamide therapy of severe systemic necrotizing vasculitis. *N Engl J Med* 1979, 301:235–238.

14. Savage COS, Winearls CG, Evans DJ, et al.: Microscopic polyarteritis: presentation, pathology and prognosis. *Q J Med* 1985, 56:467–483.

15. Guillevin L, Guittard T, Bletry O, et al.: Systemic necrotizing angiitis with asthma: causes, and precipitating factors in 43 cases. *Lung* 1987, 165:165–172.

16. Hall S, Barr W, Lie JT, et al.: Takayasu arteritis: a study of 32 North American patients. *Medicine* 1985, 64:89–99.

17. Langford CA, Talar-Williams C, Sneller MC: Use of methotrexate and glucocorticoids in the treatment of Wegener's Granulomatosis: long-term renal outcome in patients with glomerulonephritis. *Arthritis Rheum* 2000, 43:1836–1840.

18. Jennette JC, Falk RJ: Small-vessel vasculitis. *N Engl J Med* 1997, 337:1512–1523.

19. Lanham JG, Elkon KB, Pusey CD, Hughes GR: Systemic vasculitis with asthma and eosinophilia: a clinical approach to the Churg-Strauss syndrome. *Medicine* 1984, 63:65–81.

20. Chumbley LC, Harrison EG, DeRemee RA: Allergic granulomatosis and angiitis (Churg-Strauss syndrome) report and analysis of 30 cases. *Mayo Clin Proc* 1977, 52:477–484.

21. Wilson AG: Immunologic diseases of the lungs. In *Imaging of Diseases of the Chest*, edn 2. Edited by Armstrong P, Wilson AG, Dee P, Hansell DM. St. Louis: Mosby; 1995:485–567.

22. Winterbauer RH: Wegener's granulomatosis and other pulmonary granulomatosis vasculitides. In *Pulmonary and Critical Care Medicine*, vol 2. Edited by Bone RC. St. Louis: Mosby; 1993:1–13.

23. The Visual Aids Subcommittee of the Professional Education Committee of the Arthritis Foundation: *Clinical Slide Collection of the Rheumatic Diseases*. New York: The Arthritis Foundation; 1995.

24. Lebovics RS, Hoffman, GS, Leavitt RY, et al.: The management of subglottic stenosis in patients with Wegener's granulomatosis. *Laryngoscope* 1992, 102:1341–1345.

25. Rottem M, Fauci AS, Hallahan CW, et al.: Wegener granulomatosis in children and adolescents: clinical presentation and outcome. *J Pediatr* 1993, 122:26–31.

26. Gross WL: Antineutrophil cytoplasmic autoantibody testing in vasculitides. In *Rheumatic Disease Clinics of North America—Vasculitis*, vol 21. Edited by Hunder GG. Philadelphia: WB Saunders; 1995:987–1011.

27. Calabrese LH: Vasculitis: New York Rheumatism Association—Rheumatology Board Review Course, September 27, 1996.

VENOUS THROMBOEMBOLISM

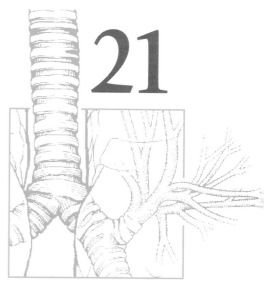

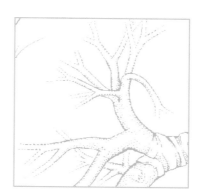

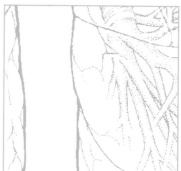

Jennifer A. Sewell &
D. Keith Payne

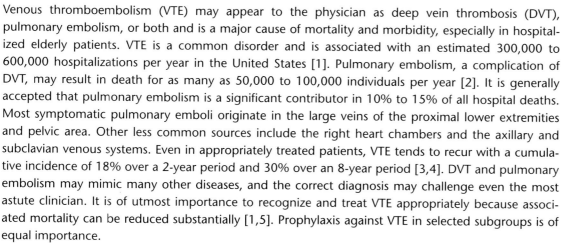

Venous thromboembolism (VTE) may appear to the physician as deep vein thrombosis (DVT), pulmonary embolism, or both and is a major cause of mortality and morbidity, especially in hospitalized elderly patients. VTE is a common disorder and is associated with an estimated 300,000 to 600,000 hospitalizations per year in the United States [1]. Pulmonary embolism, a complication of DVT, may result in death for as many as 50,000 to 100,000 individuals per year [2]. It is generally accepted that pulmonary embolism is a significant contributor in 10% to 15% of all hospital deaths. Most symptomatic pulmonary emboli originate in the large veins of the proximal lower extremities and pelvic area. Other less common sources include the right heart chambers and the axillary and subclavian venous systems. Even in appropriately treated patients, VTE tends to recur with a cumulative incidence of 18% over a 2-year period and 30% over an 8-year period [3,4]. DVT and pulmonary embolism may mimic many other diseases, and the correct diagnosis may challenge even the most astute clinician. It is of utmost importance to recognize and treat VTE appropriately because associated mortality can be reduced substantially [1,5]. Prophylaxis against VTE in selected subgroups is of equal importance.

This chapter illustrates several concepts in diagnosis, treatment, and prophylaxis of VTE. Newer diagnostic and therapeutic modalities are rapidly emerging and may significantly improve the management of VTE in the near future. Computerized tomography and magnetic resonance imaging are potentially useful tools for the diagnosis of VTE. New data suggest that a relatively simple serum test, D-dimer levels, may be useful to exclude the diagnosis of pulmonary embolism. Traditionally, patients with an acute episode of VTE have been hospitalized for extended periods of time. The use of short-course therapy along with weight-based heparin nomograms may shorten hospitalization times significantly and decrease the number of recurrent episodes. The use of low–molecular–weight heparin has made outpatient treatment of DVT practical and safe for many patients. Thrombolytic agents for the treatment of VTE continue to be a source of some controversy because no clear reduction in mortality has been shown compared with conventional therapy. New findings and controversies such as these continue to energize the field of venous thromboembolism research, introducing new data and improved tools for use by the physician in the hope of providing better patient care.

RISK FACTORS FOR VENOUS THROMBOEMBOLIC DISEASE

Stasis of blood flow

Prolonged bedrest or immobility

Congestive heart failure

Paralytic stroke

Intimal injury

Prior thromboembolism

Trauma (especially to lower extremities, pelvis, and spinal cord)

Major surgery (especially involving lower extremity, abdomen, and pelvis)

Hypercoagulable states

Primary

    Antithrombin III deficiency

    Protein C deficiency

    Protein S deficiency

    Factor V Leiden mutation

    Dysfibrinogenemia

    Homocystinuria

    Increased factor VIII levels

Secondary

    Malignancy

    Pregnancy (especially in the puerperium)

    Trauma/major surgery

    Oral contraceptives

    Nephrotic syndrome

    Myeloproliferative syndromes

    Lupus anticoagulant/antiphospholipid syndrome

    High-dose chemotherapy

    Heparin-induced thrombocytopenia and thrombosis

    Obesity

    Age >40 y

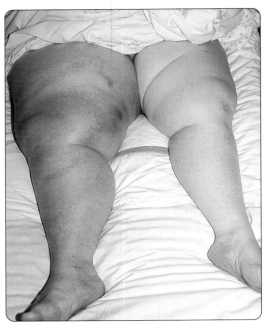

Figure 21-1.
Risk factors associated with venous thromboembolism (VTE). The great 19th century German pathologist Rudolph Virchow proposed three basic factors leading to thrombus formation. Today, "Virchow's triad"—stasis of blood flow, intimal injury, and hypercoagulability— still provides the basis for our understanding of clinically apparent risk factors for VTE. VTE is unusual in patients who do not have at least one risk factor. As the number of risk factors increases, the degree of risk also increases.

Figure 21-2.
Deep vein thrombosis (DVT). A 35-year-old woman with slightly prolonged activated partial thromboplastin time had a massively swollen leg. DVT was confirmed by noninvasive testing. The patient was also found to have a lupus anticoagulant. Several other disease processes may mimic DVT, and the clinical examination is less than 50% accurate. In symptomatic individuals, noninvasive tests such as impedance plethysmography or ultrasonography are extremely accurate (above the knees) and are usually sufficient to make the diagnosis. (See Color Plate.)

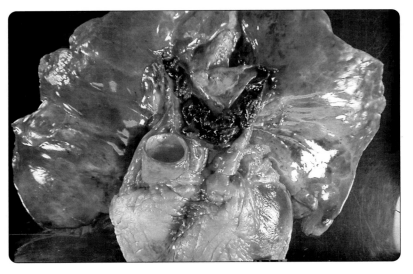

Figure 21-3.
Autopsy specimen showing saddle pulmonary embolism. *Saddle embolism* is a term used to describe embolic obstruction at the bifurcation of the main trunk of the pulmonary artery. This massive embolus resulted in acute right-sided heart failure, cardiogenic shock, and death. Appropriate prophylaxis therapy may prevent such a catastrophic sequela of deep vein thrombosis. (See Color Plate.)

CLINICAL FEATURES

SIGNS OR SYMPTOMS OBSERVED IN PATIENTS WITH THROMBOEMBOLISM

		Study	
		Stein *et al.* [6], % (*n* = 117)	Anderson *et al.* [1], % (*n* = 131)
Pulmonary embolism	Dyspnea	73	77
	Tachypnea	70	70
	Chest pain	66	55
	Cough	37	—
	Tachycardia	30	43
	Cyanosis	1	18
	Hemoptysis	13	13
	Wheezing	9	—
	Hypotension	—	10
	Syncope	—	10
	Elevated jugular venous pulse	—	8
	Temperature >38.5°C	7	—
	S-3 gallop	3	5
	Pleural friction rub	3	2
Deep vein thrombosis	Swelling	28	88*
	Pain	26	56
	Tenderness	—	55
	Warmth	—	42
	Redness	—	34
	Homan's sign	4	13
	Palpable cord	—	6

*n = 274.

Figure 21-4.
Signs and symptoms associated with acute thromboembolism. The study by Stein *et al.* [6] consisted of patients from the Prospective Investigation of Pulmonary Embolism Diagnosis (PIOPED) trial and was screened to exclude patients with preexisting cardiac or pulmonary disease. In contrast, almost one third of patients in the retrospective study by Anderson *et al.* [1] had evidence of chronic obstructive pulmonary disease and congestive heart failure. Although individual signs and symptoms are not sensitive or specific, Stein's group reported that 91% of patients with proven pulmonary embolism were found to have dyspnea, hemoptysis, or pleuritic chest pain.

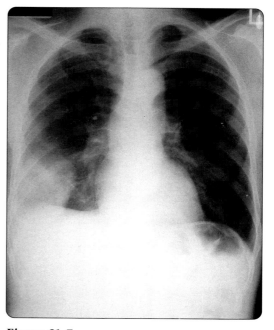

Figure 21-5.
Chest radiograph showing pulmonary infarct in the right lower lobe. This patient had low-grade fever, hemoptysis, and pleuritic chest pain. The ventilation-perfusion scan was read as high probability for pulmonary embolism. A pleural-based density in the lower lobe with the convexity directed toward the hilum signifies pulmonary infarction. This sign is also known as "Hampton's hump."

CHEST RADIOGRAPHIC FINDINGS IN PATIENTS WITH PULMONARY EMBOLISM

	COPD, % (*n* = 21)	No prior cardiopulmonary disease, % (*n* = 117)
Atelectasis or pulmonary parenchymal abnormality	76	68
Pleural effusion	52	48
Pleural-based opacity	33	35
Elevated diaphragm	14	24
Decreased pulmonary vascularity	38	21
Prominent central pulmonary artery	29	15
Cardiomegaly	19	12
Westermark's sign*	5	7
Pulmonary edema	14	4

*Westermark's sign—prominent central pulmonary artery and decreased pulmonary vascularity.
COPD—chronic obstructive pulmonary disease.

Figure 21-6.
Chest radiographic findings in patients with pulmonary embolism. Although frequently abnormal, the chest radiograph is nonspecific for the diagnosis of pulmonary embolism and cannot be used to confirm the diagnosis. The existence of underlying lung disease may also influence the chest radiographic appearance of pulmonary embolism. (*Data from* Stein [7].)

Diagnosis of Venous Thromboembolism

TESTS USED IN DIAGNOSIS OF DEEP VEIN THROMBOSIS

Test	Description
Contrast venography	Diagnostic gold standard and the only accurate method for determining the presence or absence of DVT in asymptomatic individuals. The test is technically difficult to perform and many patients experience discomfort from the procedure. Approximately 1%–2% of patients with negative studies may develop DVT from the procedure, and up to 10% of test results may be uninterpretable due to inadequate examinations or interobserver variability [8].
IPG	Inflation and deflation of a thigh cuff causes changes in electrical impedance, which are attenuated by presence of thrombus. The negative predictive value of IPG and ultrasonography are identical. Serial negative IPG or ultrasonography is comparable in accuracy to negative venography in patients with suspected DVT [9,10].
Compression ultrasound	In many centers, this is the diagnostic modality of choice. The sensitivity and specificity approach 97%–98% for symptomatic patients. The sensitivity for high-risk asymptomatic individuals is only 50%–60% [9].
Magnetic resonance imaging	Preliminary studies indicate very high sensitivity and specificity. Useful for accurate imaging of clots in all areas. Although noninvasive, the test is expensive and experience is limited [11].
D-dimer	Recent studies indicate that low levels of plasma D-dimer (<500 ng/mL) by ELISA technique may have a high negative predictive value when used in patients with suspected venous thromboembolism. The sensitivity is reported to be 95%–98% and the specificity below 50% [12]. A whole blood agglutination assay has also been reported to have a sensitivity of 97.5%. The results of a D-dimer assay in addition to noninvasive imaging may be useful in excluding thromboembolic disease with more confidence [13].

DVT—deep vein thrombosis; ELISA—enzyme-linked immunosorbent assay; IPG—impedance plethysmography.

Figure 21-7.

Tests used in the diagnosis of deep vein thrombosis. The various tests used to diagnose thrombosis in proximal thigh veins are summarized in the figure. The reliable diagnosis of calf vein thrombi is possible only with contrast venography or magnetic resonance imaging. The clinical significance of these thrombi is debatable because less than 20% migrate proximally. If calf thrombi are diagnosed, serial noninvasive testing to observe for proximal migration is prudent.

THE USE OF VENTILATION PERFUSION SCAN IN DIAGNOSING PULMONARY EMBOLISM

High probability

≥2 large segmental (>75% of a segment) perfusion defects without corresponding ventilation or radiographic abnormalities or substantially larger than matching ventilation or radiologic abnormalities

OR

≥2 moderate segmental (>25% and <75% of a segment) perfusion defects without matching ventilation or chest radiographic abnormalities plus one large unmatched segmental defect

OR

≥4 moderate segmental perfusion defects without matching ventilation or chest radiologic abnormalities

Intermediate probability

Scans that do not fall into normal, very low, low, or high probability categories

Low probability

Nonsegmental perfusion defects

OR

Single moderate mismatched segmental perfusion defect with normal chest radiograph

OR

Any perfusion defect with a substantially larger abnormality on chest radiograph

OR

Large or moderate segmental perfusion defects involving no more than four segments in one lung and no more than three segments in one lung region with matching or larger ventilation/radiographic abnormalities

OR

More than three small segmental perfusion defects (<25% of a segment) with a normal chest radiograph

Very low probability

Three or fewer small segmental perfusion defects with a normal chest radiograph

Normal

No perfusion defects present

Figure 21-8.

The use of ventilation-perfusion scan in diagnosing pulmonary embolism. The criteria used for interpreting ventilation-perfusion scans are listed in the figure. In patients suspected to have pulmonary embolism, this study is ordered routinely. The perfusion scan is usually performed first. Macroaggregates of albumin labeled with technetium-99m are injected, and images are obtained in anterior, posterior, and right and left lateral and oblique views. If the perfusion scan is normal, there is no need to perform a ventilation scan. Defects in perfusion are assessed and quantified. The ventilation scan is performed by inhalation of a radioactive gas, usually 133 Xe is mixed with air. The patient breathes this radioactive mixture until a state of equilibrium has been reached between the spirometer and lungs, then the patient breathes room air. Images taken in this wash-out phase are useful in detecting ventilation abnormalities. (*Adapted from* the PIOPED Investigators [14].)

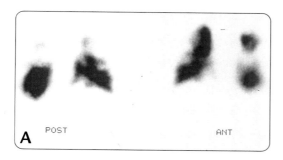

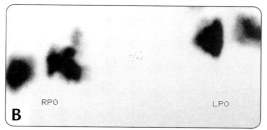

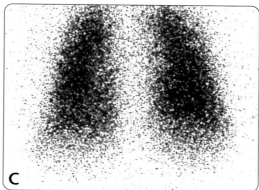

Figure 21-9.
High-probability ventilation-perfusion scan.
A and **B,** Multiple large segmental and subsegmental perfusion defects are seen bilaterally. **C,** The corresponding ventilation image was normal. The patient was treated for pulmonary embolism.

PROSPECTIVE INVESTIGATION OF PULMONARY EMBOLISM DIAGNOSIS RESULTS

Scan category	PE present	PE absent	PE uncertain	No angiogram	Total
High probability	102	14	1	7	124
Intermediate probability	105	217	9	33	364
Low probability	39	199	12	62	312
Near normal or normal	5	50	2	74	131
Total	251	480	24	176	931

PE—pulmonary embolism.

Figure 21-10.
Prospective Investigation of Pulmonary Embolism Diagnosis (PIOPED) results. This prospective study was designed to study the accuracy of ventilation-perfusion ($\dot{V}/\dot{Q}$) scan in the diagnosis of pulmonary embolism. Results of $\dot{V}/\dot{Q}$ scan were compared with pulmonary angiography, which was used as a gold standard. From the results it is obvious that more than two thirds of patients have scans of low or intermediate probability that are nondiagnostic. Although a high-probability scan usually indicates pulmonary embolism, only a minority of patients with pulmonary embolism have a high-probability scan. Near-normal lung scans make the diagnosis of pulmonary embolism very unlikely. (*Data from* the PIOPED Investigators [14].)

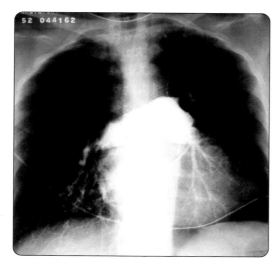

Figure 21-11.
Pulmonary angiogram showing pulmonary embolism. Pulmonary angiography remains the diagnostic gold standard for pulmonary embolism. Access to the pulmonary artery is obtained via transvenous catheter placement. The diagnosis is confirmed by persistent filling defect or abrupt cut-off of flow. Abrupt cut-off of flow to the right and left upper lobe vessels is seen in this patient.

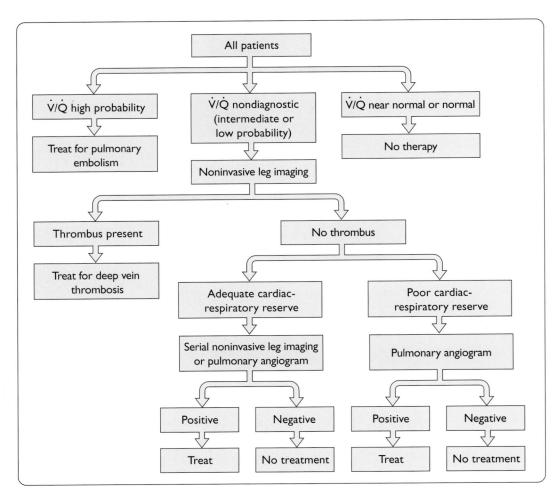

Figure 21-12.
Suggested diagnostic strategy for venous thromboembolism. The PIOPED study revealed that results of ventilation-perfusion ($\dot{V}/\dot{Q}$) scans are nondiagnostic in more than 70% of the cases. The diagnostic strategy proposed in the figure provides a rational approach to work up patients with suspected thromboembolic disease. The role of spiral CT scan in the diagnosis of pulmonary embolism remains controversial with a wide range of reported sensitivities (53%–100%) and specificities (81%–100%) [15]. (*Adapted from* Stein et al. [16].)

PROPHYLAXIS AND THERAPY OF THROMBOEMBOLIC DISEASE

GRADING METHOD FOR EVALUATING PROPHYLAXIS RECOMMENDATIONS

Level of evidence	Grade of recommendation
Level 1	Grade A
	Results come from a randomized controlled trial or meta-analysis of such trials in which the lower limit of the CI for the treatment effect exceeds the minimum clinically important benefit
Level 2	Grade B
	Results from a randomized controlled trial or meta-analysis of such trials in which the confidence limit for the treatment effect overlaps the minimum clinically important benefit
Level 3	Grade C
	Results come from nonrandomized concurrent cohort studies
Level 4	Grade C
	Results come from nonrandomized historical cohort studies
Level 5	Grade C
	Results come from case series

Figure 21-13.
Prophylaxis and therapy of thromboembolic disease. The prophylaxis and appropriate treatment for thromboembolic disease is an area of intense study and debate. The role of-therapies such as thrombolysis, low–molecular–weight heparins, and hirudin is in an evolutionary phase, and a detailed discourse is beyond the scope of this publication. Reviews on these subjects are available in the literature [17–19]. (*Adapted from* Cook et al. [20].)

RECOMMENDATIONS FOR THE PREVENTION OF VENOUS THROMBOEMBOLISM

Nature of illness/surgery	Grade/level of evidence	Recommendation
Low-risk general surgical patients undergoing minor surgery; age <40 y, no specific risk factors	Grade C/level 3 data	Early ambulation
Moderate-risk general surgical patients undergoing major operations; age >40 y, no specific risk factors	Grade A/level 1 data	Elastic stockings; IPC, LDUH every 12 h
High-risk patients undergoing major general surgical procedures; age >40 y, other risk factors present	Grade A/level 1 data	LDUH every 8 h or LMWH
		IPC would be a good choice if high-risk for wound hematoma
Very high-risk general surgical patients with multiple risk factors	Grade B/level 2 data	LDUH or LMWH or dextran plus IPC; start heparin preoperatively
		Dextran and IPC can be used intraoperatively
Hip replacement	Grade A/level 1 data	LMWH or warfarin (INR 2.0–3.0) or adjusted-dose heparin
		Start preoperatively or immediately postoperatively
		IPC and elastic stockings plus anticoagulants have added benefit
Knee replacement	Grade A/level 1 data	LMWH or IPC
Hip fracture	Grade A/level 1 data	LMWH or warfarin
Intracranial neurosurgery	Grade A/level 1 data	IPC and/or elastic stockings; LDUH acceptable; IPC plus LDUH are more efficacious and should be considered in high-risk patients
Spinal cord injury and paralysis	Grade B/level 2 data	Adjusted-dose heparin or LMWH
	Grade C/level 4	Warfarin (INR 2.0–3.0)
	Grade B/level 2	LDUH, elastic stockings, and IPC used alone are ineffective; they may be useful in combination
Multiple trauma	Grade C/levels 3,4	IPC/LMWH/warfarin when feasible
		Consider inferior vena caval filter, serial duplex/IPG
Myocardial infarction	Grade A/level 1	LDUH or full-dose anticoagulation
	Grade C/level 4	IPC/elastic stockings if heparin contraindicated
Ischemic stroke; lower extremity paralysis	Grade A/level 1 data	LDUH or LMWH
	Grade C/level 4	IPC/elastic stockings
General medical patients/congestive heart failure/chest infection	Grade A/level 1 data	LDUH or LMWH
Long-term central vein catheter	Grade A/level 1 data	Coumadin 1 mg daily

INR—International Normalized Ratio; IPC—intermittent pneumatic compression; LDUH—low-dose unfractionated heparin; LMWH—low–molecular weight heparin.

Figure 21-14.

Recommendations for prevention of venous thromboembolism (VTE). Despite widespread recognition of the risks of VTE in selected patient groups with known risk factors, prophylaxis remains underused. Effective methods of prevention are more practical and cost effective than intensive surveillance. Because VTE may be clinically silent (and suddenly fatal), it is unwise to rely on the development of compatible signs and symptoms. (*Adapted from* Clagget *et al.* [21].)

DOSAGE AND MONITORING OF ANTICOAGULANT THERAPY

After initiating heparin therapy, repeat APTT every 6 h for first 24 h and then every 24 h when therapeutic APTT is achieved

Warfarin 5 mg/d can be started on day 1 of therapy; there is no benefit from higher starting doses

Platelet count should be monitored at least every 3 d during initial heparin therapy

Therapeutic APTT should correspond to plasma heparin level of 0.2–0.4 IU/mL

Heparin is usually continued for 5–7 d

Heparin can be stopped after 4–5 d of warfarin therapy when INR is in 2.0–3.0 range

APTT—activated partial thromboplastin time; INR—International Normalized Ratio.

Figure 21-15.

Dosage and monitoring of anticoagulant therapy [22,23]. An activated partial thromboplastin time ratio of 1.5 to 2.5 has traditionally been used to define the boundaries of therapeutic heparin effects. The actual therapeutic range may vary according to the thromboplastin reagent used by a particular laboratory. Warfarin acts by inhibiting the synthesis of vitamin K-dependent coagulation factors in the liver (II, VII, IX, and X). The half-lives of these factors are relatively long (60, 6, 24, and 40 hours, respectively), thus the onset of action of warfarin is slow—3 or more days may be required to achieve a therapeutic response. Traditionally, warfarin therapy has been monitored by measuring the prothrombin time (PT). To standardize the monitoring of therapy, the INR is used by many laboratories. The PT of the patient is compared with a normal control PT value; this ratio is then plotted against the International Sensitivity Index (ISI) to calculate the INR (INR = PT ratio[isi]). The ISI is obtained by comparing the local thromboplastin reagent used for testing with a standardized international reagent [24].

Heparin Order Sheet (All blanks must be filled in by physician)

1. Make calculations using total body weight: _____ kg
2. BOLUS HEPARIN, 80 units/kg = _____ units IV
3. IV HEPARIN infusion, 18 units/kg/h = _____units/h (20,000 units heparin in 500 mL of D$_5$W, 40 units/mL)
4. WARFARIN _____mg orally everyday to start on 2nd day of heparin
5. LABORATORY: APTT, PT, CBC now
   CBC with platelet count every 3 days
   APTT 6 h after heparin bolus
   PT every day (start on 3rd day of heparin)
6. ADJUST heparin infusion based on sliding scale below:

PTT <35	80 unit/kg bolus = _____units Increase drip 4 units/kg/h = _____units/h
PTT 35–45	40 unit/kg bolus = _____units Increase drip 2 units/kg/h = _____units/h
PTT 46–70	No change
PTT 71–90	Reduce drip 2 units/kg/h = _____units/h
PTT >90	Hold heparin for 1 h, Reduce drip 3 units/kg/h = _____units/h

7. Order a PTT 6 h after any dosage change, adjusting heparin infusion by the sliding scale until PTT is therapeutic (46–70 s). When 2 consecutive PTTs are therapeutic, order PTT (and re-adjust heparin drip as needed) every 24 h.

Please make changes as promptly as possible and round off doses to the nearest mL/h (nearest 40 units/h).

Signed: _____   Date: _____

Figure 21-16.

Sample weight-based heparin order sheet with nomogram. Unfractionated heparin has been the initial therapeutic agent of choice for many years. It acts by potentiating the effect of antithrombin III against factor Xa and thrombin. Several dosing regimens have been evaluated for the treatment of acute venous thrombosis and pulmonary embolism. Weight-based dosing regimens have been shown to achieve a more rapid therapeutic response and a reduced rate of recurrent thromboembolism. Intravenous (IV) administration is preferred in acute deep vein thrombosis and pulmonary embolism, although subcutaneous dosing regimens are also effective. APTT—active partial thromboplastin time; CBC—complete blood cell count; D$_5$W—5% dextrose in water; PT—prothrombin time. (*Adapted from* Raschke *et al.* [25].)

LOW-MOLECULAR-WEIGHT HEPARIN PREPARATIONS

Product name (trade name)	Type of use	Indications	Dosage	Pregnancy category	FDA approval date
Ardeparin (Normiflo; Wyeth-Ayerst, Philadelphia, PA)	Prophylaxis	Knee replacement	50 units/kg SC q 12 h	C	January 1998
Dalteparin (Fragmin; Pharmacia, Peapack, NJ)	Prophylaxis	Abdominal surgery	2500 units SC QD	B	December 1994
		Orthopedic surgery/ high-risk patient	5000 units SC QD		
	Treatment	DVT and/or PE	200 units/kg SC QD up to 18,000 units SC QD		
Enoxaparin (Lovenox; Aventis, Parsippany, NJ)	Prophylaxis	Knee replacement/hip replacement	30 units SC q 12 h	B	March 1993
		Abdominal surgery/hip replacement/very high risk patient	40 units SC QD		
	Treatment	DVT and/or PE	1 mg/kg SC q 12 h		
Tinzaparin (Innohep; DuPont, Wilmington, DE)	Treatment	DVT and/or PE	175 units/kg SC QD	B	July 2000

Figure 21-17.

Low-molecular-weight heparin preparations. Ardeparin, dalteparin, enoxaparin, and tinzaparin are low-molecular-weight heparins approved for use in the United States. This group of agents acts by inhibition of factor Xa more than thrombin (IIa), thus they have much less effect on the activated partial thromboplastin time than unfractionated heparin. They have a longer half-life and the convenience of once or twice daily dosing. However, they are 10 to 20 times more expensive than unfractionated heparin [17].

IMPORTANT DRUG INTERACTIONS WITH WARFARIN

Drugs that decrease warfarin requirement	Drugs that increase warfarin requirement
Phenylbutazone	Barbiturates
Metronidazole	Carbamazepine
Trimethoprim-sulfamethoxazole	Rifampin
Amiodarone	Penicillin
Second- and third-generation cephalosporins	Griseofulvin
Clofibrate	Cholestyramine
Erythromycin	
Anabolic steroids	
Thyroxine	

Figure 21-18.
Important drug interactions with warfarin. The figure includes only a short list of commonly used agents that are known to have clinically significant interactions with warfarin; several other drugs have pharmacokinetic and pharmacodynamic interactions with warfarin. Careful review of medications, alcohol consumption, and dietary factors is mandatory in patients who are on warfarin therapy.

OUTPATIENT THERAPY OF DVT WITH LOW-MOLECULAR-WEIGHT HEPARIN

Confirmed diagnosis by objective criteria (Doppler ultrasonography or venography)

Obtain complete blood count with platelets, PT, and PTT; initiate any further work-up for underlying cause of thrombosis

Patient (or family member/caretaker) must demonstrate ability to give subcutaneous injections

First dose of LMWH administered at health facility

Begin oral anticoagulant

Arrange outpatient laboratory twice weekly (PT, INR, and complete blood count)

Follow up with full clinical visit within 7 days of initiating therapy, discontinue LMWH when INR ranges from 2.0 to 3.0

Consider inpatient therapy when:

    Signs or symptoms of pulmonary embolism, or confirmed PE

    Comorbid condition prompting admission

    History of heparin-induced thrombocytopenia

    History of nonadherence with medical regimen

    Inaccessible to close follow-up

    High risk for complications and bleeding

        Elderly or high risk for falls

        Low hemoglobin at diagnosis

        Active bleeding (ie, heme-positive stool)

        History of CVA within 6 weeks

        History of major surgery within 2 weeks

        Thrombocytopenia

        Any other medical condition with increased risk of bleeding

    Patients on hemodialysis

Figure 21-20.
Mechanism of action of low–molecular-weight heparins. Unfractionated heparin and low–molecular-weight heparins bind with antithrombin III. This causes an accelerated interaction between antithrombin III and factor Xa to inactivate both molecules. The inactivation of thrombin (IIa) requires the formation of a ternary heparin-antithrombin-thrombin complex. Chains of at least 18 saccharide units are required to form the complex, thus low–molecular–weight heparins have less anti-IIa activity than unfractionated heparin. (*Adapted from* Weitz [17].)

Figure 21-19.
Outpatient therapy of DVT with low-molecular-weight heparin. Studies have shown that outpatient treatment of DVT with LMWH has comparable efficacy and safety compared to inpatient treatment with heparin and/or coumadin [26–29]. LMWH has made outpatient treatment of thromboembolic disease feasible because of its ease of administration, safety, and reduced need for laboratory monitoring, as well as decreased health care costs and improved patient satisfaction. However, because of the longer half-life of LMWH, patients at high-risk for bleeding may benefit from UFH, which allows for quicker reversal of anticoagulation in the event of bleeding. Careful selection of patients who are good candidates for outpatient treatment will help lessen complications [30]. These are general recommendations only. The decision to admit or discharge early must be individualized. The outpatient treatment of patients with documented pulmonary embolism is being investigated, and studies have been promising in those with hemodynamically stable PE [31,32].

VENOUS THROMBOEMBOLIC DISEASE IN PREGNANCY

Condition	Recommendation*
Previous venous thrombosis or PE before pregnancy	Heparin 5000 U every 12 h or adjusted dose to produce a heparin level of 0.1–0.2 U/mL throughout pregnancy followed by warfarin postpartum for 4–6 wk
	OR
	Clinical surveillance combined with serial noninvasive leg testing during pregnancy followed by warfarin postpartum for 4–6 wk
Venous thrombosis or PE during pregnancy	Full-dose intravenous heparin for 5–10 d followed by subcutaneous injections every 12 h to prolong 6-h postinjection APTT into the therapeutic range until delivery; postpartum warfarin can then be used
Antiphospholipid antibody	
>1 previous pregnancy loss	Aspirin + prednisone or aspirin + heparin or aspirin alone
0–1 previous pregnancy loss	Low-dose aspirin during the 2nd and 3rd trimester
Previous venous thrombosis	Subcutaneous heparin every 12 h to prolong postinjection APTT into therapeutic range
No previous venous thrombosis	Clinical surveillance + noninvasive leg imaging
	OR
	Heparin 5000 U every 12 h throughout pregnancy

*Grading of recommendation for all is C/level IV or V.
APTT—activated partial thromboplastin time; PE—pulmonary embolism.

Figure 21-21.

Venous thromboembolic disease in pregnancy. The management of thromboembolic disease in the pregnant patient is complicated by issues of safety to the mother and fetus. Warfarin is teratogenic and should not be used in pregnant women; therefore, unfractionated heparin has been the traditional agent of choice. Low-molecular-weight heparins do not cross the placenta, and evidence suggests that they are safe during pregnancy [33]. Although there is no clear information on appropriate dosing in pregnant women, some authorities recommend periodic measurement of the anti-factor Xa levels 4 hours after injection to achieve levels between 0.5 and 1.2 units/mL [34,35].

COMPLICATIONS OF ANTICOAGULATION

	Complication	Management
Heparin	Bleeding	Stop heparin infusion. For severe bleeding, the anticoagulant effect of heparin can be reversed with intravenous protamine sulfate 1 mg/100 units of heparin bolus or 0.5 mg for the number of units given by constant infusion over the past hour; provide supportive care including transfusion and clot evacuation from closed body cavities as needed.
	Heparin-induced thrombocytopenia and thrombosis	Carefully monitor platelet count during therapy. Stop-heparin for platelet counts <75,000. Replace heparin with direct inhibitors of thrombin-like desirudin if necessary. These agents do not cause heparin-induced thrombocytopenia. Avoid platelet transfusion because of the risk for thrombosis.
	Heparin-induced osteoporosis (therapy >1 mo)	LMWHs may have lower propensity to cause osteoporosis as compared with unfractionated heparin; consider LMWH if prolonged heparin therapy is necessary.
Warfarin	Bleeding	Stop therapy. Administer vitamin K and fresh-frozen plasma for severe bleeding; provide supportive care including transfusion and clot evacuation from closed body cavities as needed
	Skin necrosis (rare)	Supportive care.
	Teratogenicity	Do not use in pregnancy or in patients planning to become pregnant.

LMWH—low–molecular-weight heparin.

Figure 21-22.

Complications of anticoagulation. Major bleeding episodes with the use of heparin are much more likely to occur in patients with identifiable risks for bleeding rather than an excessively long activated partial thromboplastin time per se. LMWH does not affect the APTT to a significant degree; therefore, the APTT need not be routinely measured. Many factors influence the prothrombin time during warfarin therapy. Weekly or biweekly measurements are necessary until the prothrombin time stabilizes. Thereafter, monthly measurements of the prothrombin time may be sufficient.

RISKS AND BENEFITS OF THROMBOLYTICS VS HEPARIN THERAPY FOR PULMONARY EMBOLISM

	Thrombolytic therapy	No difference	Heparin
Improved resolution at 2–4 h after onset of therapy			
Angiography	+	-	-
Pulmonary artery pressure	+	-	-
Echocardiography	+	-	-
Resolution at 24 h			
Lung scan	+	-	-
Angiography	+	-	-
Echocardiography	+	-	-
Pulmonary artery pressure	+	-	-
Resolution at 1 wk and 30 d (lung scan)	-	+	-
Rate of confirmed recurrent pulmonary embolism	-	+	-
Hospital mortality	-	+	-
Late mortality	-	+	-
Less severe bleeding	-	-	+
Less intracranial hemorrhage	-	-	+
Lower cost	-	-	+

+ sign indicates advantage of treatment.

Figure 21-23.
Risks and benefits of thrombolytics versus heparin therapy for pulmonary embolism. The role of thrombolytic therapy in the management of acute thromboembolic disease is unclear. Improvement in hemodynamic parameters and reduction in clot burden have been demonstrated after thrombolysis; however, no improvement in mortality has been demonstrated when compared with conventional anticoagulation. Nonetheless, in selected patients with acute pulmonary embolism and hemodynamic instability, thrombolytics may prove to be life saving. (*Adapted from* Dalen *et al.* [18].)

APPROVED THROMBOLYTICS FOR PULMONARY EMBOLISM

Streptokinase
    250,000 IU as loading dose over 30 min, followed by 100,000 U/h for 24 h
Urokinase
    4400 IU/kg as a loading dose over 10 min, followed by 4400 IU/kg/h for 12–24 h
Recombinant tissue-plasminogen activator
    100 mg as a continuous peripheral intravenous infusion administered over 2 h

Figure 21-24.
Approved thrombolytics for pulmonary embolism. All three US Food and Drug Administration–approved regimens used fixed or weight-adjusted doses. No further dosage adjustments are made. Heparin is resumed after the thrombolytic infusion when the activated partial thromboplastin time is less than 2.5 × control.

INDICATIONS AND CONTRAINDICATIONS FOR THROMBOLYTIC THERAPY IN PULMONARY EMBOLISM

Indications

Hemodynamic instability
Hypoxia on 100% oxygen
Right ventricular dysfunction by echocardiography [36]

Contraindications [37]

Relative
    Recent surgery within last 10 d
    Neurosurgery within 6 mo
    Ophthalmologic surgery within 6 wk
    Hypertension >200 mm Hg systolic or 110 mm Hg diastolic
    Hypertensive retinopathy with hemorrhages or exudates
    Cerebrovascular disease
    Major internal bleeding within the last 6 mo
    Infectious endocarditis
    Pericarditis
Absolute
    Active internal bleeding

    Previous arterial punctures within 10 d
    Bleeding disorder (thrombocytopenia, renal failure, liver failure)
    Placement of central venous catheter within 48 h
    Intracerebral aneurysm or malignancy
    Cardiopulmonary resuscitation within 2 wk
    Pregnancy and the 1st 10 d postpartum
    Severe trauma within 2 mo

Figure 21-25.
Indications and contraindications for thrombolytic therapy in pulmonary embolism. Thrombolytics may also be used to treat extensive ileofemoral venous thrombosis in selected patients with a low risk of bleeding. Some evidence exists that the incidence of postthrombotic syndrome is reduced if complete thrombolysis is achieved. Often the decision to administer thrombolytic therapy has to be individualized after careful review of potential risks and benefits.

INFERIOR VENA CAVAL FILTER DEVICES

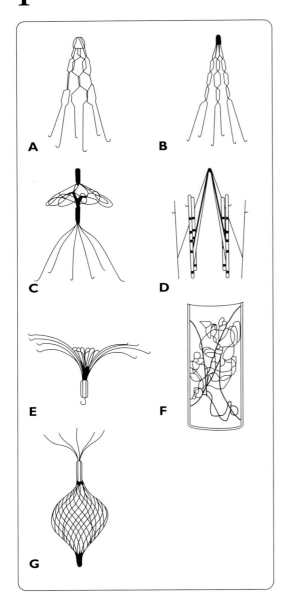

Figure 21-26.
Various inferior vena caval filters. **A**, Greenfield filter; **B**, Titanium Greenfield filter; **C**, Simon-Nitinol filter; **D**, LGM or Vena Tech filter; **E**, Amplatz filter; **F**, Bird's Nest filter; **G**, Günther filter. Surgical interruption of the inferior vena cava was first practiced more than 100 years ago. The practice is percutaneous insertion of a filter device in the inferior vena cava under fluoroscopy to prevent pulmonary embolism. (*Adapted from Becker et al.* [38].)

INDICATIONS FOR INFERIOR VENA CAVAL FILTER PLACEMENT

Anticoagulation contraindicated (*eg*, patients with multiple trauma, active bleeding)

Failure of antithrombotic therapy

Complications from anticoagulant therapy preclude further use

Prophylaxis against embolism from preexisting deep vein thrombosis in patients with poor cardiopulmonary reserve

Prophylaxis against embolism in patients at high risk to develop deep vein thrombosis

Patients with recurrent pulmonary embolism undergoing thromboendarterectomy

Figure 21-27.
Indications for inferior vena caval (IVC) filters. IVC filters are widely used, but randomized controlled trials assessing their efficacy are lacking. The procedure is not difficult to perform in experienced hands; mortality from filter placement is less than 1% [38]. Nonfatal complications that have been reported include misplacement, cellulitis, hematoma, and venous thrombosis. Proximal or distal migration of the device may also occur. Erosion of the filter into the vena cava wall has been reported; it usually occurs slowly with very few clinical complications. IVC obstruction and lower extremity venous insufficiency may occur in some patients [38,39]. If possible, anticoagulation should be used after filter placement to prevent morbidity from deep vein thrombosis in the legs and to prevent clot formation on the filter [40]. Note that IVC filters may lose their effectiveness within a few months due to the development of collateral venous circulation.

CHRONIC THROMBOEMBOLIC PULMONARY HYPERTENSION

CLINICAL FEATURES OF CHRONIC THROMBOEMBOLIC PULMONARY HYPERTENSION

Exercise intolerance

Progressive dyspnea

Chest pain

Syncope

Loud pulmonic component of S2

Fixed splitting of S2

Elevated jugular venous pulse

Lower extremity edema

Murmur of tricuspid insufficiency

Figure 21-28.
Clinical features of chronic thromboembolic pulmonary hypertension. Fewer than 1% of patients with acute pulmonary embolism develop chronic venous thromboembolism. Patients with this condition often have silent pulmonary emboli, which organize and eventually recanalize but cause substantial narrowing of the proximal pulmonary arteries. This condition results in pulmonary hypertension, right ventricular strain, and eventually right ventricular failure [41].

SUGGESTED WORK-UP FOR CHRONIC THROMBOEMBOLIC PULMONARY HYPERTENSION

Test	Result/rationale
Arterial blood gases	Hypoxemia; increase alveolar-arterial gradient at rest or exercise
Echocardiography	Right ventricular hypertrophy
Ventilation-perfusion scan	Mismatched segmental or larger perfusion defects
Right heart catheterization	Provides objective evidence of severity of pulmonary hypertension
Pulmonary angiogram	Bilateral narrowing of major pulmonary arteries is diagnostic
Computed tomographic scan of chest	Helpful in excluding other causes and may show clot in proximal divisions of the pulmonary artery
Pulmonary angioscopy	Permits direct visualization of the obstructing lesions and suitability for surgery

Figure 21-29.

Suggested work-up for chronic thromboembolic pulmonary hypertension. The ventilation-perfusion scan is usually abnormal but may understate the extent of central pulmonary vascular obstruction. Right heart catheterization and pulmonary angiography are essential to quantitate the degree of pulmonary hypertension and delineate the true extent of central pulmonary artery obstruction.

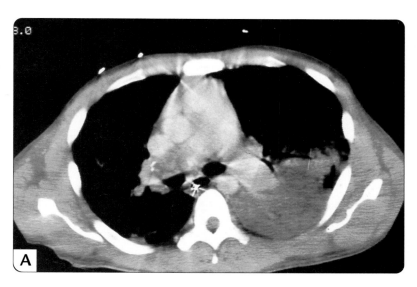

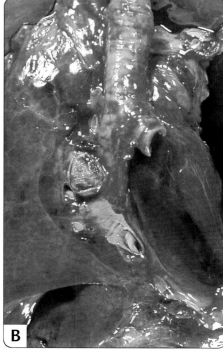

Figure 21-30.
A, Computed tomographic scan demonstrating infarcted lung on left and large clot in the right main pulmonary artery. **B,** Autopsy specimen from same patient demonstrating organized clot in right main pulmonary artery. The patient presented with chronic dyspnea and hemoptysis and later died from complications of severe pulmonary hypertension. Patients with moderate to severe pulmonary hypertension may be considered for thromboendarterectomy. The operative mortality has decreased to approximately 5% with improvement in technique. Patients may experience dramatic relief of symptoms. Life-long anticoagulation is required to prevent recurrence. (See Color Plate.)

REFERENCES

1. Anderson FA Jr, Wheeler HB, Goldberg RJ, et al.: A population based perspective on the hospital incidence and case fatality rates of deep vein thrombosis and pulmonary embolism: the Worcester DVT study. Arch Intern Med 1991, 151:933–938.

2. Dalen JE, Alpert JS: Natural history of pulmonary embolism. Prog Cardiovasc Dis 1975, 17:257–270.

3. Prandoni P, Lensing AWA, et al.: The long-term clinical course of acute deep venous thrombosis. Ann Intern Med 1996, 125:1–7.

4. Schulman S, Rhedin A-S, Lindmarker P, et al. and the Duration of Anticoagulation Trial Study Group: A comparison of six weeks with six months of oral anticoagulant therapy after a first episode of venous thromboembolism. N Engl J Med 1995, 332:1661–1665.

5. Carson JL, Kelley MA, Duff A, et al.: The clinical course of pulmonary embolism. N Engl J Med 1992, 326:1240–1245.

6. Stein PD, Terrin ML, Hales CA, et al.: Clinical, laboratory, roentgenographic, and electrocardiographic findings in patients with acute pulmonary embolism and no pre-existing cardiac or pulmonary disease. Chest 1991, 100:598–603.

7. Stein PD: Diagnosis in patients with chronic obstructive pulmonary disease. In Pulmonary Embolism. Baltimore: Williams and Wilkins; 1996:217–231.

8. Burke B, Sostman HD, Carrol BA, Witty LA: The diagnostic approach to deep venous thrombosis. Clin Chest Med 1995, 16:253–268.

9. Heijboer H, Buller HR, Lensing AWA, et al.: A comparison of real time ultrasonography with impedance plethysmography for the diagnosis of deep vein thrombosis in symptomatic outpatients. N Engl J Med 1993, 329:1365–1369.

10. Huisman MV, Buller HR, ten Cate JW, et al.: Management of clinically suspected acute venous thrombosis in outpatients with serial impedance plethysmography in a community hospital setting. Arch Intern Med 1989, 149:511–513.

11. Meaney JFM, Weg JG, Chenevert TL, et al.: Diagnosis of pulmonary embolism with magnetic resonance angiography. N Engl J Med 1997, 336:1422–1427.

12. Bounameaux H, Moerloose P, Perrier A, Reber G: Plasma measurement of D-dimer as diagnostic aid in suspected venous thromboembolism: an overview. Thromb Haemost 1994, 71:1–6.

13. Ginsberg JS, Kearon C, Douketis J, et al.: The use of D-dimer testing and impedance plethysmographic examination in patients with clinical indications of deep vein thrombosis. Arch Intern Med 1997, 157:1077–1081.

14. The PIOPED Investigators: Value of the ventilation/perfusion scan in acute pulmonary embolism: results of the prospective investigation of pulmonary embolism diagnosis (PIOPED). JAMA 1990, 263:2753–2759.

15. Rathbun SW, Raskob GE, Whitsett TL: Sensitivity and specificity of helical computed tomography in the diagnosis of pulmonary embolism: a systematic review. Ann Intern Med 2000, 132:227–232.

16. Stein PD, Hull RD, Pineo G: Strategy that includes serial non-invasive leg tests for diagnosis of thromboembolic disease in patients with suspected acute pulmonary embolism based on data from PIOPED—Prospective Investigation of Pulmonary Embolism Diagnosis. *Arch Intern Med* 1995, 155:2101–2104.

17. Weitz JI: Low molecular weight heparins. *N Engl J Med* 1997, 337:688–698.

18. Dalen J, Alpert JS, Hirsh J: Thrombolytic therapy for pulmonary embolism: is it effective? Is it safe? When is it indicated? *Arch Intern Med* 1997, 157:2550–2556.

19. Ginsberg JS: Drug therapy: management of venous thromboembolism. *N Engl J Med* 1996, 335:1816–1828.

20. Cook DJ, Guyatt GH, Laupacis A, *et al.*: Clinical recommendations using levels of evidence for antithrombotic agents. *Chest* 1995, 108:227S–230S.

21. Clagett GP, Anderson FA, Heit J, *et al.*: Prevention of venous thromboembolism. *Chest* 1995, 108:312S–334S.

22. Hull RD, Raskob GE, Lemaire J, *et al.*: Optimal therapeutic level of heparin therapy in patients with venous thrombosis. *Arch Intern Med* 1992, 152:1589–1595.

23. Harrison L, Johnston M, Massicotte MP, *et al.*: Comparison of 5 mg and 10 mg loading doses in initiation of warfarin therapy. *Ann Intern Med* 1997, 126:133–136.

24. Hirsh J, Dalen JE, Deykin D, *et al.*: Oral anticoagulants: mechanism of action, clinical effectiveness, and optimal therapeutic range. *Chest* 1995, 108: 231 S–246 S.

25. Raschke RA, Reily BM, Guidry JR, *et al.*: The weight based heparin dosing nomogram compared with a "standard care" nomogram: a randomized controlled trial. *Ann Intern Med* 1993, 119:874–881.

26. Hull RD, Raskob GE, Pineo GF, *et al.*: The treatment of proximal vein thrombosis with subcutaneous low molecular weight heparin compared with continuous intravenous heparin. The Canadian American Thrombosis Study Group. *Clin Appl Thromb Hemost* 1995, 1:151.

27. Koopman MMW, Prandoni P, Piovella F, *et al.*: Treatment of venous thrombosis with intravenous unfractionated heparin administered in the hospital as compared with subcutaneous low-molecular-weight heparin administered at home. *N Engl J Med* 1996, 334:682.

28. Levine M, Gent M, Hirsh J, *et al.*: A comparison of low-molecular-weight heparin administered primarily at home with unfractionated heparin administered in the hospital. *N Engl J Med* 1996, 334:677.

29. Boccalon H: Clinical outcome and cost of hospital vs. home treatment of proximal deep vein thrombosis with a low-molecular-weight heparin: the Vascular Midi-Pyrenees study. *Arch Intern Med* 2000, 160(12):1769–1773.

30. Yusen R: Criteria for outpatient management of proximal lower extremity deep venous thrombosis. *Chest* 1999, 115(4): 972–979

31. Kovacs MJ, Anderson D, Morrow B, Gray L, Touchie D, Wells PS: Outpatient treatment of pulmonary embolism with dalteparin. *Thromb Haemost* 2000, 83(2):209–211.

32. Well PS, Kovacs MJ, Bormanis J, *et al.*: Expanding eligibility for outpatient treatment of deep venous thrombosis and pulmonary embolism with low-molecular-weight heparin. *Arch Intern Med* 1998, 158:1809–1812.

33. Sanson BJ: Safety of low-molecular-weight heparin in pregnancy: a systematic review. *Thromb Haemost* 1999, 81(5):668–672.

34. American College of Obstetricians and Gynecologists: Thromboembolism in pregnancy. *ACOG Practice Bulletin 19.* ACOG 2000; Washington, DC.

35. Ginsberg JS, Hirsh J: Use of antithrombotic agents during pregnancy. *Chest* 1998, 114:524S.

36. Goldhaber SZ, Haire WD, Feldstein ML, *et al.*: Alteplase versus heparin in acute pulmonary embolism: randomised trial assessing right-ventricular function and pulmonary perfusion. *Lancet* 1993, 341:507–511.

37. A collaborative study by the PIOPED investigators: Tissue plasminogen activator for the treatment of acute pulmonary embolism. *Chest* 1990, 97:528–533.

38. Becker DM, Philbrick JT, Selby JB: Inferior vena cava filters: indications, safety, effectiveness. *Arch Intern Med* 1992, 152:1985–1994.

39. Greenfield LJ, Michna BA: Twelve year experience with the Greenfield filter. *Surgery* 1988, 104:706–712.

40. Decousus H, Leizorovicz A, Parent F, *et al.*: A clinical trial of vena caval filters in the prevention of pulmonary embolism in patients with proximal deep-vein thrombosis. *N Engl J Med* 1998, 338:409–415.

41. Jamieson SW, Auger WR, Fedullo PF, *et al.*: Experience and results with 150 pulmonary thromboendarterectomy operations over a 29 month period. *J Thorac Cardiovasc Surg* 1993, 106:116–127.

PRIMARY PULMONARY HYPERTENSION

22

Boaz A. Markewitz,
C. Gregory Elliott &
John R. Michael

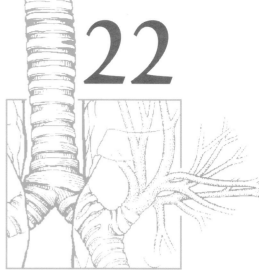

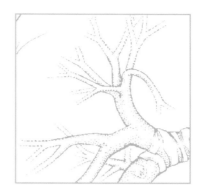

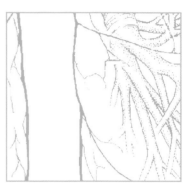

Primary pulmonary hypertension (PPH) is a rare disease characterized by an unexplained elevation in pulmonary artery pressure. Cases of patients dying with cyanosis and right heart failure from an unknown cause have been reported for more than a century; however, the last two decades have seen a refinement in our understanding of the pathology and pathogenesis of this disorder and significant advances in treatment [1,2].

Primary pulmonary hypertension is defined as a mean pulmonary artery pressure higher than 25 mm Hg at rest or 30 mm Hg with exercise in the absence of congenital or acquired pulmonary, cardiac, or collagen vascular disease [3]. In several large studies, the mean age at diagnosis has been in the 30s, with the peak incidence for women being in the 30s and for men in the 40s; the female-to-male ratio is nearly 2:1 [3–5]. This disorder has been described at both extremes of age, with the older-than-60-years group accounting for up to 9% of cases [3,4,6].

Pathologic lesions in PPH have been reported in the pulmonary arterial, capillary, and venular circulation [7,8]. These distinctions may have therapeutic importance because epoprostenol use in pulmonary veno-occlusive disease has been associated with the development of pulmonary edema [9]. PPH is primarily an arteriopathy with four reported lesions: isolated medial hypertrophy, plexiform lesions, thrombotic pulmonary arteriopathy, and isolated pulmonary arteritis [7]. While the plexiform lesion was once considered pathognomonic for PPH, it is recognized that these lesions are seen in diseases other than PPH and that PPH can be diagnosed in its absence.

The most frequent symptoms in PPH are dyspnea and fatigue; the physical findings are those of pulmonary hypertension and right heart failure. The nonspecific nature of its symptoms and the absence of heart failure until late in the disease likely account for the mean delay of 2 years from symptom onset to diagnosis [3,4,10].

The diagnostic evaluation is focused primarily on the exclusion of underlying heart and lung disease. The usual diagnostic studies include a chest radiograph, electrocardiogram (EKG), pulmonary function tests, arterial blood gas determination, ventilation-perfusion scanning, serologic studies screening for collagen vascular diseases, echocardiography, and if indicated, polysomnography or computed tomographic scan of the chest. The presence of pulmonary hypertension is usually first documented noninvasively by two-dimensional echocardiography. Right heart catheterization remains the gold standard for establishing the presence of pulmonary hypertension.

In addition to measuring pulmonary artery pressure directly, cardiac catheterization provides diagnostic, therapeutic, and prognostic information. As the catheter traverses from the central veins into the pulmonary artery, serial oxyhemoglobin measurements are made to determine if a step-up in oxygenation exists; if so, then pulmonary hypertension is secondary to hyperkinetic causes. Similarly, an elevated pulmonary capillary wedge pressure may reflect pulmonary venous hypertension and, thus, indicate that pulmonary hypertension is due to passive causes. The right atrial pressure, pulmonary artery pressure, and cardiac output quantify disease severity and anticipated mortality. Finally, the responsiveness of the pulmonary circulation to acute testing with vasodilators identifies patients who are candidates for long-term therapy with calcium channel blockers and have improved survival [11,12].

Patients diagnosed with PPH may need to make lifestyle changes. If patients are treated with vasodilators, they can engage in physical activity as long as it does not produce chest pain, significant shortness of breath, pre-syncope, or syncope. Isometric exercises, hypobaric environments (*eg*, high altitude or unpressurized airplane cabins), and medications with cardiovascular effects (*eg*, decongestants with α-adrenergic actions) should be avoided. The hemodynamic changes of pregnancy are not well-tolerated by patients with PPH; postpartum deaths have been reported. Although effective birth control is important, oral contraceptives should not be used because of their potential prothrombotic properties. Due to the development of in situ thrombi, all patients without contraindications should receive anticoagulant therapy; two studies suggest that warfarin improves survival [4,12]. Diuretics and digoxin may be used, albeit cautiously, once right heart failure has developed. Approximately 20% to 30% of patients with PPH will have a favorable response (*ie*, decrease in pulmonary artery pressure and pulmonary vascular resis-

tance; an increase or no change in cardiac index, with no decrease in mean arterial pressure or arterial oxygen saturation) to acute vasodilation [12–14]. Chronic therapy with calcium channel antagonists should be limited to acute "responders." Patients with New York Heart Association functional class III or IV despite maximal therapy are candidates for continuous epoprostenol therapy, regardless of their acute responsiveness to vasodilators. This treatment modality appears to improve survival in "responders" and "nonresponders" to vasodilators, which suggests that its mechanism of action may include effects independent of its action on vascular tone [15–18]. The inadvertent cessation of continuous intravenous epoprostenol therapy can lead to an acute life-threatening worsening of pulmonary hypertension. Patients who do not respond to epoprostenol or deteriorate with escalating doses are candidates for transplantation.

CLASSIFICATION

A. CLASSIFICATION OF PULMONARY HYPERTENSION

Pulmonary arterial hypertension

Pulmonary venous hypertension

Pulmonary hypertension associated with disorders of the respiratory system and hypoxemia

Pulmonary hypertension caused by chronic thrombotic and embolic disease

Pulmonary hypertension caused by disorders directly affecting the pulmonary vasculature

B. PULMONARY ARTERIAL HYPERTENSION: DIAGNOSTIC CATEGORIES

Primary pulmonary hypertension
  Sporadic
  Familial
Pulmonary hypertension related to:
  Collagen vascular disease
  Congenital systemic to pulmonary shunts
  Portal hypertension
  HIV infection
  Drugs/toxins
    Anorexigens
    Other
  Persistent pulmonary hypertension of the newborn
  Other

Figure 22-1.
A and **B**, Classification of pulmonary hypertension. The World Health Organization's World Symposium on Primary Pulmonary Hypertension (1998) recommended significant changes to the nomenclature and pathologic classification of pulmonary hypertension. Previous classifications of pulmonary hypertension based on pathophysiology (*ie*, passive, hyperkinetic, vaso-occlusive) or anatomic site (*ie*, disorders of the left heart, pulmonary veins, pulmonary capillaries, pulmonary arteries) have been replaced by a diagnostic classification system that allows for categorization by common clinical features. This change was motivated in part by recognition of the clinical parallels between primary pulmonary hypertension and pulmonary hypertension related to select conditions, such as collagen vascular diseases [19].

PATHOLOGIC CLASSIFICATION OF PULMONARY VASCULAR DISEASE

Vasculature
  Vessels
    Arteries
    Capillaries
    Veins
    Lymphatics
    Bronchial vessels
  Components
    Intima
    Media
    Adventitia
    Complex vascular lesions
    Inflammatory cells
  Quantification
Lung tissue
  Components
    Airway
    Alveoli
    Interstitium
    Pleura

Figure 22-2.

Pathologic classification of pulmonary hypertension. The pathologic classification adopted by the World Health Organization shifts the focus from a graded classification method to a descriptive system in which the structures listed in this figure are described comprehensively. It is recommended that the percentage of abnormal vessels and the changes in cellular components, pattern (*ie*, eccentric, concentric), and matrix be made explicit. In addition, the occurrence of complex vascular lesions, such as plexiform lesions, and presence and location of inflammatory cells should be detailed. Although the entire pulmonary circulation, from artery to vein, may be involved in primary pulmonary hypertension (PPH), most patients have an arteriopathy. No diagnostic histologic lesions are unique to PPH [19].

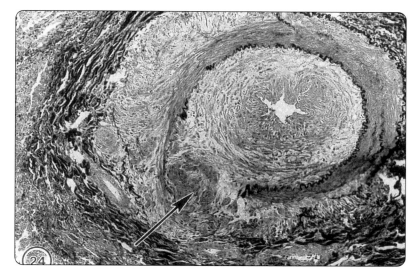

Figure 22-3.

The plexiform lesion. Pathologic lesions in primary pulmonary hypertension (PPH) have been reported in the pulmonary arterial, capillary, and venular circulation. However, PPH is primarily an arteriopathy with four reported lesions: plexiform lesions, isolated medial hypertrophy, thrombotic pulmonary arteriopathy, and isolated pulmonary arteritis. The plexiform lesions in PPH, unlike those seen in pulmonary hypertension related to other conditions, represent monoclonal endothelial cell expansion. This monoclonal cell growth may be a consequence of abnormal growth or apoptosis gene expression in endothelial cells [20,21]. *Arrow* points to early plexiform lesion. (*Adapted from* Pietra [7].)

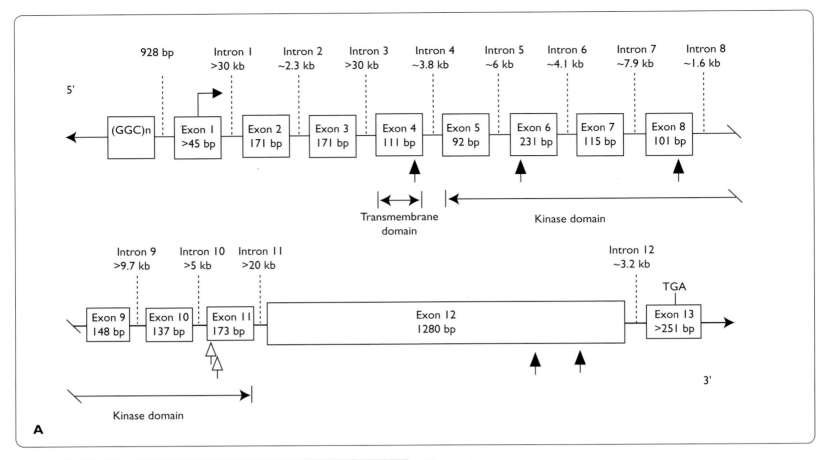

B. RESULTING DNA SEQUENCE VARIATIONS FROM MUTATIONS

Family	Exon	DNA sequence variation
PPH001, 008, 021	11	1471 → T
PPH010	8	1099-1103delGGGGA
PPH015	12	2579delT
PPH017	4	507-510delCTTTinsAAA
PPH018	12	2617C → T
PPH019	11	1472G → A
PPH022	6	690-691delAinsT

Figure 22-4.

Genetics of primary pulmonary hypertension. Primary pulmonary hypertension (PPH) occurs in familial and sporadic forms. At least 6% of patients in the National Institutes of Health PPH registry had one or more family members affected with PPH. Familial PPH is an autosomal dominant disease with incomplete penetrance and genetic anticipation. It has been mapped to locus PPH1 on chromosome 2q33. Familial PPH results from mutations in BMPR2, which encodes for a transforming growth factor-β type II receptor, bone morphogenetic protein receptor type II. The sporadic form of the disease is associated with similar mutations in more than 25% of cases [22–25]. **A,** Intron/exon structure of the human BMPR2 gene with sizes as indicated. *Filled arrows* indicate mutation sites that cause premature termination of BMPR2; *unfilled arrows* denote mutations in exon 11 resulting in a change in the amino acid sequence. **B,** Resulting DNA sequence variations from mutations. (Adapted from Deng *et al.* [23].)

WORLD HEALTH ORGANIZATION RISK FACTORS FOR PULMONARY ARTERY HYPERTENSION

Drugs and toxins
Definite
Aminorex
Fenfluramine
Dexfenfluramine
Toxic rapeseed oil
Very likely
Amphetamines
L-tryptophan
Possible
Meta-amphetamines
Cocaine
Chemotherapeutic agents
Unlikely
Antidepressants
Oral contraceptives
Estrogen therapy
Cigarette smoking
Demographic and medical conditions
Definite
Gender
Possible
Pregnancy
Systemic hypertension
Unlikely
Obesity
Diseases
Definite
HIV infection
Very likely
Portal hypertension/liver disease
Collagen vascular diseases
Congenital systemic-pulmonary cardiac shunts
Possible
Thyroid disorders

Figure 22-5.

Risk factors for pulmonary arterial hypertension. Numerous agents and conditions have been suggested as having a causal or facilitating role in pulmonary arterial hypertension. Appetite suppressants in particular have been implicated in several outbreaks. Fenfluramine and dexfenfluramine may cause pulmonary arterial hypertension through effects on potassium channels [26]. The mechanism(s) for many of the other listed conditions is unknown. It is likely that genetic susceptibility plays a major causal role in many, if not most, patients [19].

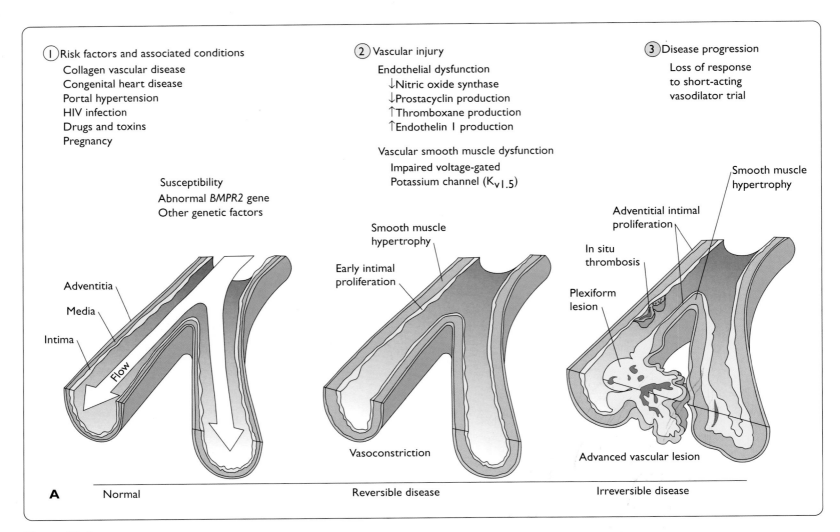

1 Risk factors and associated conditions
Collagen vascular disease
Congenital heart disease
Portal hypertension
HIV infection
Drugs and toxins
Pregnancy

Susceptibility
Abnormal *BMPR2* gene
Other genetic factors

Adventitia
Media
Intima
Flow

2 Vascular injury
Endothelial dysfunction
↓Nitric oxide synthase
↓Prostacyclin production
↑Thromboxane production
↑Endothelin 1 production

Vascular smooth muscle dysfunction
Impaired voltage-gated
Potassium channel ($K_{v1.5}$)

Smooth muscle
hypertrophy

Early intimal
proliferation

Vasoconstriction

3 Disease progression
Loss of response
to short-acting
vasodilator trial

Smooth muscle
hypertrophy

Adventitial intimal
proliferation

In situ
thrombosis

Plexiform
lesion

Advanced vascular lesion

A   Normal   Reversible disease   Irreversible disease

Figure 22-6.

Pathogenesis. The pathogenesis of primary pulmonary hypertension (PPH) is not completely understood. **A,** Injury to the pulmonary vasculature (eg, from anorexigens, scleroderma, left-to-right cardiac shunts) in susceptible individuals seems to progress to the extreme pathologic changes characteristic of this disorder. An alteration in the levels or actions of molecules that regulate pulmonary vascular tone and endothelial or smooth muscle cell growth may be involved. Heightened vascular tone and vascular remodeling may be joined events responding to the same molecular signals. For example, factors responsible for increasing vascular tone may also increase smooth muscle mitogenesis (eg, endothelin-1), and conversely, vasodilators may inhibit smooth muscle growth (eg, nitric oxide). An imbalance in the levels of these competing processes may contribute to the development of PPH [27–32].

(Continued on next page)

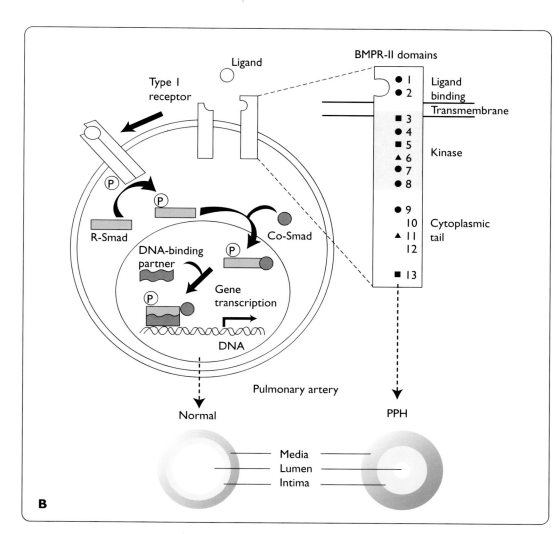

Figure 22-6. *(Continued)* **B,** The exact mechanism by which defects in the transforming growth factor-beta (TGF-β) signaling pathway lead to the vascular lesions characteristic of PPH are uncertain. The TGF-β family of peptides regulates numerous cellular functions in many tissues; in vascular endothelial cells one of their actions is growth inhibition. Loss of this inhibitory action confers a growth advantage with dysregulated cellular proliferation. In this pathway, a ligand binds to BMPR-II, which then forms a heteromeric complex with a type I receptor on the cell surface. The type II receptors activate the type I receptor serine kinases, which then leads to phosphorylation of a group of intracellular signal mediators called Smads. The Smad complex regulates transcription in target genes. The numbers 1 to 13 refer to mutation sites in BPMR-II [22–25,33]. (Panel A *adapted from* Gaine [27]. Panel B *adapted from* Thomson *et al.* [22].)

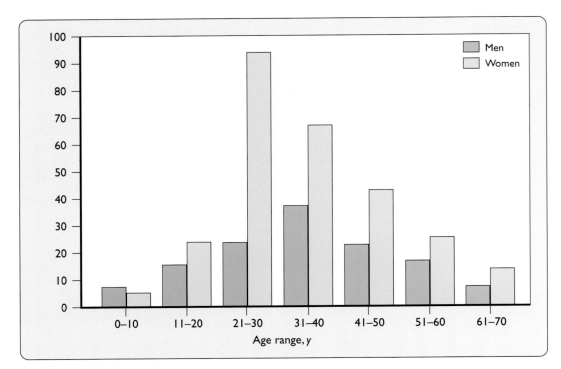

Figure 22-7.
Patient distribution. Three large US reports (data compiled in figure) show similar age and gender distributions for patients with primary pulmonary hypertension (PPH) [3–5]. The mean age at diagnosis ranged from 29.8 to 36.4 years. The National Institutes of Health patient registry reported a female-to-male ratio of 1.7:1 and a racial distribution similar to that of the general population [3].

SYMPTOMS IN PATIENTS WITH PRIMARY PULMONARY HYPERTENSION

Symptom	Initial symptoms, %	Symptoms present at diagnosis, %
Dyspnea	60	98
Fatigue	19	73
Syncope	8	36
Chest pain	7	47
Near syncope	5	41
Palpitations	5	33
Peripheral edema	3	37

Figure 22-8.
Symptoms in patients with primary pulmonary hypertension. The most common reason patients with primary pulmonary hypertension seek medical advice is dyspnea, a nearly universal symptom as the disease progresses. The mechanism for this symptom is unclear. Near-syncope and syncope, often related to activity, result from inadequate cardiac output [2,3]. Other occasional complaints not listed here include cough, hoarseness, and hemoptysis. Seventy-five percent of female patients and 64% of male patients were in the New York Heart Association functional class III or IV on enrollment in the National Institutes of Health patient registry [3]. (*Data from* Rich et al. [3].)

PHYSICAL FINDINGS IN PATIENTS WITH PRIMARY PULMONARY HYPERTENSION

Findings	Patients, %
Increase in P_2	93
Tricuspid regurgitation	40
Right-sided S_4	38
Peripheral edema	32
Right-sided S_3	23
Cyanosis	20
Pulmonic insufficiency	13

Figure 22-9.
Physical findings in patients with primary pulmonary hypertension. The physical examination is nonspecific, revealing signs of pulmonary hypertension and right ventricular failure. In the National Institutes of Health study, the presence of an S_3 gallop and tricuspid regurgitation were associated with an increase in right atrial pressure and a decrease in cardiac index; the finding of pulmonary insufficiency was associated with a higher mean pulmonary artery pressure [3]. The physical examination helps exclude secondary causes of pulmonary hypertension by an absence of crackles, wheezes, and clubbing. (*Data from* Rich et al. [3].)

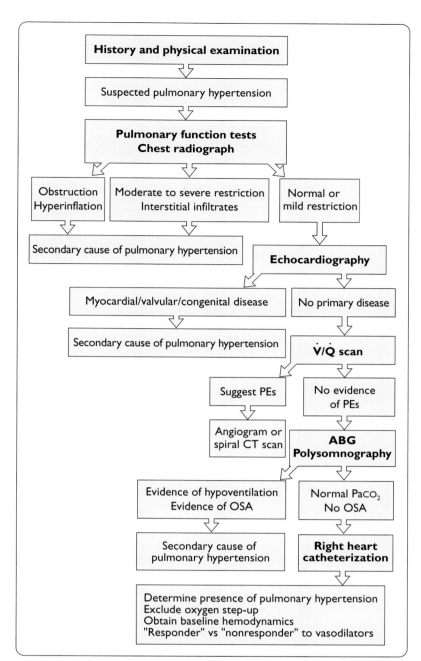

Figure 22-10.

Diagnostic evaluation. Primary pulmonary hypertension (PPH) is a diagnosis of exclusion arrived at through a series of studies. The exact order of tests is not as important as excluding underlying heart and lung disease. Echocardiography is the central noninvasive study when pulmonary hypertension is suspected because it can be used to estimate systolic pulmonary artery pressure and exclude valvular and myocardial disease. Pulmonary artery catheterization is required to establish the diagnosis; however, it can be difficult to perform in the presence of a dilated right ventricle with severe tricuspid regurgitation and a reduced cardiac output. ABG—arterial blood gases; CT—computed tomography; OSA—obstructive sleep apnea; PE—pulmonary edema; V̇/Q̇—ventilation-perfusion.

ABNORMAL FINDINGS IN COMMON TESTS FOR PATIENTS WITH PRIMARY PULMONARY HYPERTENSION

Chest radiograph	Prominent main pulmonary artery, enlarged hilar vessels, decreased peripheral vessels (pruning)
Pulmonary function tests	Mild restriction, decreased D$_{LCO}$
Arterial blood gases	Hypoxemia, hypocarbia
Electrocardiogram	RAD, RVH
$\dot{V}/\dot{Q}$ scan	Normal or small patchy abnormalities
Pulmonary arteriogram	Dilated proximal vessels, which taper rapidly; pruning of distal vessels
Doppler echocardiography	RAE, RVE+H, tricuspid regurgitation, pulmonary insufficiency, paradoxic septal motion, partial systolic closure of pulmonary valve
Exercise test	Decreased $\dot{V}O_2$ max, high VE, low anaerobic threshold, decreased max O_2 pulse, increased A-a gradient
Serology	ANA, anti-Ku antibodies

A-a—*alveolar-arterial*; ANA—*antinuclear antibodies*; D$_{LCO}$—*diffusing capacity of lung for carbon monoxide*; RAD—*right access deviation*; RAE—*right arterial enlargement*; RVE+H—*right ventricular enlargement and hypertrophy*; RVH—*right ventricular hypertrophy*; VE—*minute ventilation*; $\dot{V}O_2$ max—*maximum oxygen consumption*; $\dot{V}/\dot{Q}$—*ventilation-perfusion.*

Figure 22-11.

Abnormal findings in common tests for patients with primary pulmonary hypertension. The chest radiograph is abnormal in most patients, showing cardiac enlargement, prominent central vessels, and diminished peripheral vessels [3,4]. In chest radiographs of patients with veno-occlusive disease, basilar vascular markings and septal lines may be increased [34]. The concomitant presence of prominent main and hilar pulmonary vessels and decreased peripheral vessels is associated with a higher mean pulmonary artery pressure and decreased cardiac index [3]. Pulmonary function studies are useful primarily for excluding obstructive or severe restrictive lung disease [3,10]. Exercise capacity correlates with pulmonary hemodynamics and may be used as an independent predictor of survival [15,35].

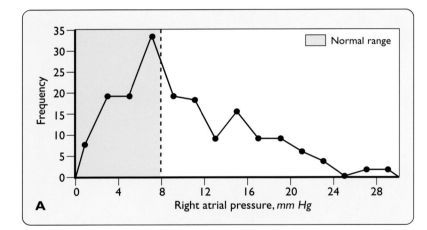

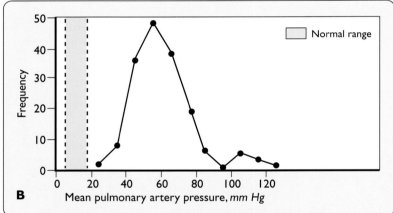

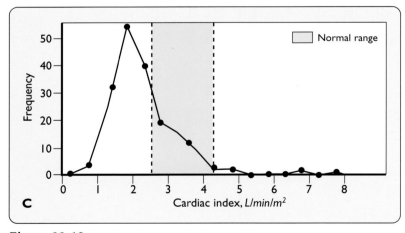

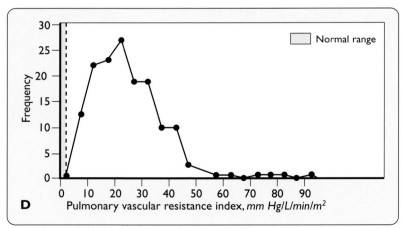

Figure 22-12.

A–D, Hemodynamics. By the time patients are diagnosed with primary pulmonary hypertension (PPH), their hemodynamic variables are profoundly altered. The mean pulmonary artery pressure is elevated several fold; higher pressures are associated with more disabling symptoms and a worse prognosis [3,4,10,11]. In the National Institutes of Health registry, the pulmonary vascular resistance was increased 15-fold on average; on average the right atrial pressure was increased in 72% of patients and the cardiac index decreased in 71% of patients [3]. Although left-sided filling pressures are usually normal, profound dilation of the right ventricle can increase left ventricular filling pressures. In addition, the pulmonary capillary wedge pressure can be variable and elevated in patients with pulmonary veno-occlusive disease. (*Adapted from* Rich *et al.* [3].)

TREATMENT

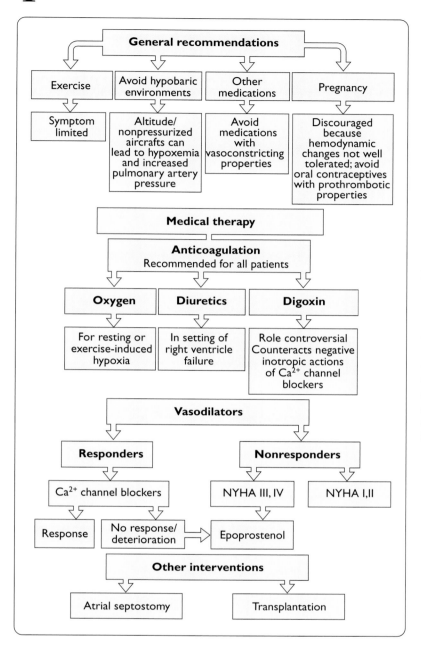

Figure 22-13.

Treatment flow diagram. Although primary pulmonary hypertension (PPH) remains an incurable disease, significant strides have been made in its treatment. Patients need to be educated to avoid factors that can worsen their already deranged pulmonary hemodynamics. Medical therapy needs to be individualized. All patients without contraindication should be anticoagulated as two noncontrolled studies suggest it prolongs survival [4,12]. Supplemental oxygen is reserved for patients with resting or exercise-induced hypoxemia. Right ventricular failure and high dose calcium channel blockers can lead to salt and water retention. The consequences of increased fluid volume include hepatic congestion, ascites, and peripheral edema; diuretics can be used judiciously to reduce congestive symptoms without compromising the function of the preload-dependent right ventricle. Digoxin has been recommended in patients on a high dose of calcium channel blockers to counteract their negative inotropic actions [12,36]. Vasodilators are advocated for PPH on the premise that vasoconstriction contributes to the heightened pulmonary vascular resistance. Approximately 25% to 30% of patients will have an acute favorable response to vasodilators and are candidates for long-term treatment with calcium channel blockers (nifedipine and diltiazem are the most widely used agents) [12,14]. The medications are given at doses that maximize hemodynamic improvement without adversely effecting systemic blood pressure, cardiac output, or gas exchange. Their therapeutic efficacy and dose over time can be adjusted based on symptoms, serial echocardiograms and cardiac catheterization. The doses used often exceed that which is required to control hypertension or anginal symptoms. Patients who deteriorate on calcium channel blockers or nonresponders with New York Heart Association functional class III or IV are candidates for chronic therapy with epoprostenol. Patients without a response to epoprostenol are candidates for lung or heart-lung transplantation.

A. ASSESSMENT OF VASODILATOR RESPONSIVENESS

Pulmonary artery pressure	Decreases by more than 20%–25%
Pulmonary vascular resistance	Decreases by more than 30%–35%
Cardiac output	Increases
Mean arterial pressure	Minimal decrease
Systemic arterial oxygen saturation	No change or improved

B. VASODILATORS USED TO TEST FOR ACUTE RESPONSIVENESS

Epoprostenol (IV infusion)	2–20 ng/kg/min
Adenosine (IV infusion)	50–350 µg/kg/min
Inhaled nitric oxide	5–40 ppm

IV—intravenous.

Figure 22-14.

Acute testing—defining vasodilator responsiveness and drug regimens. Calcium channel blockers can cause life-threatening adverse events in patients with primary pulmonary hypertension (PPH) so they should not be used empirically, but limited to patients with a favorable acute hemodynamic response. Unfortunately, there is no universally agreed on definition for a favorable response. The desired pattern is of a reduction in pulmonary artery pressure and pulmonary vascular resistance with an increase in cardiac output and no deterioration in gas exchange or decrease in systemic blood pressure. **A,** Given the spontaneous variability in pulmonary hemodynamics the mean pulmonary artery pressure and pulmonary vascular resistance should decrease at least 10 mm Hg (or 20%) and 20%, respectively, to increase confidence that the findings are drug effects [2,13,14,37–40]. **B,** Acute hemodynamic testing with invasive monitoring is performed with short-acting vasodilators. The calcium channel blockers have been supplanted by inhaled nitric oxide, epoprostenol, and adenosine. The acute vasodilator is titrated up until the patient has symptoms of intolerance or the systolic blood pressure falls. Consideration should be given to sending patients to specialized centers experienced with these tests.

PROGNOSIS

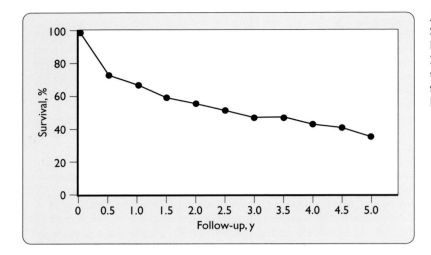

Figure 22-15.
Survival of patients with primary pulmonary hypertension. In the National Institutes of Health patient registry, the estimated median survival was 2.8 years. Patients may live longer, particularly with more aggressive medical therapy [11]. The majority of deaths were from progressive right ventricular failure and a significant number of patients had sudden death. (*Adapted from* D'Alonzo *et al.* [11].)

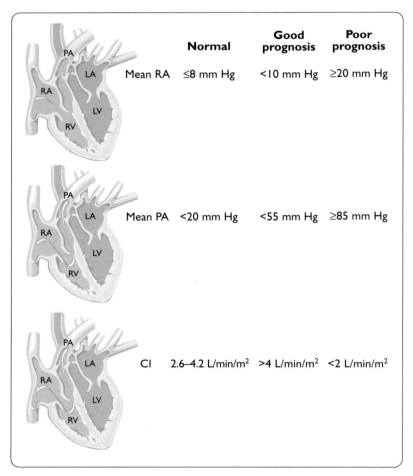

Figure 22-16.
Hemodynamic predictors of survival. Hemodynamic, clinical, and therapeutic variables can be used to predict patient survival. The probabilities of survival duration are related to mean right atrial (RA) and pulmonary artery (PA) pressures and the cardiac index (CI). The patient's New York Heart Association functional class, exercise tolerance, and response to vasodilators also correlate with survival [2,11,12]. LA—left atrium; LV—left ventricle; RV—right ventricle.

Figure 22-17.
Effect of therapy on survival. Long-term treatment with nifedipine or diltiazem can enhance survival. Anticoagulation, regardless of the patient's response to vasodilators, improves survival; this effect is even more pronounced in the nonresponder group [4,12]. (*Adapted from* Rich *et al.* [12].)

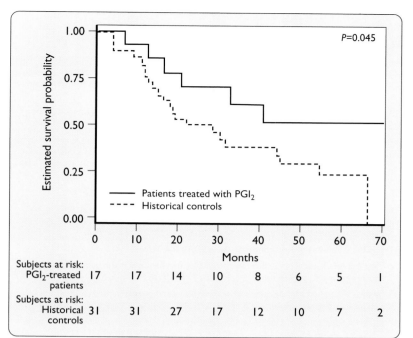

Subjects at risk:
| PGI₂-treated patients | 17 | 17 | 14 | 10 | 8 | 6 | 5 | 1 |

| | | | | | | | | |

Subjects at risk:
| Historical controls | 31 | 31 | 27 | 17 | 12 | 10 | 7 | 2 |

Figure 22-18.

Effect of epoprostenol on survival. Treatment with continuous intravenous epoprostenol improves exercise tolerance, pulmonary hemodynamics (an effect that is sustained over time), and survival [15–17,41]. The long-term effects on pulmonary hemodynamics are seen even in patients without an acute response to vasodilators [15–17]. This suggests that the effect of epoprostenol may be mediated through a mechanism other than vasodilation, such as inhibiting platelet aggregation or altering vascular remodeling. Continuous infusion of epoprostenol, for example, favorably affects the balance between endothelin-1 (a potent vasoconstrictor and smooth muscle mitogen) clearance and release, in patients with primary pulmonary hypertension [18]. (*Adapted from* Barst et al. [16].)

HEMODYNAMIC EFFECTS OF LONG-TERM EPOPROSTENOL

Variable	Baseline	Epoprostenol*
Mean arterial pressure	102 ± 18	87 ± 10
Right atrial pressure	15 ± 6	9 ± 7
Mean pulmonary artery pressure	67 ± 10	52 ± 12
Pulmonary vascular resistance	16.7 ± 5.4	7.9 ± 3.8
Cardiac output	3.76 ± 1.19	6.29 ± 1.97
Systemic arterial oxygen saturation	91 ± 5	93 ± 6
Mixed venous oxygen saturation	53 ± 8	64 ± 10

Significant difference compared with baseline.

Figure 22-19.

Hemodynamic effects of long-term epoprostenol. Long-term treatment (*ie*, ≥12 weeks) with intravenous epoprostenol improves right ventricular hemodynamic indices [15,17,41]. Over time, increasing doses of epoprostenol are required. The major limitation of this therapy relates to side effects from the delivery system, which include line infection, sepsis, thrombosis, and inadvertent cessation of delivery due to mechanical malfunctions [15–17]. Aerosolization of prostacyclin and an analog, iloprost, has been described and may offer an alternative delivery method in the future [42]. (There is a significant difference for all values on epoprostenol compared with baseline.) (*Adapted from* McLaughlin et al. [17].)

POTENTIAL FUTURE THERAPIES

Prostacyclin analogues
   Beraprost (oral)
   Iloprost (inhaled)
   Uniprost (subcutaneous)
Endothelin receptor antagonists
   Dosentan
   TBC11251
   ZD 1611
Serotonin receptor antagonists
   Ketanserin
Gene therapy
   Prostacyclin synthase
   Inducible nitric oxide
   BMPR2 receptor

Thromboxane synthase inhibitor/thromboxane antagonist
   Terbogrel
Anticoagulants
   Glycoprotein IIb/IIIa platelet receptor antagonists
   Heparins

Ion channel activators
   DHEA

Anti-inflammatory/antineoplastic agents?

Figure 22-20.

Potential future therapies. Although there has been significant progress in treating patients with primary pulmonary hypertension (PPH), therapeutics have limitations. Drug side effects, systemic vascular actions, and complications from delivery systems carry significant morbidity. The increasing knowledge in the pathogenesis of PPH offers new avenues for medical intervention.

REFERENCES

1. Fishman AP: A century of primary pulmonary hypertension. In *Primary Pulmonary Hypertension: Lung Biology in Health and Disease*, vol 99. Edited by Rubin LJ and Rich S. New York: Marcel Dekker; 1997:1–17.

2. Rubin LJ: Primary pulmonary hypertension. *N Engl J Med* 1997, 336:111–117.

3. Rich S, Dantzker DR, Ayres SM, et al.: Primary pulmonary hypertension: a national prospective study. *Ann Intern Med* 1987, 107:216–223.

4. Fuster V, Steele PM, Edwards WD, Gersh BJ, McGoon MD, Frye RL: Primary pulmonary hypertension: natural history and the importance of thrombosis. *Circulation* 1984, 70:580–587.

5. Glanville AR, Burke CM, Theodore J, Robin ED: Primary pulmonary hypertension: length of survival in patients referred for heart-lung transplantation. *Chest* 1987, 91:675–681.

6. Braman SS, Eby E, Kuhn C, Rounds S: Primary pulmonary hypertension in the elderly. *Arch Intern Med* 1991, 151:2433–2438.

7. Pietra GG: The pathology of primary pulmonary hypertension. In *Primary Pulmonary Hypertension: Lung Biology in Health and Disease*, vol 99. Edited by Rubin LJ and Rich S. New York: Marcel Dekker; 1997:19–61.

8. Pietra GG: Histopathology of primary pulmonary hypertension. *Chest* 1994, 105:2S–6S.

9. Rubin LJ, Mendoza J, Hood M, et al.: Treatment of primary pulmonary hypertension with continuous prostacyclin (epoprostenol): results of a randomized trial. *Ann Intern Med* 1990, 112:485–491.

10. Brenot F: Primary pulmonary hypertension: case series from France. *Chest* 1994, 105:33S–36S.

11. D'Alonzo GE, Barst RJ, Ayres SM, et al.: Survival in patients with primary pulmonary hypertension: results from a national prospective registry. *Ann Intern Med* 1991, 115:343–349.

12. Rich S, Kaufmann E, Levy PS: The effect of high doses of calcium-channel blockers on survival in primary pulmonary hypertension. *N Engl J Med* 1992, 327:76–81.

13. Rich S, Kaufmann E: High dose titration of calcium channel blocking agents for primary pulmonary hypertension: guidelines for short-term drug testing. *J Am Coll Cardiol* 1991, 18:1323–1327.

14. Weir EK, Rubin LJ, Ayres SM, et al.: The acute administration of vasodilators in primary pulmonary hypertension: experience from the National Institutes of Health registry on primary pulmonary hypertension. *Am Rev Respir Dis* 1989, 140:1623–1630.

15. Barst RJ, Rubin LJ, Long WA, et al.: A comparison of continuous intravenous epoprostenol (prostacyclin) with conventional therapy for primary pulmonary hypertension. *N Engl J Med* 1996, 334:296–301.

16. Barst RJ, Rubin LJ, McGoon MD, Caldwell EJ, Long WA, Levy PS: Survival in primary pulmonary hypertension with long-term continuous intravenous prostacyclin. *Ann Intern Med* 1994, 121:409–415.

17. McLaughlin VV, Genthner DE, Panella MM, Rich S: Reduction in pulmonary vascular resistance with long-term epoprostenol (prostacyclin) therapy in primary pulmonary hypertension. *N Engl J Med* 1998, 338:273–277.

18. Langleben D, Barst RJ, Badesch D, et al.: Continuous infusion of epoprostenol improves the net balance between pulmonary endothelin-1 clearance and release in primary pulmonary hypertension. *Circulation* 1999, 99:3266–3271.

19. Rich S: Primary pulmonary hypertension. *Executive Summary from the World Symposium.* World Health Organization; 1998.

20. Lee S-D, Shroyer KR, Markham NE, Cool CD, Voelkel NF, Tuder RM: Monoclonal endothelial cell proliferation is present in primary but not secondary pulmonary hypertension. *J Clin Invest* 1998, 101:927–934.

21. Yeager ME, Halley GR, Golpon HA, Voelkel NF, Tuder RM: Microsatellite instability of endothelial cell growth and apoptosis genes within plexiform lesions in primary pulmonary hypertension. *Circ Res* 2001, 88:e2–e11.

22. Thomson JR, Machado RD, Pauciulo MW, et al.: Sporadic primary pulmonary hypertension is associated with germline mutations of the gene encoding BMPR-II, a receptor member of the TGF-b family. *J Med Genet* 2000, 37:741–745.

23. Deng Z, Morse JH, Slager SL, et al.: Familial primary pulmonary hypertension (gene PPH1) is caused by mutations in the bone morphogenetic protein receptor-II gene. *Am J Hum Genet* 2000, 67:737–744.

24. Lane KB, Machado RD, Pauciulo MW, et al., and The International PPH Consortium: Heterozygous germline mutations in BMPR2, encoding a TGF-β receptor, cause familial primary pulmonary hypertension. *Nature Genet* 2000, 26:81–84.

25. Scott J: Pulling apart pulmonary hypertension. *Nature Genet* 2000, 26:3–4.

26. Weir EK, Reeve HL, Huang JMC, et al.: Anorexic agents aminorex, fenfluramine, and dexfenfluramine inhibit potassium current in rat pulmonary vascular smooth muscle and cause pulmonary vasoconstriction. *Circulation* 1996, 94:2216–2220.

27. Gaine S: Pulmonary hypertension. *JAMA* 2000, 284:3160–3168.

28. Voelkel NF, Tuder RM: Cellular and molecular mechanisms in the pathogenesis of severe pulmonary hypertension. *Eur Respir J* 1995, 8:2129–2138.

29. Herve P, Launay J-M, Scrobohaci M-L, et al.: Increased plasma serotonin in primary pulmonary hypertension. *Am J Med* 1995, 99:249–254.

30. Giaid A, Yanagisawa M, Langleben D, et al.: Expression of endothelin-1 in the lungs of patients with pulmonary hypertension. *N Engl J Med* 1993, 328:1732–1739.

31. Christman BW, McPherson CD, Newman JH, et al.: An imbalance between the excretion of thromboxane and prostacyclin metabolites in pulmonary hypertension. *N Engl J Med* 1992, 327:70–75.

32. Egermayer P, Town GI, Peacock AJ: Role of serotonin in the pathogenesis of acute and chronic pulmonary hypertension. *Thorax* 1999, 54:161–168.

33. Zimmerman CM, Padgett RW: Transforming growth factor b signaling mediators and modulators. *Gene* 2000, 249:17–30.

34. Rich S, Pietra GG, Kieras K, Hart K, Brundage BH: Primary pulmonary hypertension: radiographic and scintigraphic patterns of histologic subtypes. *Ann Intern Med* 1986, 105:499–502.

35. Rhodes J, Barst RJ, Garofano RP, Thoele DG, Gersony WM: Hemodynamic correlates of exercise function in patients with primary pulmonary hypertension. *J Am Coll Cardiol* 1991, 18:1738–1744.

36. Rich S, Brundage BH: High-dose calcium channel-blocking therapy for primary pulmonary hypertension: evidence for long-term reduction in pulmonary arterial pressure and regression of right ventricular hypertrophy. *Circulation* 1987, 76:135–141.

37. Rubin LJ: Primary pulmonary hypertension. *Chest* 1993, 104:236–250.

38. Galie N, Ussia G, Passarelli P, Parlangeli R, Branzi A, Magnani B: Role of pharmacologic test in the treatment of primary pulmonary hypertension. *Am J Cardiol* 1995, 75:55A–62A.

39. Kneussl MP, Lang IM, Brenot FP: Medical management of primary pulmonary hypertension. *Eur Respir J* 1996, 9:2401–2409.

40. Rich S, D'Alonzo GE, Dantzker DR, Levy PS: Magnitude and implications of spontaneous hemodynamic variability in primary pulmonary hypertension. *Am J Cardiol* 1985, 55:159–163.

41. Shapiro SM, Oudiz RJ, Cao T, et al.: Primary pulmonary hypertension: improved long-term effects and survival with continuous intravenous epoprostenol infusion. *J Am Coll Cardiol* 1997, 30:343–349.

42. Olschewski H, Ghofrani A, Schmehl T, et al.: Inhaled iloprost to treat severe pulmonary hypertension: an uncontrolled trial. *Ann Intern Med* 2000, 132:435–443.

THE HIGH-RISK SURGICAL PATIENT

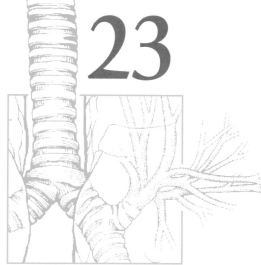

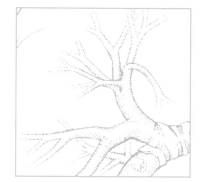

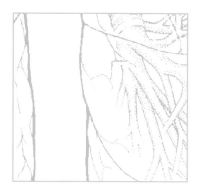

Ann S. Kirby &
Sean Keenan

Defining the "high-risk" surgical patient is not as straightforward a task as it appears. "High-risk" may be applied to either the surgery or the patient. In the early literature on the perioperative period, it was applied to the surgery and the overall status of the patient, and reflected the increased risk of morbidity and mortality documented through retrospective chart reviews. The more recent literature concentrates on univariate and multifactorial patient-based risk indexes that have been validated prospectively in clinical studies. This chapter briefly reviews some of the important historical ground-work that has led us to where we are today in risk assessment and management of these complex cases.

The complications of high-risk surgery fall into many categories, but the most common and severe—after death—are cardiac and respiratory complications. This chapter concentrates primarily on these outcomes, focusing on the noncardiac surgical patient. Cardiac surgical patients are discussed briefly and separately because they comprise an important group of patients in the critical care environment. In addition, this chapter reviews some of the literature that discusses perioperative anesthetic technique and its effect on the outcome in the high-risk surgical patient. Also discussed is the literature that assesses the role of perioperative invasive Swan-Ganz catheter monitoring in the high-risk surgical patient. Several excellent in-depth reviews of the literature are available [1–5].

RISK ASSESSMENT

CRITERIA FOR HIGH-RISK CLASSIFICATION

Previous severe cardiorespiratory illness, *eg*, acute myocardial infarction, chronic obstructive pulmonary disease, stroke

Extensive ablative surgery planned for carcinoma, *eg*, esophagectomy and total gastrectomy, or prolonged surgery (>8 h)

Severe multiple trauma, *eg*, involving more than three organs or two systems, or in the opening of two body cavities

Massive acute blood loss (>8 U), resulting in a blood volume <1.5 L/m^2 or hematocrit <20%

Age >70 y and evidence of limited physiologic reserve of one or more vital organs

Shock, indicated by mean arterial pressure <60 mm Hg, central venous pressure <15 cm H$_2$O, and urinary output <20 mL/h

Septicemia, positive blood culture or septic focus, indicated by leukocyte count >13,000, spiking fever to 101° F for 48 h, and hemodynamic instability

Respiratory failure, indicated by Pao$_2$ <60 on Fio$_2$ >0.4, Qs/Qt >30%, with mechanical ventilation needed for more than 48 h

Acute abdominal catastrophe with hemodynamic instability, as seen in pancreatitis, gangrenous bowel, peritonitis, perforated viscus, or gastrointestinal bleeding

Acute renal failure, indicated by blood urea nitrogen >50 mg/dL, creatinine >3 mg/dL

Late-stage vascular disease involving aortic disease

Fio$_2$—percentage of inspired oxygen; Qs/Qt—shunt fraction.

Figure 23-1.
Criteria for high-risk classification. In the 1970s and early 1980s, the criteria identified as important in predicting adverse outcomes perioperatively included patient and surgical characteristics. These outcomes, although commonly cardiac, included all adverse events. Although helpful epidemiologically, this information did not lead to useful intervention for risk assessment and management of patients, but identified areas for subsequent research.

CARDIAC ASSESSMENT

CARDIAC RISK INDICES

Multifactorial indices using multivariate analysis to identify factors correlating with cardiac complications/death

17 studies (>100 patients)

Dripps [6]

Goldman *et al.* [7]

Detsky *et al.* [8]

Larsen *et al.* [9]

Figure 23-2.
Cardiac risk indices in the preoperative patient. In 1977, the first large, well-designed prospective study using multifactorial indices to assess cardiac risk in the noncardiac patient was done by Goldman *et al.* [7]. Several other multivariate analyses validated this technique and led to the widespread use of risk indices.

A. GOALS OF PREOPERATIVE EVALUATION

Identify health issues that may increase perioperative morbidity or mortality

Stratify patients according to risk of perioperative cardiac complications or death

Modify risk factors, if possible

Optimize postoperative care

B. GOALS OF RISK STRATIFICATION

Accurately predict the risk of perioperative myocardial infarction or death

Assess need for preoperative investigations

Assess need for interventions to reduce the perioperative risk

Provide informed consent to patient

Reduce long-term cardiac complications

Figure 23-3.
A, Goals of preoperative evaluation. The goals of cardiac evaluation must incorporate the full spectrum of perioperative care. **B,** Risk stratification is an important objective in this evaluation, as an educated discussion with the patient follows naturally and truly informed consent for the planned procedure is obtained.

THE NEED FOR STRATIFICATION IN PERIPHERAL VASCULAR SURGERY

Characteristics of peripheral vascular surgery

10% of all surgeries

High-risk procedures:

3.1% incidence of postoperative myocardial infarction

5.2% overall perioperative mortality

2.7% mortality from cardiac events

Indications for stratification

Higher prevalence coronary artery disease

Hemodynamically stressful surgery

THE BURDEN OF DISEASE

In 1988:

27 million noncardiac surgeries (United States)

8 million with CAD/cardiac risk factors

50,000 postoperative myocardial infarctions

20,000 postoperative deaths

Projected for 2015:

Estimated 37 million surgeries

40% of cases with CAD/risk factors for CAD

CAD—coronary artery disease.

Figure 23-4.
The need for stratification in peripheral vascular surgery. A specific example of a patient group that is appropriate for risk stratification is the peripheral vascular surgical group, which has been clearly identified with a higher cardiac morbidity rate than other surgical groups [10]. (*Adapted from* Warner *et al.* [10].)

Figure 23-5.
The burden of disease. The importance of cardiac evaluation is due to the burden of disease in the population, *ie*, the prevalence of cardiac disease and its associated morbidity in an aging population. It is predicted that in the year 2015, an estimated 37 million surgeries will be performed, and 40% of this population will have coronary artery disease. Perioperative cardiac morbidity is the leading cause of death postoperatively; thus, an increasing number of high-risk patients will require noncardiac surgery and appropriate perioperative assessment and management. (*Adapted from* Mangano [2].)

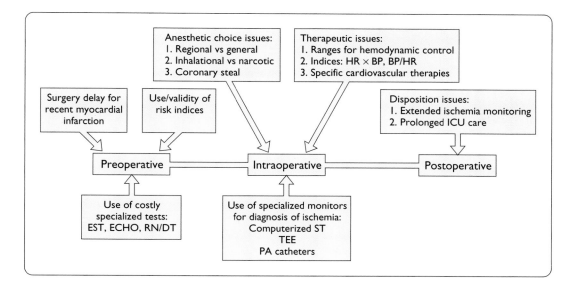

Figure 23-6.
Cardiovascular tests, procedures, and care regimen dilemmas for the three perioperative periods. The diagnostic and therapeutic dilemmas of managing the high-risk surgical patient, outlined here lead naturally to assessment and intervention during three phases: the preoperative, intraoperative, and postoperative periods. BP—blood pressure; DT—dipyridamole thallium; ECHO—echocardiogram; EST—exercise stress test; HR—heart rate; ICU—intensive care unit; PA—pulmonary artery; RN—radionuclear; TEE—transesophageal echocardiography. (*Adapted from* Mangano [2].)

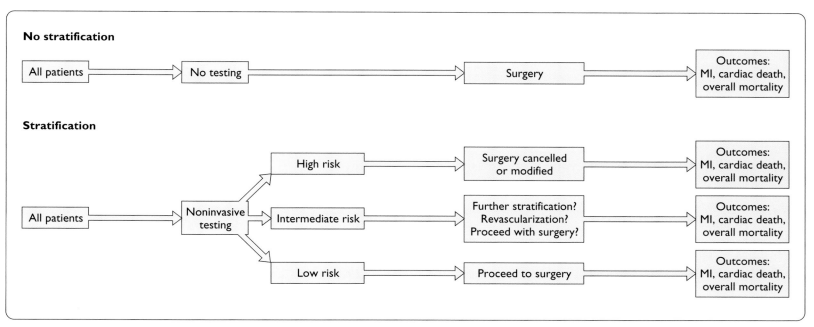

Figure 23-7.
Goal of cardiac risk stratification. The preoperative evaluation of patients allows the physician to carry out risk stratification and to identify patients who may benefit from short- or long-term intervention. For example, patients identified as low-risk can go to the operating room without intervention, whereas patients identified as high-risk may need to be considered for coronary revascularization first to avoid the risks of unnecessary testing and delays in surgery. At the very least, truly informed consent can be obtained. Risk stratification can be based on univariate predictors, such as a recent (within 6 months) myocardial infarction (MI), congestive heart failure, unstable angina, or a positive stress test, which have all been shown to be independent risk factors for postoperative cardiac complications.

AMERICAN SOCIETY OF ANESTHESIOLOGISTS PHYSICAL STATUS SCALE

I. Healthy individual
II. Mild systemic disease
III. Severe systemic disease
IV. Incapacitating systemic disease
V. Moribund patient not expected to survive 24 h
VI. Added to any class for emergency surgery

Figure 23-8.
American Society of Anesthesiologists (ASA) physical status scale. Multifactorial risk indices allow better prediction of complications in patients by covering a wide spectrum of diseases and surgical procedures. Altogether 17 studies of multifactorial indexes are available, the most validated remain the 1) ASA classification [11], 2) Goldman scale [7], and 3) Detsky modification [8]. The ASA classification has withstood the test of time and remains the anesthetist's standard assessment tool. (*Adapted from* Faigal and Blaisdell [11].)

THE GOLDMAN CARDIAC RISK INDEX

		Points
History	Age >70 y	5
	Myocardial infarction <6 mo	10
Physical examination	Significant aortic stenosis	8
	S3 gallop or jugular venous distention	11
Electrocardiogram	Any rhythm other than sinus	7
	>5 premature ventricular contractions/min	7
Poor general medical condition	PO_2 <60, PCO_2 >50, K^+<3, BUN>50, creatinine >260 mmol/L, bedridden	3
Operation	Emergency	4
	Intrathoracic or intra-abdominal aortic	3
		Total: 53 points

Goldman classification (*n*)	Points	MI/APE, *n* (%)	Cardiac deaths, *n* (%)
1 (537)	0–5	4 (0.7)	1 (0.2)
2 (316)	6–12	16 (5)	5 (2)
3 (130)	13–25	15 (11)	3 (2)
4 (18)	>25	4 (22)	10 (56)

APE—acute perioperative event; BUN—blood urea nitrogen; MI—myocardial infarction.

Figure 23-9.
The Goldman cardiac risk index. The Goldman cardiac risk index, developed in 1977, has been prospectively validated several times and is used routinely by internists managing patients perioperatively. It is least useful for patients with peripheral vascular disease, who are at significant risk for cardiac complications [4,12]. (*Adapted from Goldman et al. [7].*)

A. DETSKY MODIFIED MULTIFACTORIAL RISK INDEX

		Points
Coronary artery disease	Myocardial infarction <6 mo	10
	Myocardial infarction >6 mo	5
Canadian Cardiovascular Society angina	Class III	10
	Class IV	20
	Unstable angina <6 mo	10
Alveolar pulmonary edema	Within 1 wk	10
	Ever	5
Suspected critical aortic stenosis		20
Arrhythmias	Rhythm other than sinus or sinus plus APBs	5
	>5 PVC before surgery	5
Poor general medical status (as per original CRI)		5
Age >70 y		5
Emergency operation		10
		Total: 120 points

	Relative risk of complications during:		
Class (likelihood ratio)	Major surgery	Minor surgery	All surgery
I (0–15)	0.42	0.39	0.43
II (15–30)	3.58	2.75	3.38
III (>30)	14.93	12.20	10.60

APBs—atrial premature beats; CRI—cardiac risk index; PVC—premature ventricular contractions.

Figure 23-10.
A, Detsky modified multifactorial risk index. The Detsky modification, although more complex than the Goldman cardiac risk index (*see* Fig. 23-9), takes coronary artery disease into account and incorporates pretest probability and likelihood ratios.

(*Continued on next page*)

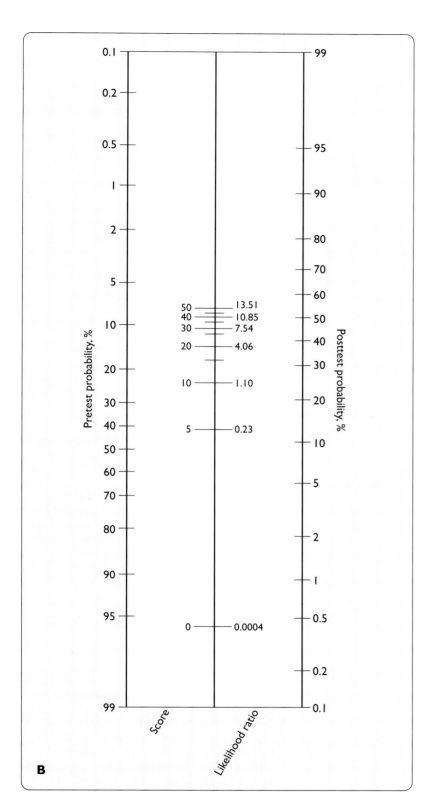

Figure 23-10. *(Continued)*
B, Pretest probability as defined by the surgical procedural risks associated with institutions. A line is drawn from the pretest probability through the index score/likelihood ratio, giving a posttest probability for a specific patient. Ultimately, these scales allow the physician to stratify patients into low-, intermediate-, or high-risk groups, and identify patients who may require further evaluation, possible intervention, or reconsideration of surgery. (Panel A *adapted from* Detsky *et al.* [8].)

Preoperative Monitoring

THALLIUM MYOCARDIAL IMAGING

Six early studies of DTI:
    High sensitivity (90%–100%)
    Good specificity (53%–80%)
Two studies cast doubt on usefulness of DTI:
    Mangano *et al.* [19]
    Baron *et al.* [20]
Low sensitivity: - LR 1.05/1.06
Low specificity: + LR 0.9–0.91
Combined data: - LR 0.87 + LR 1.3
No added benefit of DTI over chance alone

DTI—dipyridamole thallium imaging; LR—likelihood ratio.

Figure 23-11.

Thallium myocardial imaging. Cardiac evaluation includes assessment of left ventricular ejection fraction, exercise stress testing, pharmacologic stress testing, thallium imaging, dobutamine stress echocardiography, and monitoring for silent ischemia. These tests are valuable only if they predict the presence or absence of postoperative risk. There is little evidence that preoperative evaluation of ejection fraction results in any intervention that may change the preoperative outcome [13,14]. Evaluation for cardiac ischemia using exercise testing coronary angiography is warranted in patients who would require clinical assessment independent of their need for surgery, ie, patients with unstable angina or a recent myocardial infarction [15]. In asymptomatic patients, particularly patients with peripheral vascular disease, it is less clear that this information is helpful in guiding perioperative intervention [16,17]. Monitoring for silent ischemia has not proven useful yet in the preoperative assessment of patients [18], although it clearly predicts postoperative cardiac morbidity when demonstrated during or after surgery. Thallium imaging initially showed promise in predicting the outcome in selected populations; however, more rigorous studies by Mangano *et al.* [19] and Baron *et al.* [20] demonstrated low sensitivity and low specificity for this test and, thus, have cast doubt on its usefulness. Dobutamine echocardiography may prove to be a useful prediction tool in the future; its ability to predict outcome in a defined population is supported by one well-designed study in the peripheral vascular surgery population [21].

DOES PREOPERATIVE MANAGEMENT REDUCE RISK?

No studies show clinical benefit from
    Nitrates
    Optimization of hemodynamics
    β-blockers
    Afterload reduction

Figure 23-12.

The role of preoperative management in risk reduction. Unfortunately, few good studies exist that demonstrate any benefit from preoperative medical management strategies. The use of β-blockers preoperatively has been shown to reduce silent ischemia intraoperatively; however, this has not resulted in any identifiable benefit postoperatively and is therefore not currently recommended. The only group to show some benefit from preoperative optimization of hemodynamics through invasive monitoring and intervention consists of patients undergoing major peripheral vascular procedures [22]. Further evaluation is needed prior to making any generalized recommendations. There is no clear evidence of benefit from perioperative nitrate use or afterload reduction; however, this does not preclude their use based on clinical judgment and experience.

Intraoperative Factors

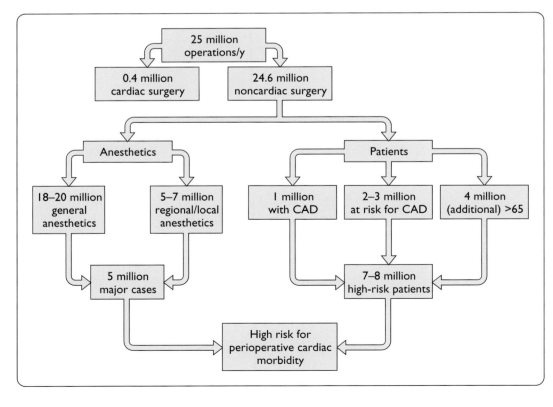

Figure 23-13.

Estimates of surgical data in the United States, 1988. The total number of high-risk surgical patients was estimated to be 7 to 8 million. Six million (30%) were older than 65 years of age. Of these, 1 million had coronary artery disease (CAD) and 2 to 3 million were at risk for CAD, resulting in 4 million patients older than 65 years of age considered high-risk because of CAD. The choice of anesthetic may play an important role, at least theoretically. Unfortunately, no studies have shown a significant difference in outcome of cardiac complications for regional versus general anesthesia [23,24], although regional anesthesia has benefits in the pulmonary disease population. It is expected that these differences will be demonstrable in the future; practice patterns are already changing to accommodate these clinical impression. In addition, there is no good evidence of any difference in outcome between inhalational versus narcotic anesthesia. Again, this does not preclude its use based on clinical judgment. (*Adapted from* Mangano [2].)

INDICATIONS FOR PERIOPERATIVE HEMODYNAMIC MONITORING

Aortic peripheral vascular surgery in high-risk patients

Hip fracture surgery in high-risk patients

Elderly or high-risk patients undergoing major surgery

Figure 23-14.

Indications for perioperative hemodynamic monitoring. Although some studies recommend intraoperative hemodynamic monitoring, no evidence is available that clearly supports this strategy or shows an improvement in outcome. At least one large multicenter trial is underway, and many other less rigorous trials have produced conflicting results.

INTRAOPERATIVE RISK FACTORS

	Study	
Factor	**Supported**	**Refuted**
Classic risk factors		
Anesthetic	Rao [25]	Driscoll [37], Knapp [47], Topkins [48], Arkins [29], Mauney [31], Tarhan [26], Goldman [27], Steen [28], Djokovic [33], von Knorring [43]
Site of surgery	Tarhan [26], Goldman [27], Steen [28], Rao [25], Larsen [9]	Driscoll [37], Topkins [48], Cooperman [49], von Knorring [43], Foster [50]
Duration of anesthesia/ surgery	Arkins [29], Cogbill [30], Mauney [31], Goldman [27], Steen [28]	Driscoll [37], Topkins [48], Tarhan [26], Djokovic [33], von Knorring [43], Rao [25]
Emergency surgery	Arkins [29], Vacanti [32], Goldman [27], Djokovic [33], Larsen [9]	Rao [25]
Dynamic risk factors		
Hypertension	Plumlee [34], Steen [28]	Goldman [27], Riles [41], Schoeppel [44], Rao [25]
Hypotension	Wroblewski [35], Wasserman [36], Driscoll [37], Chamberlain [38], Mauney [31], Plumlee [34], Goldman [27,39], Steen [28], Mahar [40], Riles [41], Eerola [42], von Knorring [43], Schoeppel [44], Rao [25]	Nachlas [51]
Tachycardia	Rao [25]	—
Myocardial ischemia	Smith [45]	—
Ventricular dysfunction	Rao [25]	—
Dysrhythmias	Sapala [46], Steen [28]	Goldman [52], Rao [25]

Figure 23-15.

Perioperative cardiac morbidity. Even the documentation of adverse intraoperative events has not necessarily led to the prediction of adverse postoperative outcomes. Practice patterns depend on personal and institutional preferences and guidelines. (*Adapted from* Mangano [2].)

Postoperative Management

SUMMARY OF CLINICAL DATA OF SERIES 2

	Nonrandomized (n = 45)	CVP-control (n = 30)	PA-control (n = 30)	PA-protocol (n = 28)
Age, y	56.9 ± 2.5	55.2 ± 3.0	53.4 ± 2.5	56.4 ± 3.1
Sex, males/females, %	45/55	64/36	39/61	75/25
Hospital days	21.9 ± 1.7	22.2 ± 2.8	25.2 ± 3.4	19.3 ± 2.4
ICU days	14.0 ± 1.7	11.5 ± 1.7	15.8 ± 3.1	10.2 ± 1.6*
Ventilator days	6.5 ± 1.3	4.6 ± 1.4	9.4 ± 3.4	2.3 ± 0.5*
Intraoperative deaths, n	0	0	1	0
Postoperative deaths, n (%)	17 (38%)	7 (23%)	10 (33%)	1 (4%)†

*P<0.05 compared with its control group.
†P<0.01 compared with its control group.
CVP—central venous pressure; PA—pulmonary artery.

Figure 23-16.
Postoperative care optimization interventions. The standard of care for the postoperative high-risk surgical patient includes a sophisticated nursing and monitoring environment associated with an increased level of care. Unfortunately, evidence in the literature supporting an improved outcome in mortality using this strategy is lacking. However, this has become the accepted standard of care across North America. There is some evidence in the literature of reduced morbidity—ie, decreased duration of hospital and intensive care unit stay, and decreased duration of ventilation—in this population. However, evidence of reduced mortality is not as clear [53,54]. Research efforts are focused on evaluating the efficacy and effectiveness of invasive monitoring and optimization/supranormalization of hemodynamic parameters, in addition to the standard supportive and interventional care provided in the high-risk surgical population. The outcomes being evaluated include morbidity in addition to mortality because morbidity is recognized as a more appropriate outcome to measure in this population. Invasive monitoring, at the very least, may help the physician stratify patients by prognosis, because survivors are noted to have increased oxygen delivery, oxygen consumption, and cardiac index compared with nonsurvivors [53,55], reflecting the expected compensatory increases to meet increased metabolic needs. Although some evidence exists to support invasive monitoring and supranormalization of oxygen parameters, some of it is conflicting. Before this strategy can be recommended as standard of care, further evaluation needs to be done. A large multicenter trial that may help elucidate these issues further in the high-risk surgical population is underway in Canada. (*Adapted from* Shoemaker et al. [53].)

PULMONARY ASSESSMENT

POTENTIAL PULMONARY COMPLICATIONS

Respiratory failure requiring:
  Prolonged intubation (>48 h)
  Reintubation
Respiratory arrest
Lobar collapse
Atelectasis
Pneumonia
Pneumothorax
Bronchopleural fistula
Pleural space infection

Figure 23-17.
Potential pulmonary complications. The incidence of postoperative pulmonary complication varies from 4% to 54%, depending on the population studied and the definition used [56–60]. The inclusion of minor complications, specifically atelectasis on radiograph alone, accounts for the higher estimates. The complications that are of primary interest to the critical care physician are listed in the figure.

RISK FACTORS FOR POSTOPERATIVE PULMONARY COMPLICATIONS

Patient-related factors

Chronic obstructive pulmonary disease

Hypercapnia (>45 mm Hg)

Asthma

Obesity

Smoking

Hypoventilation/sleep apnea

Age

Non–patient-related factors

Type of anesthesia

Type of surgery

Type of incision

Cardioplegic agents

Nasogastric tube

Figure 23-18.

Risk factors for postoperative pulmonary complications. To decrease the likelihood of complications, the critical care physician must first be able to identify those factors that place the patient at increased risk. Risk factors can be considered to be either patient- or procedure-derived. Knowing what risk factors are present in an individual allows the physician to plan specific perioperative care, including modification of potentially reversible risk factors, patient education, and arrangement of the appropriate level of postoperative monitoring.

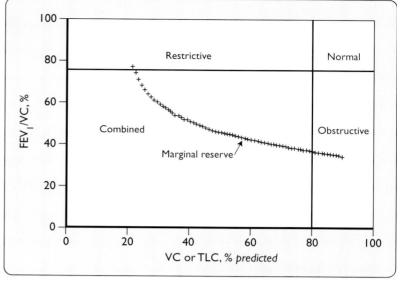

Figure 23-19.

Relative risk of surgery in patients with lung disease. Decreased pulmonary reserve leaves patients with an advanced obstructive or restrictive lung disease at increased risk of pulmonary complications. FEV₁—forced expiratory volume in 1 second; TLC—total lung capacity; VC—pulmonary capillary blood volume. (*Adapted from* Hodgkin [61].)

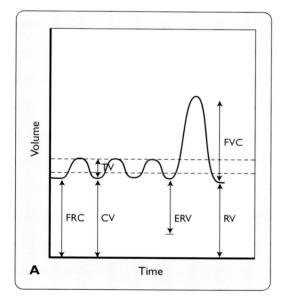

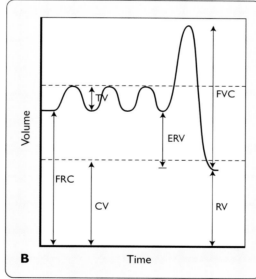

Figure 23-20.

A and **B**, Postoperative decrease in functional residual capacity (FRC) (*panel A*) compared with preoperative situation (*panel B*). The normal lung has a large pulmonary reserve and can withstand a transient loss of lung function. The supine position and general anesthesia lead to a decrease in FRC. As the FRC decreases, it nears the level of the closing volume (*ie*, the lung volume at which small airways close). If the FRC drops below the closing volume, the small airways will close during normal tidal breathing and atelectasis, with its associated pulmonary shunt, will result. In obese patients [62–64] and those with chronic obstructive pulmonary disease (COPD) [65], there is already a tendency to airway closure during tidal breathing, which places these patients at significantly increased risk of atelectasis. Nonresectional thoracic surgery, cardiac surgery, and abdominal surgery all increase the tendency to a reduction in FRC and the risk of atelectasis. CV—closing volume; ERV—expiratory reserve volume; FVC—forced vital capacity; RV—residual volume; TV—tidal volume. (*Adapted from* Cordarco and Golish [66].)

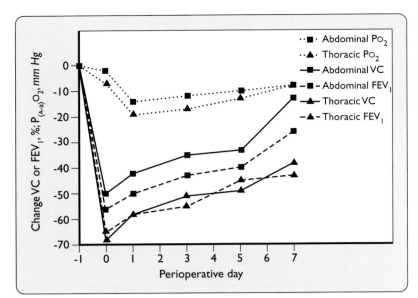

Figure 23-21.
Average change in spirometric values and $P_{(A-a)}O_2$ after abdominal and thoracic surgery. Diaphragmatic function has been shown to be inhibited for many days after upper abdominal surgery [67,68] independent of associated incisional pain. It is possible that patients undergoing laparoscopic surgery may be less prone to this phenomenon [69–71]. Potentially reversible factors occurring postoperatively include pain and body position. FEV_1—forced expiratory volume in 1 second; VC—pulmonary capillary blood volume. (*Adapted from* Bryant *et al.* [72].)

Preoperative Assessment

PATIENT FACTORS CONTRIBUTING TO INCREASED PULMONARY COMPLICATIONS

History

Prior lung disease (COPD, ILD)—decreased respiratory reserve

Asthma—brochospasm, atelectasis secondary to mucus plugging, pneumothorax

Obesity—increased atelectasis postoperatively

Smoking history—increased secretions, atelectasis

OSA—increased likelihood of respiratory arrest without precautions

Inability to protect airway (bulbar weakness secondary to stroke, motor neuron disease)—increased likelihood of aspiration

Physical examination

Upper airway—gag reflex, airway caliber (sleep apnea?)

Neck circumference—OSA

Obesity—atelectasis, OSA

Signs of COPD

Wheezing—increased likelihood of postoperative bronchospasm

COPD—chronic obstructive pulmonary disease; ILD—interstitial lung disease; OSA—obstructive sleep apnea.

Figure 23-22.
Patient factors contributing to increased pulmonary complications. Understanding the pathophysiology behind pulmonary complications allows the physician to approach preoperative patient assessment in a logical manner. A patient history and physical examination comprise the first step. By combining findings from these two procedures with knowledge of the proposed surgical procedure, the physician can decide whether to obtain pulmonary function tests.

A. AMERICAN COLLEGE OF PHYSICIANS GUIDELINES FOR PREOPERATIVE SPIROMETRY

Lung resection

Coronary artery bypass graft and smoking history or dyspnea

Upper abdominal surgery and smoking history or dyspnea

Lower abdominal surgery and uncharacterized pulmonary disease*, particularly if the surgical procedure will be prolonged or extensive

Other surgery and uncharacterized pulmonary disease*, particularly in those who might require strenuous postoperative rehabilitation

*Uncharacterized pulmonary disease is defined by the authors as pulmonary symptoms or a history of pulmonary disease and no pulmonary function tests within 60 d.

B. INDICATIONS FOR PREOPERATIVE PULMONARY FUNCTION TESTS

Suggestive history—prior symptomatic lung disease

Suggestive physical examination wheezing, signs of chronic obstructive pulmonary disease

Lung resectional surgery

Figure 23-23.
A, American College of Physicians guidelines for preoperative spirometry. A study found that a large proportion of preoperative pulmonary function tests are ordered inappropriately [73]. **B,** We suggest that clinicians follow the American College of Physicians Guidelines [74] or the alternative approach illustrated in *panel B*. Arterial blood gases may be obtained in patients with abnormal spirometry. Patients with suspected obstructive sleep apnea should undergo a formal sleep study [75].

PERIOPERATIVE ACTION PLAN FOR PATIENTS WITH INCREASED RISK OF PULMONARY COMPLICATIONS

Stop smoking

Consider need for weight loss

Control bronchospasm

Discuss method of anesthesia with anesthesiologist

Educate patient

For patients with sleep, ensure nasal continuous positive airway pressure is available in recovery room

Control pain

Consider requirement for monitoring during intermediate care or intensive care

Figure 23-24.

Perioperative action plan for patients with increased risk of pulmonary complications. Once the risk profile of the specific patient has been identified, patient factors that are reversible preoperatively should be addressed: smoking cessation, as much weight loss as possible, and optimization of pulmonary status in patients with underlying lung disease. The proposed surgical procedure should be reviewed to consider such factors as the use of regional anesthesia, the planned incision, and the type of surgical procedure (*ie*, open versus laparoscopic surgery). The importance of preoperative patient education with regard to deep breathing exercises and incentive spirometry has been shown to be beneficial [58,60]. Patients with obstructive sleep apnea or believed to be at risk for sleep apnea should be treated perioperatively with nasal continuous positive airway pressure to prevent an adverse outcome [75]. Pain control will allow patients to perform deep breathing exercises adequately to minimize atelectasis and associated pulmonary complications. Perhaps most important of all is the need to provide the appropriate level of postoperative monitoring and patient care. Patients at high risk may require postoperative intensive care and prolonged ventilation. Those at a lower risk may benefit from physiotherapy and respiratory therapy in an intermediate care unit.

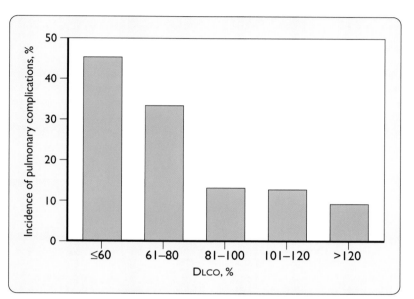

Figure 23-25.

Prevalence of mortality after major pulmonary resection. Patients selected for resectional lung surgery are unique. Not only are they at increased risk due to incisional pain and diaphragmatic dysfunction [76], they will also lose a portion of their lung as a result of the procedure. In addition, most of these patients have a history of smoking, which results in abnormal baseline pulmonary function. The importance of baseline lung function is illustrated by the relationship between diffusing capacity and pulmonary complications. D_{LCO}—diffusing capacity of lung for carbon monoxide. (*Adapted from* Wait [71].)

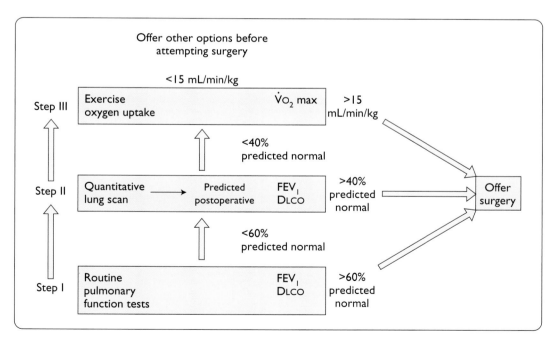

Figure 23-26.

Evaluation of cardiopulmonary operability. A stepwise approach to assessing patients for resectional surgery has been advocated with an emphasis on the utility of exercise testing in patients otherwise considered borderline [77,78]. D_{LCO}—diffusing capacity of lung for carbon monoxide; FEV_1—forced expiratory volume in 1 second; $\dot{V}O_2$—oxygen consumption per unit time. (*Adapted from* Marshall and Olsen [79].)

Postoperative Management

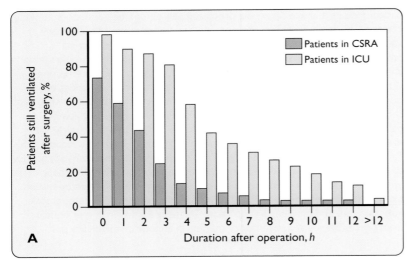

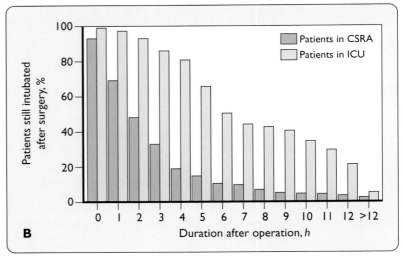

Figure 23-27.

A and **B**, Ventilatory (*panel A*) and airway (*panel B*) status of postoperative patients. The care of patients undergoing cardiac surgery has changed significantly over the past 5 to 10 years. In the current environment of cost containment, these patients are likely to receive immediate postoperative care in a cardiac surgical recovery area (CSRA), where a major emphasis has been placed on rapidly weaning cardiac patients from mechanical ventilation and rapid discharge from the intensive care unit (ICU) [80]. Previously, the popularity of high-dose narcotic anesthesia and the belief that complete

postoperative rest improved the outcome of surgery resulted in patients commonly being ventilated longer than 24 to 48 hours [81]. More recently, however, a different approach to anesthesia has been adopted that incorporates lower doses of narcotic utilization of shorter acting sedation agents, most commonly propofol [82,83]. As demonstrated in the figures, this change in approach has resulted in a shortened duration of ventilation and time to extubation [83], leading to patients bypassing admission to the intensive care unit postoperatively in some centers. (*Adapted from* Chong *et al.* [83].)

REFERENCES

1. Goldman L: Cardiac risks and complications of noncardiac surgery. *Ann Intern Med* 1983, 98:504–513.

2. Mangano DT: Perioperative cardiac morbidity. *Anesthesiology* 1990, 72:153–184.

3. Mangano DT, Goldman L: Preoperative assessment of patients with known or suspected coronary disease. *N Engl J Med* 1995, 33:1730–1736.

4. Wong T, Detsky A: Preoperative cardiac risk assessment for patients having peripheral vascular surgery. *Ann Intern Med* 1992, 116:743–753.

5. Gass GD, Olsen GD: Preoperative pulmonary function testing to predict postoperative morbidity and mortality. *Chest* 1986, 89:127–135.

6. Dripps RD: The role of anesthesia in surgical mortality. *JAMA* 1961, 178:261–266.

7. Goldman L, Caldera DL, Neustrum SR, *et al.*: Multifactorial index of cardiac risk in noncardiac surgical procedures. *N Engl J Med* 1977, 297:845–850.

8. Detsky AS, Abrams HB, McLaughlin JR, *et al.*: Predicting cardiac complications in patients undergoing non-cardiac surgery. *J Gen Intern Med* 1986, 1:211–219.

9. Larsen SF, Olesen KH, Jacobsen E, *et al.*: Prediction of cardiac risk in noncardiac surgery. *Eur Heart J* 1987, 8:179–185.

10. Warner MA, Shield SE, Chute CG: Major morbidity and mortality within 1 month of ambulatory surgery and anesthesia. *JAMA* 1993, 270:1437–1441.

11. Faigal DW, Blaisdell WP: The estimation of surgical risk. *Med Clin North Am* 1979, 63:1131–1143.

12. Schueppert MT, Kresowik TF, Corry DC: Selection of patients for cardiac evaluation before peripheral vascular operations. *J Vasc Surg* 1996, 23:802–809.

13. Garson MC, Hurst JM, Hertzig VS, *et al.*: Cardiac prognosis in noncardiac geriatric surgery. *Ann Intern Med* 1985, 103:832–837.

14. Ruddy TD, McPhail NV, Calvin JE, *et al.*: Comparison of exercise testing, dipyridamole thallium imaging and gated blood pool scanning for the prediction of cardiac complications following vascular surgery [abstract]. *J Am Coll Cardiol* 1989, 13:149A.

15. Gianrossi R, Detrano R, Mulvihill D, *et al.*: Exercise-induced ST depression in the diagnosis of multivessel coronary disease: a meta-analysis. *Circulation* 1989, 80:87–98.

16. Cutler BS, Wheeler HB, Paraskos JA, Cardullo PA: Applicability and interpretation of electrocardiographic stress testing in patients with peripheral vascular disease. *Am J Surg* 1981, 141:501–506.

17. Kaaja R, Sell H, Erkola O, Harjula A: Predictive value of annual electrocardiographic monitored exercise testing before abdominal aortic or peripheral vascular surgery. *Angiology* 1993, Jan:11–15.

18. Mangano DT, Browner WS, Hollenberg M, *et al.*: Association of perioperative myocardial ischemia with cardiac morbidity and mortality in men undergoing noncardiac surgery. *N Engl J Med* 1990, 323:1781–1788.

19. Mangano DT, London MJ, Tubau JF, *et al.*: and the Study of Perioperative Ischemia Research Group: Dipyridamole-thallium scintigraphy as a screening test: a re-examination of its predictive potential. *Circulation* 1991, 84:493–502.

20. Baron JF, Mundler O, Bertrand M, *et al.*: Dipyridamole-thallium scintigraphy and gated radionuclide angiography to assess cardiac risk before abdominal aortic surgery. *N Engl J Med* 1994, 330:663–669.

21. Poldermans D, Fioretti PM, Forster T, *et al.*: Dobutamine stress echocardiography for assessment of perioperative cardiac risk in patients undergoing major vascular surgery. *Circulation* 1993, 8:1506–1512.

22. Berlauk JF, Abrams JH, Gilmour IJ, *et al.*: Preoperative optimisation of cardiovascular hemodynamics improves outcome in peripheral vascular surgery: a prospective randomised clinical trial. *Ann Surg* 1991, 214:289–299.

23. Cohen MM, Duncan PG, Tate RB: Does anesthesia contribute to operative mortality? *JAMA* 1988, 260:2859–2863.

24. Yeager MP, Glass DD, Neff RK, *et al.*: Epidural anesthesia and analgesia in high risk surgical patients. *Anesthesiology* 1987, 66:729–736.

25. Rao TK, Jacobs KH, El-Etr AA: Reinfarction following anesthesia in patients with myocardial infarction. *Anesthesiology* 1983, 59:499–505.

26. Tarhan S, Moffitt E, Taylor WF, Guiliani ER: Myocardial infarction after general anesthesia. *JAMA* 1972, 220:1451–1454.

27. Goldman L, Caldera DL, Nussbaum SR, *et al.*: Multifactorial index of cardiac risk in noncardiac surgical procedures. *N Engl J Med* 1977, 297:845–850.

28. Steen PA, Tinker JH, Tarhan S: Myocardial reinfarction after anesthesia and surgery. *JAMA* 1978, 239:2566–2570.

29. Arkins R, Smessaertt AA, Hicks RG: Mortality and morbidity in surgical patients with coronary-artery disease. *JAMA* 1964, 190:485–488.

30. Cogbill CL: Operation in the aged. *Arch Surg* 1967, 94:2202–2205.

31. Mauney MF Jr, Ebert PA, Sabiston DC Jr: Postoperative myocardial infarction: a study of predisposing factors, diagnosis, and mortality in a high risk group of surgical patients. *Ann Surg* 1970, 172:497–503.

32. Vacanti CJ, VanHouten RJ, Hill RC: A statistical analysis of the relationship of physical status to postoperative mortality in 68,388 cases. *Anesth Analg* 1970, 49:565–566.

33. Djokovic JL, Hedley-Whyte J: Prediction of outcome of surgery and anesthesia in patients over 80. *JAMA* 1979, 242:2301–2306.

34. Plumlee JE, Boettner RB: Myocardial infarction during and following anesthesia and operation. *South Med J* 1972, 65:886–889.

35. Wroblewski F, La Due JS: Myocardial infarction adds a postoperative complication of major surgery. *JAMA* 1952, 150:1212–1216.

36. Wasserman F, Bellet S, Saichek RP: Postoperative myocardial infarction: report of twenty-five cases. *N Engl J Med* 1955, 252:967–974.

37. Driscoll AC, Hobika JH, Etsten BE, Proger S: Clinically unrecognized myocardial infarction following surgery. *N Engl J Med* 1961, 264:633–639.

38. Chamberlain DA, Seal-Edmonds J: Effects of surgery under general anaesthesia on the electrocardiogram in ischemic heart disease and hypertension. *Br Med J* 1964, 2:784–787.

39. Goldman L, Caldera DL: Risks of general anesthesia and elective operation in the hypertensive patient. *Anesthesiology* 1979, 50:285–292.

40. Mahar LJ, Steen PA, Tinker JH, et al.: Perioperative myocardial infarction in patients with coronary artery disease with and without aorta-coronary bypass grafts. *J Thorac Cardiovasc Surg* 1978, 76:533–537.

41. Riles TS, Kopelman I, Imparato AM: Myocardial infarction following carotid endarterectomy: a review of 683 operations. *Surgery* 1979, 85:249–252.

42. Eerola M, Eerola R, Kaukinen S, Kaukinen L: Risk factors in surgical patients with verified preoperative myocardial infarction. *Acta Anaesthesiol Scand* 1980, 24:219–223.

43. von Knorring J: Postoperative myocardial infarction: a prospective study in a risk group of surgical patients. *Surgery* 1981, 90:55–60.

44. Schoeppel LS, Wilkinson C, Waters J, Meyers NS: Effects of myocardial infarction on perioperative cardiac complications. *Anesth Analg* 1983, 62:493–498.

45. Smith JS, Cahalan MK, Benefiel DJ, et al.: Intraoperative detection of myocardial ischemia in high-risk patients: electrocardiography versus two-dimensional trans-esophageal echocardiography. *Circulation* 1985, 72:1015–1021.

46. Sapala JA, Ponka JL, Duvernoy WFC: Operative and nonoperative risks in the cardiac patient. *J Am Geriatr Soc* 1975, 23:529–534.

47. Knapp RB, Topkins MJ, Artusio JF Jr: The cerebrovascular accident and coronary occlusion in anesthesia. *JAMA* 1962, 182:332–334.

48. Topkins MJ, Artusio JF: Myocardial infarction and surgery: a five-year study. *Anesth Analg* 1964, 43:716–720.

49. Cooperman M, Pflug B, Martin EW Jr, Evans WE: Cardiovascular risk factors in patients with peripheral vascular disease. *Surgery* 1978, 84:505–509.

50. Foster ED, Davis KB, Carpenter JA, et al.: Risk of noncardiac operation in patients with defined coronary disease: The Coronary Artery Surgery Study (CASS) Registry Experience. *Ann Thorac Surg* 1986, 41:42–50.

51. Nachlas MM, Abrams SJ, Goldberg MM: The influence of arteriosclerotic heart disease on surgical risk. *Am J Surg* 1961, 101:447–455.

52. Goldman L, Caldera DL, Southwick FS, et al.: Cardiac risk factors and complications in non-cardiac surgery. *Medicine* 1978, 57:357–370.

53. Shoemaker CW, Appel PL, Kram HB, et al.: Prospective trial of supranormal values of survivors as therapeutic goals in high-risk surgical patients. *Chest* 1988, 94:1176–1186.

54. Boyd O, Grounds M, Bennett ED: A randomized clinical trial of the effect of deliberate perioperative increase of oxygen delivery on mortality in high risk surgical patients. *JAMA* 1993, 270:2699–2707.

55. Shoemaker CW, Appel PL, Kram HB: Hemodynamic and oxygen transport responses in survivors and nonsurvivors of high-risk surgery. *Crit Care Med* 1993, 21:977–990.

56. Calligaro KD, Azurin DJ, Dougherty MJ, et al.: Pulmonary risk factors of elective abdominal aortic surgery. *J Vasc Surg* 1993, 18:914–921.

57. Kroenke K, Lawrence VA, Theroux JF, et al.: Postoperative complications after thoracic and major abdominal surgery in patients with and without obstructive lung disease. *Chest* 1993, 104:1445–1451.

58. Hall JC, Tarala R, Harris J, et al.: Incentive spirometry versus routine chest physiotherapy for prevention of pulmonary complications after abdominal surgery. *Lancet* 1991, 337:953–956.

59. Hall JC, Tarala RA, Hall JL, Mander J: A multivariate analysis of the risk of pulmonary complications after laparotomy. *Chest* 1991, 99:923–927.

60. Celli BR, Rodriguez KS, Snider GL: A controlled trial of intermittent positive pressure breathing, incentive spirometry, and deep breathing exercises in preventing pulmonary complications after abdominal surgery. *Am Rev Respir Dis* 1984, 130:12–15.

61. Hodgkin JE: Evaluation before thoracotomy. *West J Med* 1975, 122:104–109.

62. Pasulka PS, Bistrian BR, Benotti PN, Backburn GL: The risks of surgery in obese patients. *Ann Intern Med* 1986, 104:540–546.

63. Jackson MCV: Preoperative pulmonary evaluation. *Arch Intern Med* 1988, 148:2120–2127.

64. Brooks-Brun JA: Postoperative atelectasis and pneumonia: risk factors. *Am J Crit Care* 1995, 4:340–349.

65. Fraser RS, Pare JAP, Fraser RG, Pare PD: *Synopsis of Diseases of the Chest.* Philadelphia: WB Saunders; 1994:653–671.

66. Cordarco EM, Golish JA: Surgical risks, preoperative assessment, and preventive strategies for the critically ill patient. In *The High Risk Patient: Management of the Critically Ill.* Edited by Cann CC. Media, PA: Williams and Wilkins; 1995.

67. Ford GT, Whitelaw WA, Rosenal TW, et al.: Diaphragmatic function after upper abdominal surgery in humans. *Am Rev Respir Dis* 1983, 127:431–436.

68. Ford BT, Rosenal TW, Clergue F, Whitelaw WA: Respiratory physiology in upper abdominal surgery. *Clin Chest Med* 1993, 14:237–252.

69. Wittgen CM, Andrus CH, Fitzgerald SD, et al.: Analysis of the hemodynamic and ventilatory effects of laparoscopic cholecystectomy. *Arch Surg* 1991, 126:997–1001.

70. Frazee RC, Roberts JW, Okeson GC, et al.: Open versus laparoscopic cholecystectomy: a comparison of postoperative pulmonary function. *Ann Surg* 1991, 213:651–654.

71. Wait J: Southwestern Internal Medicine conference: preoperative pulmonary evaluation. *Am J Med Sci* 1995, 310:118–125.

72. Bryant LR, et al.: Lung perfusion scanning for estimation of postoperative pulmonary function. *Arch Surg* 1972, 184:52.

73. Preoperative pulmonary function testing: American College of Physicians position statement. *Ann Intern Med* 1990, 112:793–794.

74. Rennotte MT, Baele P, Aubert G, Rodenstein DO: Nasal continuous positive airway pressure in the perioperative management of patients with obstructive sleep apnea submitted to surgery. *Chest* 1995, 107:367–374.

75. Maeda H, Nakahara K, Ohno K, et al.: Diaphragm function after pulmonary resection. *Am Rev Respir Dis* 1988, 137:678–681.

76. Epstein SK, Faling LJ, Daly BDT, Celli BR: Predicting complications after pulmonary resection: preoperative exercise testing vs a multifactorial cardiopulmonary risk index. *Chest* 1993, 104:694–700.

77. Bollinger CT, Jordan P, Soler M, et al.: Exercise capacity as a predictor of postoperative complications in lung resection candidates. *Am J Respir Crit Care Med* 1995, 151:1472–1480.

78. Cheng DCH: Early extubation after cardiac surgery decreases intensive care unit stay and cost. *J Cardiothorac Vasc Anesth* 1995, 9:460–464.

79. Marshall MC, Olsen GN: The physiologic evaluation of the lung resection candidate. *Clin Chest Med* 1993, 14:305–320.

80. Samuelson PN, Reves JG, Kirklin JK, et al.: Comparison of sufentanil and enfluranenitrous oxide anesthesia for myocardial revascularization. *Anesth Analg* 1986, 65:217–226.

81. Westaby S, Pillai R, Parry A, et al.: Does modern cardiac surgery require late intensive care? *Eur J Cardiothorac Surg* 1993, 7:313–318.

82. Butler J, Chong GL, Pillai R, et al.: Early extubation after coronary artery bypass surgery: effects on oxygen flux and haemodynamics. *J Cardiovasc Surg* 1992, 33:276–280.

83. Chong JL, Grebenik C, Sinclair M, et al.: The effect of a cardiac surgical recovery area on the timing of extubation. *J Cardiothorac Vasc Anesth* 1993, 7:137–141.

ACUTE RESPIRATORY FAILURE

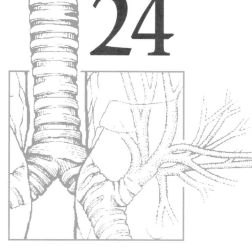
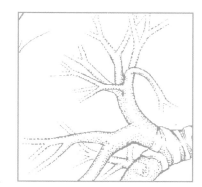

24

David Leasa & Frank Rutledge

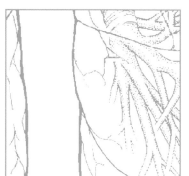

Acute respiratory failure is an impairment in the respiratory system's ability to maintain adequate arterial blood gases, resulting in an abnormally low Pao_2 and an abnormally high $Paco_2$. It is a potentially life-threatening condition.

Acute respiratory failure exists when the derangement of respiratory function occurs rapidly enough to create an emergent threat to the patient's life. In contrast, chronic respiratory failure exists when the abnormalities develop gradually and are tolerated for weeks or longer, without an immediate threat to the patient's life.

Clinical hallmarks of acute respiratory failure include dyspnea, air hunger, agitation, confusion, disorientation, panic, and obtundation. Physical findings include tachycardia, hypertension, diaphoresis, cyanosis, tachypnea, and active use of the accessory muscles of respiration. Acute respiratory failure can be categorized as one of two types: hypercarbic or hypoxemic. Although multiple causes exist, the pathophysiology can be explained through the functional component of the respiratory system that is deranged: the extrapulmonary ventilatory "pump" or the pulmonary parenchyma.

Oxygen therapy and mechanical ventilation are paramount in preserving gas exchange in the event of the failing physiology. However, attention must also be directed at reversing the factors that precipitated initial deterioration in lung or "pump" function. Not uncommonly, pre-existing chronic respiratory disease places the patient at significant risk for acute-on-chronic respiratory failure.

Specific common causes of acute respiratory failure include acute respiratory distress syndrome, head and thoracic trauma, myocardial ischemia and congestive heart failure, neuromuscular disease, obstructive airway disease (*eg*, emphysema and severe asthma), and pneumonia. This chapter provides a brief pictorial account of a few aspects of acute respiratory failure and attempts to capture common concepts that would be useful for teaching the topic.

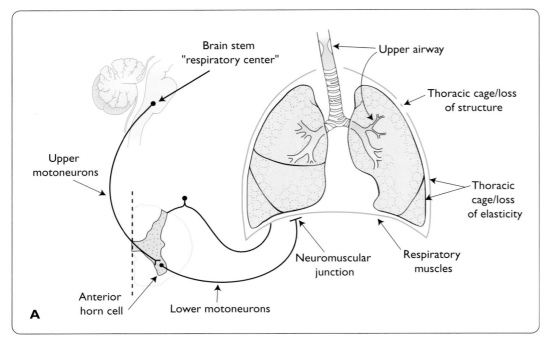

Figure 24-1.
A and **B**, Hypercarbic respiratory failure ("pump failure"). The pathophysiology of respiratory failure may be approached in terms of the component of the system that is malfunctioning—the "ventilatory pump" or the lung parenchyma, although components of both may be evident in a single patient. Hypercarbic respiratory failure is primarily failure to provide adequate alveolar ventilation. (*Adapted from* Nunn [1].)

B. HYPERCARBIC RESPIRATORY FAILURE ("PUMP FAILURE")

Features

Disease involving the extrapulmonary compartment

Impaired alveolar ventilation

Associated respiratory acidosis

Gas exchange abnormalities

Hypercarbia predominance

± Hypoxemia

Malfunctioning component— ventilatory pump

Brain stem "respiratory center" (*eg*, narcotic overdose)

Upper motoneurons (*eg*, cervical spine trauma)

Anterior horn cell (*eg*, poliomyelitis)

Lower motoneurons (*eg*, ascending polyradiculopathy)

Neuromuscular junction (*eg*, myasthenia gravis)

Respiratory muscles (*eg*, myopathy)

Thoracic cage/loss of elasticity (*eg*, kyphoscoliosis)

Thoracic cage/loss of structure (*eg*, "flail" chest wall)

Upper airway (*eg*, laryngospasm)

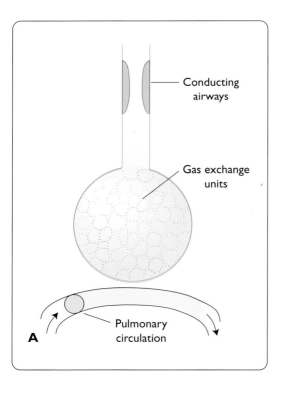

B. HYPOXEMIC RESPIRATORY FAILURE ("LUNG FAILURE")

Features

Disease involving the pulmonary compartment

Decrease in the gas exchange between the distal airway alveolus and the pulmonary capillary blood

Pao_2 <60 mm Hg on Fio_2 >0.60

Associated metabolic (lactic) acidosis

Gas exchange abnormalities

Hypoxemia predominance

± Hypercarbia

Malfunctioning component—lung parenchyma

Conducting airways (*eg*, severe asthma)

Gas exchange units (*eg*, pneumonia, acute respiratory distress syndrome)

Pulmonary circulation (*eg*, thromboembolism)

Fio_2—*fractional inspired oxygen.*

Figure 24-2.
A and **B**, Hypoxemic respiratory failure ("lung failure"). Hypoxemic respiratory failure is primarily failure to adequately oxygenate the blood.

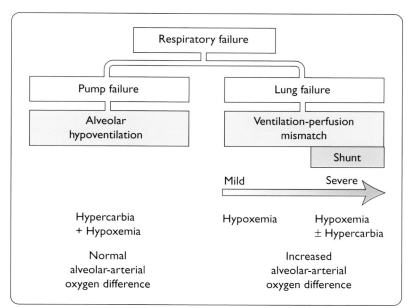

Figure 24-3.

Lung and pump failure and their effect on gas exchange. Hypercarbic respiratory failure results from disease states causing a decrease in minute ventilation or an increase in physiologic dead space, such that alveolar ventilation is inadequate to meet metabolic demands. Acute hypercarbic respiratory failure is considered present when $PaCO_2$ is at least 50 mm Hg and the arterial pH is less than 7.30. Chronic hypercarbic respiratory failure is characterized by $PaCO_2 \geq 50$ mm Hg, but with an arterial pH ≥ 7.30. The degree of hypoxemia associated with pure hypoventilation can be estimated from the alveolar gas equation, assuming that the alveolar-arterial difference for the PO_2 will be minimal or normal. Hypoxemic respiratory failure most commonly results from pulmonary conditions that cause ventilation/perfusion mismatch. Mild to moderate ventilation/perfusion mismatch results in hypoxemia, with a low or normal $PaCO_2$. Severe ventilation/perfusion mismatch results in hypoxemia and hypercarbia, as the increased ventilatory demand cannot be met. Shunting might be viewed as an extreme ventilation/perfusion abnormality, in which lung units are perfused but not ventilated. Hypoxemic respiratory failure is considered present when arterial oxygen saturations of less than 90% are observed, despite an inspired oxygen fraction above 0.60.

A. HYPOXEMIA RESPONSIVE TO O₂ IN THE ABSENCE OF PARENCHYMAL DISEASE ON CHEST RADIOGRAPH

	$\dot{V}/\dot{Q}$ mismatch	Diffusion-perfusion defect
Example	Obstructive disease of the lung	Pulmonary vascular dilations of HPS*
	Thromboembolic disease	
Diagnostic tests	Spirometry with obstructive pattern	Low DLCO
	$\dot{V}/\dot{Q}$ lung scan	Orthodeoxia
	Pulmonary angiogram	"Bubble" echocardiography†

*May also act like arteriovenous shunting if hepatocellular dysfunction is severe.
†Echocardiography with bubble study demonstrating delayed microbubble opacification of the left atrium.
DLCO—diffusing capacity of the lungs for carbon monoxide; HPS—hepatopulmonary syndrome;
   $\dot{V}/\dot{Q}$—ventilation-perfusion.

Figure 24-4.

A and **B**, Hypoxemia responsive to O₂ (*panel A*) and poorly responsive to O₂ (*panel B*) in the absence of parenchymal disease on chest radiograph. A differential diagnosis for hypoxemia, in the absence of evidence of parenchymal disease on chest radiograph, can be generated through the understanding of gas exchange pathophysiology.

B. HYPOXEMIA POORLY RESPONSIVE TO O₂ IN THE ABSENCE OF PARENCHYMAL DISEASE ON CHEST RADIOGRAPH

	Intrapulmonary shunt			Intracardiac shunt
	Arteriovenous shunt	Inapparent airspace disease	Inapparent dependent atelectasis	
Example	HHT	Early PCP	After surgery	ASD
Diagnostic tests	"Bubble" echocardiography*	HRCT of the lungs (*see* Fig. 25-5B)	CT scan of the lungs (*see* Fig. 25-6)	"Bubble" echocardiography†
	HRCT of the lungs with contrast			Cardiac catheterization
	Pulmonary angiogram			

*Echocardiography with bubble study demonstrating delayed microbubble opacification of the left atrium.
†Echocardiography with bubble study demonstrating immediate microbubble opacification of the left atrium.
ASD—atrial septal defect; HHT—hereditary hemorrhagic telangiectasia; HRCT—high-resolution computerized tomography; PCP—Pneumocystis carinii pneumonia.

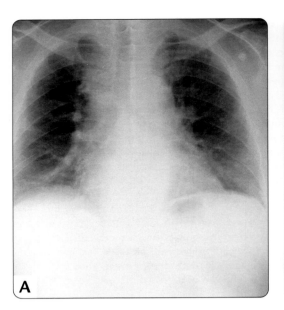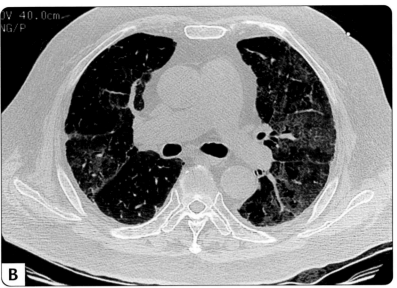

Figure 24-5.
A and **B**, Chest radiographs without apparent parenchymal disease to account for severe hypoxemia in an immunocompromised patient. High-resolution computed tomography of the lungs reveals extensive "ground glass" changes (alveolitis). Lung biopsy allowed a diagnosis of *Pneumocystis carinii* pneumonia.

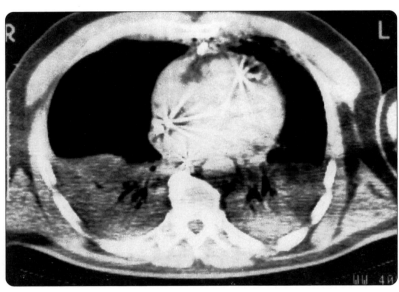

Figure 24-6.
Thoracic computed tomographic scan identifying the cause of hypoxemia. In patients requiring mechanical ventilation, the dependent (dorsal) lung regions bear a greater degree of atelectasis. This patient developed acute hypoxemic respiratory failure after cardiac surgery, and a conventional supine chest radiograph failed to explain the cause. (*From* Brussel *et al.* [2]; with permission.)

ACUTE RESPIRATORY DISTRESS SYNDROME

THE DEFINITION OF ALI AND ARDS

	Timing	Oxygenation	Chest radiograph	Pulmonary artery wedge pressure
ALI criteria	Acute onset	Pa_{O_2} ≤300 mm Hg (regardless of PEEP level)	Bilateral infiltrates (seen on frontal chest radiograph)	≤18 mm Hg when measured (or no clinical evidence of left atrial hypertension)
ARDS criteria	Acute onset	Pa_{O_2}/Fi_{O_2} ≤200 mm Hg (regardless of PEEP level)	Bilateral infiltrates (seen on frontal chest radiograph)	≤18 mm Hg when measured (or no clinical evidence of left atrial hypertension)

ALI—acute lung injury; ARDS—acute respiratory distress syndrome; Fi_{O_2}—fractional inspired oxygen; PEEP—positive end-expiratory pressure.

Figure 24-7.
The definition of acute lung injury and ARDS, according to the American-European Consensus Conference on ARDS. Acute lung injury is defined as a syndrome of acute and persistent inflammation of the lung with increased permeability that is associated with a characteristic constellation of clinical, radiologic, and physiologic abnormalities. ARDS represents the most severe end of this spectrum. (*Adapted from* Bernard *et al.* [3].)

ETIOLOGY OF ACUTE LUNG INJURY AND ACUTE RESPIRATORY DISTRESS SYNDROME

Direct lung injury

Aspiration pneumonitis

Other causes of pneumonitis: oxygen, smoke inhalation, radiation, bleomycin

Infectious pneumonia: community-acquired, nosocomial, opportunistic

Trauma: lung contusion, penetrating chest injury

Near-drowning

Fat embolism

After relief of upper airway obstruction

After bone marrow and lung transplantation

After lung re-expansion

Distant injury

Tissue inflammation, necrosis, infection ("sepsis syndrome")

Multiple trauma, major burns

Shock, hypoperfusion

Acute pancreatitis

Transfusion-associated lung injury

After cardiopulmonary bypass

Drug overdose: tricyclic antidepressants, cocaine

Neurogenic: intracerebral bleed, seizure

Figure 24-8.
The etiologies of acute lung injury and acute respiratory distress syndrome. To date, more than 60 distinct causes have been identified. (*Adapted from* Bigatello and Zapol [4].)

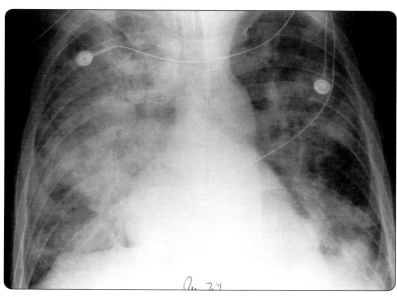

Figure 24-9.
An anteroposterior chest radiograph (supine) of a 60-year-old man with urosepsis and acute respiratory distress syndrome. The patchy, widespread opacities reflect diffuse air space disease and edema.

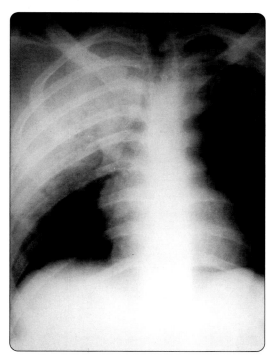

Figure 24-10.
An anteroposterior chest radiograph of a 25-year-old man with pulmonary contusion secondary to blunt thoracic trauma. The major changes are usually directly deep to the traumatized areas and are apparent soon after trauma. Radiologic resolution typically occurs rapidly, with improvement within 48 hours and complete clearing in 4 days.

THE QUALITY OF THE EVIDENCE AND THE GRADING OF RECOMMENDATIONS IN ARDS

Quality of evidence

Level 1: Randomized, prospective, controlled investigations of ARDS

Level 2: Nonrandomized, concurrent-cohort, historical-cohort investigations and case series of patients with ARDS

Level 3: Randomized, prospective, controlled investigations of sepsis or other relevant conditions with potential applications to ARDS

Level 4: Case reports of ARDS

Grading of recommendations

Grade A: Supported by at least two level-1 investigations

Grade B: Supported by one level-1 investigation only

Grade C: Supported by level-2 investigation only

Grade D: Supported by at least one level-3 investigation

Ungraded: No available clinical investigations

ARDS—acute respiratory distress syndrome.

Figure 24-11.
The quality of the evidence and the grading of recommendations in acute respiratory distress syndrome. Many therapeutic strategies in the treatment of acute respiratory distress syndrome have not been tested rigorously and remain controversial. The quality of the available evidence needs to be scientifically graded. (*Adapted from* Kollef and Schuster [5,6].)

Strategy	Recommended	Grade
Volume-cycled, assist-control mode using low-stretch ventilation (tidal volumes ≤6 mL/kg predicted body weight; plateau pressures ≤30 cm H_2O) (*See* Fig. 24-16.)	Yes	B
Lateral decubitus positioning in unilateral lung disease for persistent hypoxemia	Yes	C
PEEP to maintain Sao_2 88% to 95% and Fio_2 ≤0.60 (*See* Fig. 24-14.)	Yes	C
Open-lung approach (higher levels of PEEP and lung recruitment maneuvers)	?*†‡	B
Pressure-control inverse-ratio ventilation	?*†	C
High frequency jet ventilation	No	B
High frequency oscillatory ventilation	?*†	C
Prone position ventilation (*See* Fig. 24-19.)	?* †‡	C
Extracorporeal membrane oxygenation (ECMO)	No†	B
Extracorporeal carbon dioxide removal (ECCO$_2$-R)	No†	B
Partial liquid ventilation	?*	C
Airway pressure-release ventilation	?*	C
Tracheal gas insufflation (washes out dead space)	?* †	C
Prophylactic PEEP (>5 H_2O)	No	B
Noninvasive mask positive pressure ventilation (NIPPV)	Yes (in selected cases)	B

Inconclusive, needs further study.
†*May be considered a rescue therapy (for inadequate oxygenation, severe hypercarbia, or high airway pressures)*
‡*Large level 1 study being conducted.*
Fio_2—*fractional inspired oxygen; PEEP—positive end-expiratory presure; Sao$_2$—arterial oxygen percent saturation.*

Figure 24-12.

Ventilator management of acute respiratory distress syndrome. Mechanical ventilation is supportive in acute respiratory distress syndrome, maintaining acceptable gas exchange until lung recovery can occur. Conventional strategies have combined volume-cycled mechanical ventilation, to achieve a normal alveolar minute ventilation, with the addition of positive end-expiratory pressure, to ensure arterial oxygenation with minimal oxygen toxicity. (*Adapted from* Kollef and Schuster [5–7].)

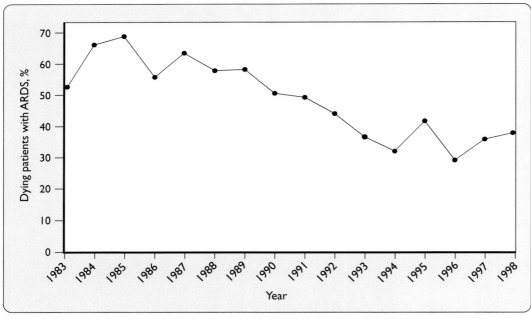

Figure 24-13.

Survival of patients with acute respiratory distress syndrome (ARDS). There is evidence that mechanical ventilation strategies and better supportive care may reduce ARDS mortality, at least in one center, from 60% in the 1980s to between 30% and 40% in the mid-1990s. Lung-protective ventilatory strategies aim to avoid the consequence of volutrauma and barotrauma that may amplify the injury to the alveolar-capillary membrane [8–10].

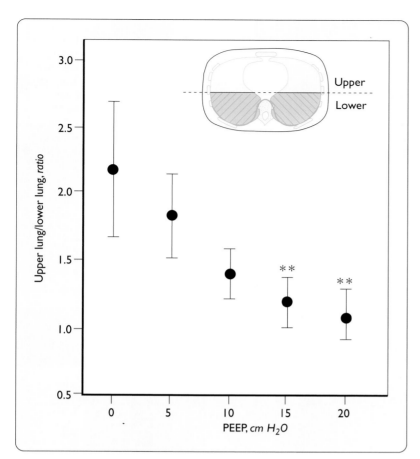

Figure 24-14.
The benefits of positive end-expiratory pressure (PEEP). In acute respiratory distress syndrome (ARDS), the lungs exhibit significant heterogeneity, which produces an uneven distribution of ventilation. In the patient requiring mechanical ventilation, the dependent (dorsal) lung regions bear a greater degree of atelectasis. This condition is best illustrated on thoracic computed tomographic scan (see Fig. 24-6). PEEP makes gas distribution more homogeneous in ARDS and improves oxygenation by recruiting lung units that remain closed at low lung volumes. In the supine patient with acute diffuse lung injury, insufflated gas preferentially distributes to the open lung units of the upper (ventral) regions. The greater hydrostatic pressures within the lower (dorsal) regions results in fewer and smaller open lung units at functional reserve capacity. PEEP recruits the closed lung units in the lower regions and "stretches" the open lung units within the upper regions. The consequence of increased PEEP is a more homogeneous distribution of insufflated gas throughout the lung. *Double asterisks* denote significant change from baseline. (*Adapted from* Gattinoni et al. [11].)

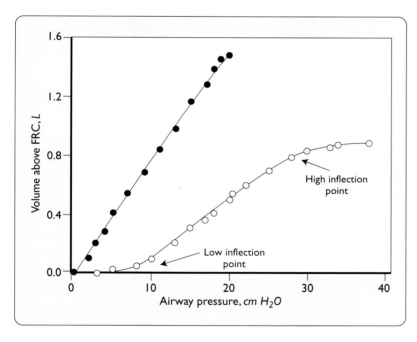

Figure 24-15.
Lung-protective, pressure-limited strategy for patients with acute respiratory distress syndrome (ARDS). A pressure-volume curve in a patient with ARDS is illustrated, compared with normal. The slope of the curve is flat at low and high airway pressures. A lower inflection point represents considerable recruitment of previously collapsed lung units; the upper inflection point represents a state of near maximal inflation. Precision adjustment of the peak inspiratory pressure, tidal volume, and positive end-expiratory pressure (PEEP) may be accomplished by recording this type of pressure-volume curve of the respiratory system. The goals are to ventilate the patient between the lower and upper inflection points with a small tidal volume (<6 mL/kg) to limit peak airway pressures (<40 cm H_2O). PEEP levels should be sufficient to prevent alveolar collapse and airway closure. The subsequent hypercarbia of this strategy is labeled "permissive hypercarbia" and is generally well-tolerated without treatment. FRC—functional reserve capacity. (*Adapted from* Bigatello and Zapol [4].)

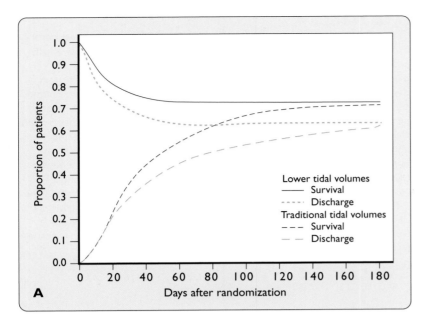

A

Figure 24-16.
A and **B**, The probability of survival and of being discharged home and breathing without assistance in patients with acute lung injury and acute respiratory distress syndrome (ARDS). A ventilation strategy using lower tidal volume (6 mL/kg of predicted body weight) compared with traditional tidal volumes (12 mL/kg of predicted body weight) resulted in decreased mortality, more days without ventilator need, and fewer incidences of multiple system organ failure (MSOF). Levels of systemic cytokines were also in the lower tidal volume group. (*Adapted from* The Acute Respiratory Distress Syndrome Network [12].)

B. PROBABILITY OF SURVIVAL

Variable	Lower tidal volume group	Traditional tidal volume group	*P* value
Death before discharge home and breathing without assistance, %	31.0	39.8	0.007
Breathing without assistance by day 28, %	65.7	55.0	<0.001
No. of ventilator-free days, days 1 to 28 (mean ± SD)	12 ± 11	10 ± 11	0.007
No. of days without failure of nonpulmonary organs or systems, days 1 to 28 (mean ± SD)	15 ± 11	12 ± 11	0.006
Change in log-transformed plasma interleukin-6 levels, in pg/mL, from day 0 to 3 (mean ± SD)	2.5 ± 0.7 to 2.0 ± 0.5	2.5 ± 0.7 to 2.3 ± 0.7	<0.001

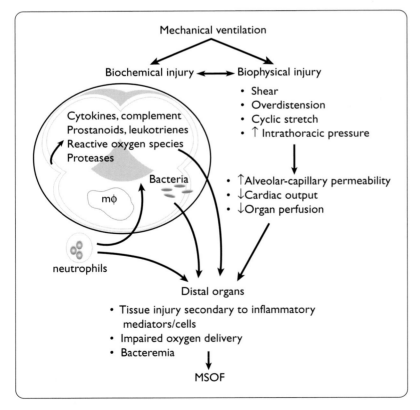

Figure 24-17.
Mechanical ventilation can have systemic effects and lead to the development of multisystem organ failure (MSOF) by several biophysical and biochemical (release of mediators) mechanisms [13,14]. The lungs of patients with ARDS are asymmetrical along the vertical axis with a small nondependent lung region continuously open to ventilation and a dependent consolidated, atelectatic region. In between, there is a region that can be recruited or derecruited depending on the particular ventilatory strategy used. Mechanical ventilation can lead to injury caused by overdistention of the small, relatively normal alveolar regions and repeated recruitment or derecruitment of alveolar units (shear stresses) that may be exacerbated with ventilation at low PEEP levels. Mechanical stress-induced inflammation of the lung may lead to an increase in cytokine levels in the lung and in the systemic circulation. Mechanical stress-induced inflammation of the lung may also partially explain the development of MSOF in many patients with ARDS. The decrease in mortality observed in a recent study that used a lung-protective strategy may be related to reduced MSOF (*see* Fig. 24-16).

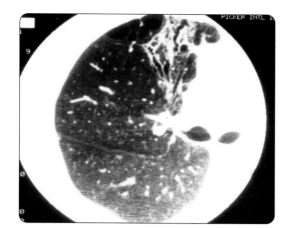

Figure 24-18.
Computed tomographic image of the thorax of an acute respiratory distress syndrome survivor revealing emphysema-like lesions (bullae). These lesions are possibly related to regional overdistention of the nondependent lung during the acute illness, *ie*, ventral areas when supine.

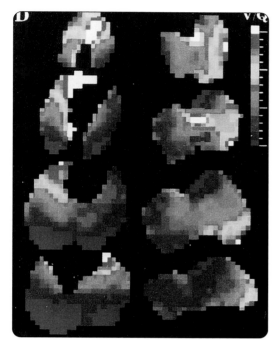

Figure 24-19.
Prone-position ventilation. Arterial oxygenation may improve, sometimes considerably, when patients with acute respiratory distress syndrome (ARDS) are turned from the supine to the prone position. When supine, in the setting of lung injury, the transpulmonary pressure (P_{tp}) is not sufficient to exceed the critical opening pressure (P_{op}) in the most dependent dorsal lung regions, *ie*, in regions where regional ventilation ($\dot{V}_r$) is reduced or absent and atelectasis, shunt, and ventilation/perfusion heterogeneity ($\dot{V}_r/\dot{Q}_r$) are most severe. The prone position, on the other hand, generates a transpulmonary pressure sufficient to exceed airway opening pressure in dorsal lung regions without adversely affecting the ventral lung regions. The result is increased dorsal $\dot{V}$ with reduced shunt and improved oxygenation. Reconstructed tomographic images of the relative $\dot{V}_r/\dot{Q}_r$ in the supine and prone positions of a dog with oleic-acid–induced lung injury is illustrated. The four transverse slices are approximately 4 cm apart and are oriented cranial to caudal (*top* to *bottom*). The *purple areas* represent absent $\dot{V}_r$ but maintained $\dot{Q}_r$ (*ie*, $\dot{V}_r/\dot{Q}_r = 0$ or shunt). (*See* Color Plate.) (*From* Lamm et al. [15]; with permission.)

Treatment	Class	Proposed mechanism of action	Recommended	Grade
Early fluid restriction/diuresis	S	Reduce the amount of extravascular lung water and alveolar flooding	Yes*	B
Surfactant replacement therapy	S	Replace dysfunctional surfactant; improve alveolar stability	No*	B**
Early corticosteroids	MI	Alter early host inflammatory cascade	No	A
Late corticosteroids	MI	Alter late host fibroproliferative response to injury	No*†	C
N-acetylcysteine	MI	Scavenger of oxygen-free radicals	No	B
Ketoconazole	MI	Inhibitor of thromboxane and leukotriene synthesis	No‡	B
Ibuprofen	MI	Inhibitor of protaglandin pathways	No	D
Alprostadil (prostaglandin E_1)	MI	Blocks platelet aggregation, modulates inflammation, vasodilator	No	B
Lisofylline	MI	Phosphodiesterase inhibitor; inhibits chemotaxis/activation of PMNs	No	B
Antiendotoxins and anticytokines	MI	Antagonists of the mediators of sepsis	No	D
Selective digestive decontamination	MI	Reduce risk of nosocomial infection	No	D
Inhaled nitric oxide	S	Modulation of hypoxic pulmonary vasoconstriction	No†	B
Supernormal oxygen transport	S	Oxygen consumption supply dependency in ARDS	No	D
Almitrine	S	Physiologic improvement in oxygenation	?§	C
Recombinant human activated protein C	MI	Antithrombotic, anti-inflammatory, profibrinolytic	Yes¶	D

*Large level 1 study being conducted.
†May be considered a rescue therapy (nonresolving ARDS or inadequate oxygenation).
‡Use for prophylaxis to be determined.
§Inconclusive, needs further study.
¶In ARDS caused by sepsis.
**Lack of efficacy in level 1 study, but dose, delivery methodology, and choice of surfactant questioned.
ARDS—acute respiratory distress syndrome; MI—modulator of inflammation; PMNs—polymorphonuclear leukocytes; S—supportive therapy.

Figure 24-20.
Pharmacologic management of acute respiratory distress syndrome (ARDS). Pharmacologic modalities in patients with ARDS can be considered supportive therapies or modulators of inflammation. Unfortunately, anti-inflammatory therapies, to date, have been discouraging in disease prevention and in survival improvement. (*Data from* Kolleff and Schuster [5,6], Hudson [16], and Ware and Matthay [7].)

MECHANICAL VENTILATION IN ACUTE RESPIRATORY FAILURE

CONSIDERATIONS TO INITIATE MECHANICAL VENTILATION IN ACUTE RESPIRATORY FAILURE

Figure 24-21.
Considerations to initiate mechanical ventilation in acute respiratory failure. Mechanical ventilation is indicated in situations in which established or impending respiratory failure exists [17].

Rapidly worsening physiologic variables
  Hypotension
  Tachycardia
  Tachypnea
  Hypoxemia
  Hypercarbia
  Acidosis
Evidence of compromised cardiac function
Impending fatigue of the respiratory muscles
  Presence of severe dyspnea and diaphoresis
  Prominent use of accessory muscles
  Paradoxic movement of the abdomen
  Upward trends in respiratory rate
  Upward trends in arterial carbon dioxide tension
Inability to protect airway and/or expectorate secretions
Increasing confusion, restlessness, and/or exhaustion

OBJECTIVES OF MECHANICAL VENTILATION IN ACUTE RESPIRATORY FAILURE

Improve pulmonary gas exchange
   Reverse hypoxemia
   Relieve acute respiratory acidosis
Correct incomplete lung inflation
   Increase lung volume
      Prevent and reverse atelectasis
      Improve lung compliance
   Prevent further lung injury
Permit lung and airway healing
Improve cardiac function
   Reduce myocardial oxygen demand
Relieve respiratory distress
   Decrease oxygen cost of breathing
   Reverse respiratory muscle fatigue
Avoid iatrogenic injury (*See* Fig. 24-24)
   Endotracheal tube complications (*See* Fig. 24-23)
   Complications of positive pressure ventilation
      Pressure-induced alveolar injury (barotrauma)
      Volume-induced alveolar injury (volutrauma)
      Reduced cardiac output
      Oxygen toxicity
      Ventilator-associated pneumonia (*See* Fig. 24-25)

Figure 24-22.

Objectives of mechanical ventilation in acute respiratory failure. Mechanical ventilation supports the failing cardiopulmonary system until its function can improve (either spontaneously or as a result of other therapy). Physiologic and clinical objectives guide its application; however, the potential for iatrogenic injury must be considered. (*Data from* Tobin [18] and Slutsky [19].)

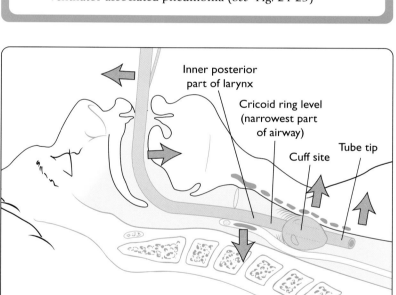

Figure 24-23.

Prolonged endotracheal intubation placing predictable forces on the airway. *Arrows* indicate forces acting to restore an elastic tracheal tube to its original shape when inserted in the patient's airway. (*Adapted from* Lindholm [20].)

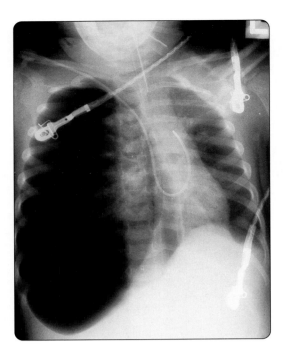

Figure 24-24.
Anteroposterior chest radiograph (supine) of an 18-year-old man with a closed head injury. A pulmonary artery catheter was inserted via the right subclavian approach. The right-sided pneumothorax is under tension, and the mediastinal structures are shifted to the left.

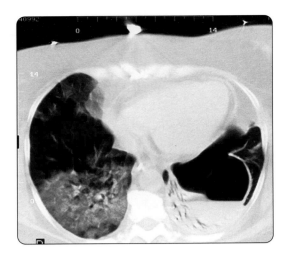

Figure 24-25.
Infected pneumatocele in the left lower lobe of a patient with acute respiratory distress syndrome.

REFERENCES

1. Nunn JF: Causes of failure of ventilation. In *Applied Respiratory Physiology.* London: Butterworth & Co.; 1987:381.

2. Brussel T, Hachenberg T, Roos N, *et al.*: Mechanical ventilation in the prone position for acute respiratory failure after cardiac surgery. *J Cardiothorac Vasc Anesth* 1993, 7:541–546.

3. Bernard GR, Artigas A, Brigham KL, *et al.*: The American-European Consensus Conference on ARDS: definitions, mechanisms, relevant outcomes, and clinical trial coordination. *Am J Respir Crit Care Med* 1994, 149:818–824.

4. Bigatello LM, Zapol WM: New approaches to acute lung injury. *Br J Anaesth* 1996, 77:99–109.

5. Kollef MH, Schuster DP: The acute respiratory distress syndrome. *N Engl J Med* 1995, 332:27–37.

6. Kollef MH, Schuster DP: Acute respiratory distress syndrome. *Dis Mon* 1996, 5:275–326.

7. Ware LB, Matthay MA: The acute respiratory distress syndrome. *N Engl J Med* 2000, 342:1334–1349.

8. Sessler CN, Bloomfield GL, Fowler AA: Current concepts of sepsis and acute lung injury. *Clin Chest Med* 1996, 17:213–235.

9. Milberg JA, Davis DR, Steinberg KP, Hudson LD: Improved survival of patients with ARDS: 1983–1993. *J Am Med Assoc* 1995, 273:306–309.

10. Steinberg KP, Hudson MA: Acute lung injury and acute respiratory distress syndrome. The clinical syndrome. *Clin Chest Med* 2000, 21:401–417.

11. Gattinoni L, Pelosi P, Crotti S, Valenza F: Effects of positive end-expiratory pressure on regional distribution of tidal volume and recruitment in adult respiratory distress syndrome. *Am J Respir Crit Care Med* 1995, 151:1807–1814.

12. The Acute Respiratory Distress Syndrome Network: Ventilation with lower tidal volumes as compared with traditional tidal volumes for acute lung injury and the acute respiratory distress syndrome. *N Engl J Med* 2000, 342:1301–1308.

13. Slutsky AS: Lung injury caused by mechanical ventilation. *Chest* 1999, 116:9S–15S.

14. Ranieri VM, Suter PM, Tortorella D, *et al.*: The effect of mechanical ventilation on pulmonary and systemic release of inflammatory mediators in patients with acute respiratory distress syndrome. *JAMA* 1999, 282:54–61.

15. Lamm WJ, Graham MM, Albert RK: Mechanism by which the prone position improves oxygenation in acute lung injury. *Am J Respir Crit Care Med* 1994, 150:184–193.

16. Hudson LD: New therapies for ARDS. *Chest* 1995, 108:795–915.

17. Ponte J: Assisted ventilation: 2. Indications for mechanical ventilation. *Thorax* 1990, 45:885–890.

18. Tobin MJ: Mechanical ventilation. *N Engl J Med* 1994, 300:1056–1061.

19. Slutsky AS: Mechanical ventilation. *Chest* 1993, 104:1833–1859.

20. Lindholm CE: Den iatrogent fororsakade trakealstenosens etiologi. *Lakartidningen* 1977, 74:2344.

MANAGEMENT OF OXYGEN DELIVERY IN THE CRITICALLY ILL PATIENT

Claudio M. Martin & Christopher J. Davreux

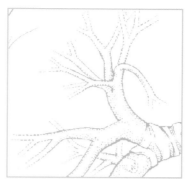
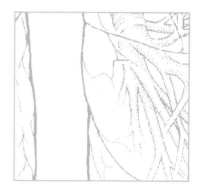

25

Supranormal oxygen delivery or goal-directed hemodynamic therapy in critically ill patients is a controversial topic. The former term was used by Abraham *et al.* [1] to describe the observation made by their research group that survivors of critical illnesses had higher than normal values for cardiac index, oxygen delivery, and oxygen consumption. This research resulted in the concept embodied by the latter term, that therapy should be directed at achieving these hemodynamic goals, which were associated with improved survival.

Although the results of clinical trials of supranormal oxygen delivery have been inconclusive, there is physiologic validity to the concept. There is no doubt that inadequate hemodynamic resuscitation may produce widespread tissue hypoxia resulting in tissue injury. The question is not whether patients should be resuscitated, but what the goals of resuscitation should be.

This chapter reviews some of the theoretic relationships between oxygen delivery and tissue injury. The results of clinical trials will be summarized, and their limitations will be discussed. Finally, a practical approach to the critically ill patient is presented. Unfortunately, there is no level-1 evidence available to support these recommendations, as recent reviews have found [2,3]. Thus, there is still a great need for physiologic studies to identify potential therapies and clinical trials to determine which interventions are truly effective.

DIAGNOSIS

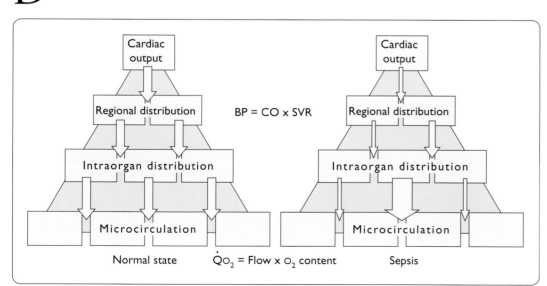

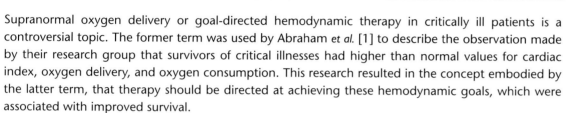

Figure 25-1.

Cardiac output and tissue oxygen saturation under normal versus hypovolemic conditions. Shock usually means that hypotension is present, but the increased cardiac output (CO) in sepsis usually results in a normal blood pressure (BP). A patient in hypovolemic shock due to a 30% volume loss can exhibit normal blood pressure because vasoconstriction occurs. Thus, centrally measured values for cardiac output and blood pressure may be misleading. If the *left panel* represents the normal state, the *right panel* shows changes that could occur in response to a decrease in cardiac output. Vascular resistance is determined mostly at the level of the small arterioles, so normal blood pressure is maintained by increasing vascular resistance. Increased resistance may result in a redistribution of blood as part of the normal response or as a result of abnormal vascular regulation. However, adequate tissue oxygen delivery requires an appropriate distribution of blood flow at all levels of the circulation. Thus, a more accurate definition of shock is the presence of tissue dysoxia when oxygen delivery is not adequately matched to tissue oxygen demand. $\dot{Q}_{O_2}$—tissue oxygen delivery; SVR—systemic vascular resistance.

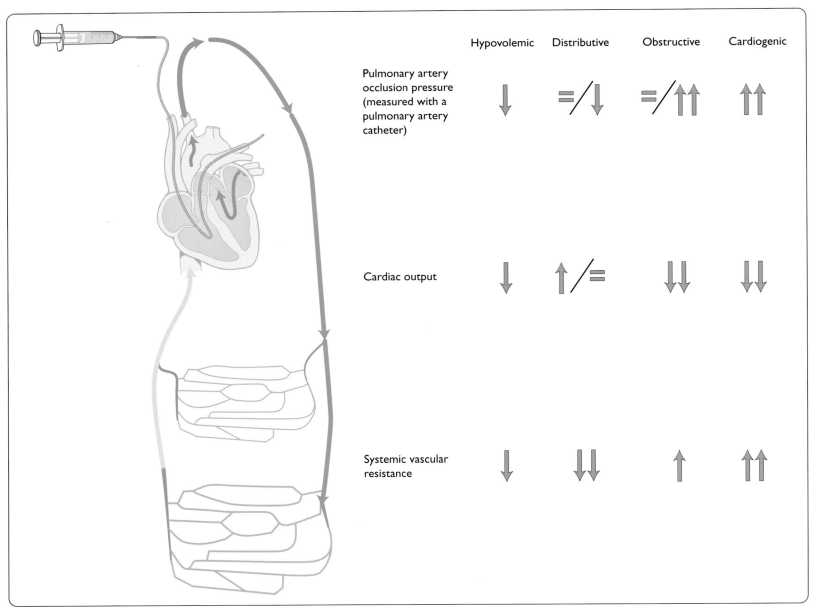

	Hypovolemic	Distributive	Obstructive	Cardiogenic
Pulmonary artery occlusion pressure (measured with a pulmonary artery catheter)	↓	=/↓	=/↑↑	↑↑
Cardiac output	↓	↑/=	↓↓	↓↓
Systemic vascular resistance	↓	↓↓	↑	↑↑

Figure 25-2.

Differential diagnosis of shock. Hypovolemic shock (due to hemorrhage and volume depletion) has a low arterial opening pressure (PaOP) and cardiac output with high systemic vascular resistance (SVR) because vasoconstriction occurs in an attempt to maintain blood pressure. Distributive shock (due to sepsis or anaphylaxis) has normal or slightly low PaOP, high or normal cardiac output, and a very low SVR. Obstructive shock (due to tamponade or pulmonary embolism) has a normal to high PaOP, low cardiac output, and increased SVR. Cardiogenic shock (due to myocardial dysfunction or acute mechanical dysfunction) has a high PaOP, very low cardiac output, and high SVR.

ETIOLOGY

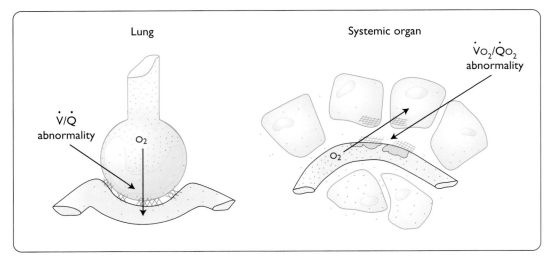

Lung   Systemic organ

Figure 25-3.

Ventilation-perfusion ($\dot{V}/\dot{Q}$) abnormality at the level of the alveolar and local tissue. The mismatch that occurs between tissue oxygen delivery ($\dot{Q}O_2$) and tissue demand (DO_2) is analogous to the $\dot{V}/\dot{Q}$ ratio mismatch that occurs in the lungs. Although local injury can contribute to the tissue $\dot{Q}O_2/DO_2$ mismatch, many other factors, such as abnormal regulation of blood flow, are likely to be involved. The balance may be stressed further by increases in DO_2, as occurs in hypermetabolic states such as sepsis or trauma. (*Adapted from* Dorinsky and Gadek [4].)

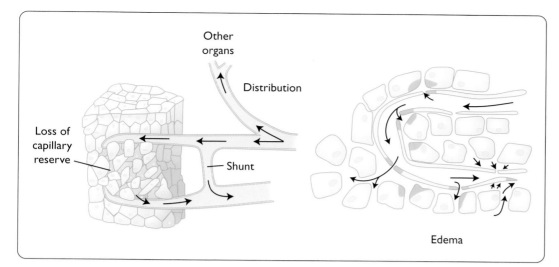

Figure 25-4.
Blood flow mechanisms responsible for a tissue oxygen delivery ($\dot{Q}_{O_2}$)/tissue demand (D_{O_2}) mismatch. $\dot{Q}_{O_2}/D_{O_2}$ mismatch may be due to alterations in blood flow at various levels of the circulation, resulting in loss of convective oxygen flux. The diffusive component of oxygen delivery may be blocked by tissue edema. Cellular metabolic defects may impair cellular oxygen metabolism. (*Adapted from* Durinsky and Gadek [4].)

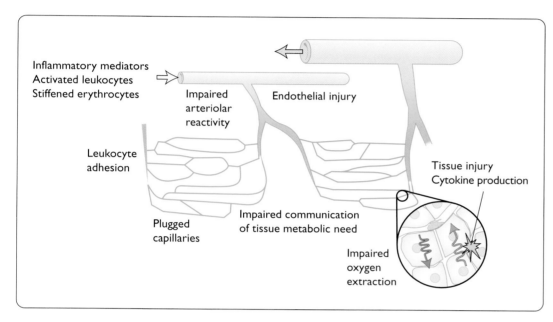

Figure 25-5.
Circulatory dysfunction in multiple organ dysfunction syndrome. Work in many laboratories has shown that abnormalities in the circulation occur at multiple sites and may be initiated or caused by many different mechanisms. These changes include altered vascular responsiveness at all levels of the arterial tree [5,6]. Changes in physical properties of erythrocytes and leukocytes may result in microvascular plugging [7–9]. Endothelial injury results in increased vascular permeability and decreased cross-sectional area, which further impedes blood flow and oxygen transfer [10,11]. Endothelial injury may also contribute to the abnormal regulation of microvascular blood flow. Circulating inflammatory mediators play an important role in the initiation and propagation of these changes [12]. Despite these advances in understanding the pathophysiology of oxygen delivery and tissue injury, there is still a lack of strong clinical evidence for the role of tissue injury in patient management procedures.

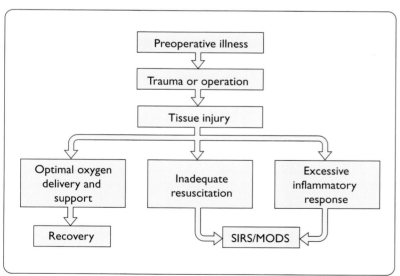

Figure 25-6.
Risk factors for systemic inflammatory response syndrome (SIRS) and multiple organ dysfunction syndrome (MODS). Surgery, trauma, or an acute condition such as gastrointestinal bleeding, are all associated with variable degrees of tissue injury. If adequate resuscitation is provided, the patient may recover without additional morbidity. However, inadequate resuscitation may result in further tissue injury, increasing the risk for SIRS and MODS. Resuscitation usually takes place during the initial patient stabilization period. The focus is on restoring intravascular volume and blood pressure. However, observations that hemodynamic parameters such as reduced cardiac output and oxygen delivery are associated with mortality show that resuscitation of critically ill patients should extend beyond the initial management phase. Hemodynamic resuscitation therefore encompasses the early period, during which treatment is usually directed to blood pressure, and a later, ongoing phase during which treatment is designed primarily to ensure adequate oxygen delivery with respect to oxygen demand. The overall goal is to improve survival by minimizing the amount of hypoxic tissue injury and MODS. Tissue injury can occur as a result of inadequate hemodynamic resuscitation or as a direct result of excessive production of cellular and humoral inflammatory mediators. When MODS occurs as a complication of sepsis or SIRS, it is termed secondary; primary MODS develops as a result of the initial injury (*eg*, severe chest or abdominal trauma).

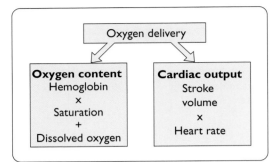

Figure 25-7.
Calculation of oxygen delivery. Oxygen delivery is determined by the equation in the figure. Examination of the individual components can be used to guide therapy.

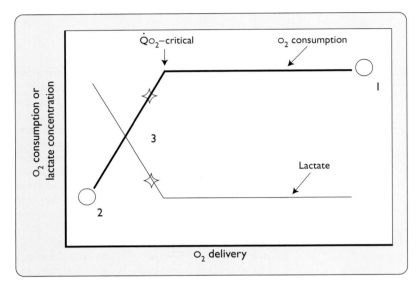

Figure 25-8.
Effect of oxygen delivery on oxygen consumption. Oxygen delivery ($\dot{Q}O_2$) is usually in excess of oxygen consumption (*1*). Thus, if delivery decreases, oxygen demands can be met by increasing oxygen extraction. Eventually, the ability to increase oxygen extraction is reached, and oxygen consumption becomes dependent on delivery (*2*). The inflection point is termed the *critical oxygen delivery level* ($\dot{Q}O_2$–critical). The goal of therapy should be to increase oxygen delivery (*3*), preferably to a point above the critical value. However, measurement of the critical point is impossible. Most patients who have been resuscitated and who are hemodynamically stable probably do not have an oxygen supply dependency that is detectable when whole-body oxygen consumption is measured [13,14]. Animal studies have shown that large increases in lactate occur at the critical point. Thus, small elevations of lactate may indicate regional insufficiencies in oxygen delivery. (Lactate levels may also increase in response to changes in cellular metabolism or decreased clearance.)

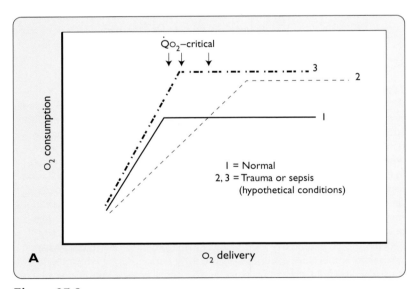

Figure 25-9.
Effect of disease on the oxygen consumption–delivery ($\dot{Q}O_2$) curve. The shape of the oxygen consumption and delivery curve can change in disease states. It also varies between different organs (and probably within different regions of an organ). **A,** Thus, in patients with sepsis or trauma, oxygen consumption might be increased, and higher oxygen delivery might be required to remain above the critical point. **B,** However, because we are unable to monitor oxygen metabolism in individual organs, it is possible that some organs or tissues are below the critical point at relatively high

levels of total body oxygen delivery. The whole-body relationship is composed of the sum of the individual organs or regions, so supply dependency in an organ may be masked. Mathematical modelling has shown that the critical $\dot{Q}O_2$ is determined by matching oxygen delivery to oxygen demand [15,16]. As heterogeneity between oxygen demand and supply increases, the curve becomes more curvilinear and the critical $\dot{Q}O_2$ increases.

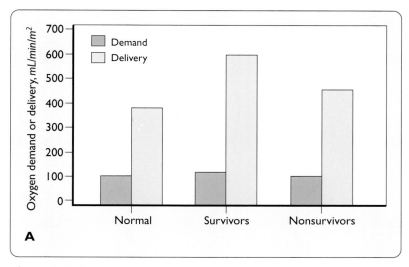

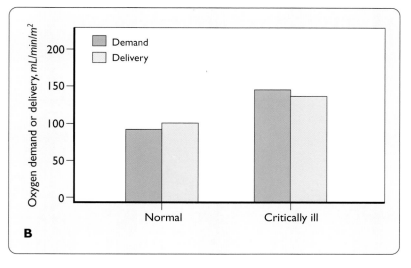

Figure 25-10.

Changes in oxygen delivery during and after disease. **A**, Supranormal oxygen delivery was initially based on the observation by Abraham et al. [1] that survivors of critical illnesses have higher cardiac output (4.5 L/min/m²), oxygen delivery (DO_2 >600 mL/min/m²), and oxygen uptake (170 mL/min/m²) than nonsurvivors. The increase in DO_2 represents as appropriate increase to meet the need of a hypermetabolic state induced by the stress of a critical illness. This increase in demand can be supported by an increase in oxygen delivery and oxygen extraction. **B**, In certain tissues, such as the heart, oxygen supply is closely linked with oxygen demand. Increases in demand may exceed increases in supply, and tissue hypoxia will develop. Despite the physiologic appeal of this goal-directed therapy, controversy exists regarding its clinical benefit.

CLINICAL TRIALS

CLINICAL TRIALS OF SUPRANORMAL OXYGEN THERAPY

Study	Patients	Outcome	Interventions	Therapy target*	Mortality rates for control/treatment groups
Shoemaker et al. [20]	High-risk surgery	Hospital mortality	Fluids/dobutamine	4.5/600/170	0.28/0.04
Boyd et al. [17]	High-risk surgery	28-d mortality	Dopexamine	—/600/—	0.22/0.06
Tuchschmidt et al. [19]	Sepsis	14-d mortality	Various	6.0/—/—	0.72/0.50
Yu et al. [18]	Sepsis	30-d mortality	Various	—/600/—	0.34/0.34
Hayes et al. [23]	High-risk surgery, sepsis	Hospital mortality	Dobutamine	4.5/600/170	0.34/0.54
Yu et al. [22]	Sepsis, hypovolemia, ARDS	30-d mortality	Various	—/600/—	0.62/0.14
Gutteriez et al. [25]	Critically ill	Mortality	Various	Gastric intramucosal pH	0.58/0.42
Gattinoni et al. [21]	Critically ill	6-mo mortality	Various	Various	0.48/0.49
Fleming et al. [24]	Trauma	Mortality	Fluids/packed cells/ dobutamine	4.5/670/166	0.44/0.24
Yu et al. [26]	Sepsis	Hospital mortality	Fluids/inotropes	—/600/—	0.52/0.21
Lobo et al. [27]	High-risk surgery	60-d mortality	Fluids/dobutamine	—/600/—	0.50/0.16

*The therapy targets are shown as cardiac index/oxygen delivery/oxygen consumption. ARDS—acute respiratory distress syndrome.

Figure 25-11.

Clinical trials of supranormal oxygen therapy. Various clinical trials have examined the role of therapy that is guided by hemodynamic or tissue perfusion parameters. The figure shows seven clinical trials of supranormal oxygen therapy [17–23] that were included in a recent meta-analysis [3]. Other studies add some useful information. A study of trauma patients used an inadequate randomization procedure but showed a trend toward reduced mortality and significant reductions in organ failures, ventilation days, and intensive care unit days [24]. Another study used treatment guided by gastric tonometry and found a survival benefit [25].

PATIENT MANAGEMENT

Monitoring Systems

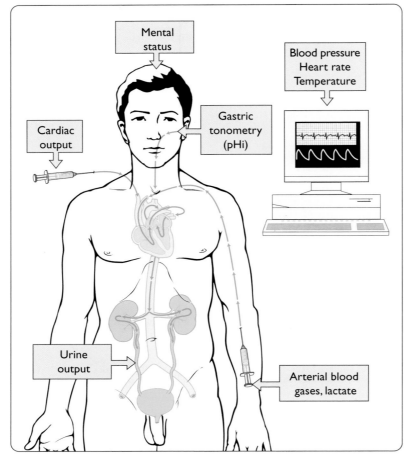

Figure 25-12.
Monitoring requirements for the critically ill patient. The first requirement to manage critically ill patients is adequate monitoring, including thorough physical assessment of mental status, temperature, and urine output, all of which are useful indicators of hemodynamic status. Direct hemodynamic measurements include heart rate and blood pressure. Cardiac output and vascular filling pressures should also be monitored in unstable patients because blood pressure alone may be misleading. Laboratory investigations should include arterial blood gases and lactate. Gastric tonometry is a newer monitoring technique that may provide information about splanchnic perfusion. pHi—intramucosal pH.

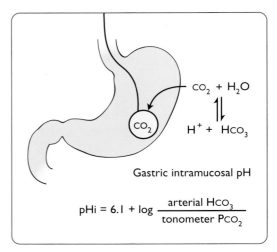

Figure 25-13.
Gastric tonometry. Gastric tonometry is a new technique that has not been evaluated fully. The figure shows the principle of its operation and how gastric intramucosal pH (pHi) is calculated. The technique has been validated in animal models and found to be unreliable when the rate of blood flow is low or absent. Various technical issues need to be considered, such as the effect of endogenous gastric acid secretion and the timing of the sample. Some investigators believe that the gradient between the tonometer and arterial P_{CO_2} is more valuable. However, studies using gastric pHi have shown that low abnormal values during the first 12 hours of intensive care predict a poor outcome compared with values that are normal or improve with the initial treatment [25,28].

Therapeutic Options

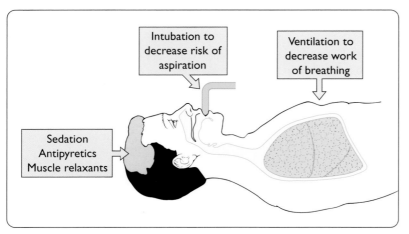

Figure 25-14.
The fundamentals of resuscitation. The fundamentals of resuscitation start with the ABCs (airway, breathing, circulation). Aspiration is common in seriously ill patients and can lead to lung injury and multiple organ dysfunction syndrome. Therefore, the airway should be protected by early intubation in most patients. Mechanical ventilation reduces the work of breathing and permits the cardiac output to be directed to other vital tissues. Up to 30% of cardiac output can be consumed by the muscles of respiration in a patient with respiratory failure. In most cases, treatment to reduce oxygen demand should be considered. Treatment options include antipyretics, adequate sedation, and muscle relaxants.

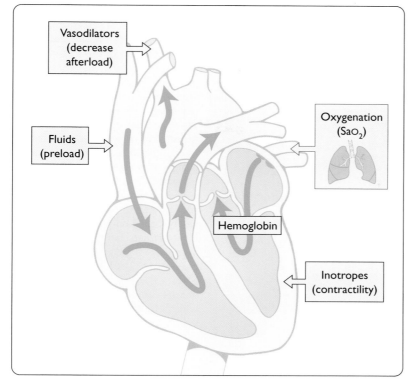

Figure 25-15.
The various approaches available for increasing oxygen delivery. The arterial oxygen percent saturation (SaO₂) should be maintained at 90% or higher. This level is usually best accomplished with adequate levels of fractional inspired oxygen and positive end-expiratory pressure (PEEP). However, high PEEP, airway pressures, and tidal volumes may all be deleterious. Because the use of pressure is limited, low volume ventilation may be the preferred approach to achieve adequate oxygenation and ventilation. However, there is insufficient data to make a clear recommendation. Fluid, transfusions, and vasoactive therapy can also be used (see Figs. 25-16 to 25-18).

PLASMA EXPANDERS

Crystalloid
    Inexpensive, simple
Colloid
    Maintain oncotic pressure
    Require less infused volume
Hypertonic solutions
    May be useful for specific conditions
Oxygen carrier solutions
    Investigational

Figure 25-16.
Plasma expanders. Plasma expanders should be used to increase the left ventricular end diastolic pressure until the stroke volume has been maximized. The choice of crystalloid or colloid is controversial because a clear benefit has not been shown for either [29,30]. A recent Cochrane review [31] suggested an increased mortality with the use of albumin. Although the use of albumin subsequently changed, the results and conclusions from the Cochrane review have been widely criticized [32]. A smaller infusion volume is required with colloid, so it may be advantageous when a rapid response is needed. Studies have not looked at long-term outcomes adequately, although an animal study showed less tissue injury with colloid therapy in sepsis [11]. In certain situations, such as hemorrhagic shock, hypertonic solutions may be useful; unfortunately, proper clinical trials using these solutions have not been done. Hemoglobin solutions that are entering clinical trials act as colloids but may also transport oxygen.

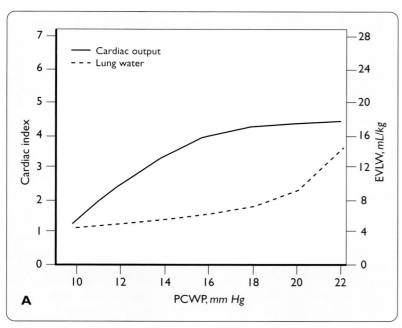

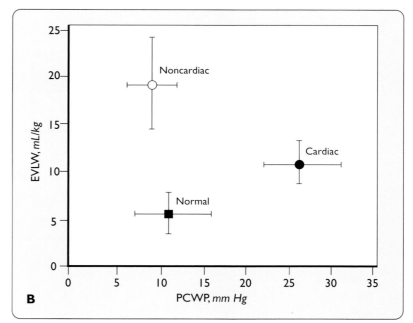

Figure 25-17.
The fluid paradox. **A,** Fluid paradox is the problem posed by using fluids to increase vascular volume and oxygen delivery while trying to keep the hydrostatic pressure low to decrease pulmonary edema. **B,** In patients with noncardiac pulmonary edema, slight increases in filling pressure cause large changes in extravascular lung water (EVLW; pulmonary edema). Two studies suggested that survival is associated with reduced filling pressures or fluid balance [33,34]. A small prospective study found improved survival when fluid management was guided by lung water measurement [35]. If the lung water measurement was high, vasoactive therapy was used to treat hypotension; if it was low or normal, fluid administration was the first choice. PCWP—pulmonary capillary wedge pressure. (Part B *adapted from* Brigham *et al.* [36].)

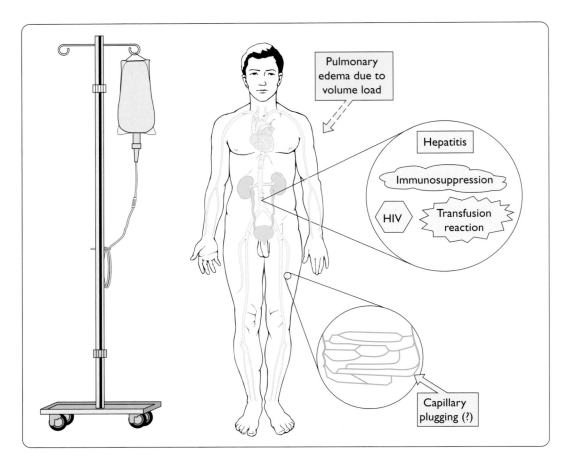

Figure 25-18.
Adverse effects of blood transfusion. Increasing hemoglobin with transfusions will increase the oxygen content of the blood, but the efficacy of transfused blood in increasing oxygen uptake (to meet oxygen demand) has never been proven. Studies in patients with sepsis [37] or acute respiratory distress syndrome [14] have not shown increased oxygen uptake after blood transfusion. We examined the effect of blood transfusion in stable septic patients [28]. No change in systemic oxygen uptake was noted, but gastric intramucosal pH decreased in some patients. More recent studies demonstrate that an order for blood transfusions should not be based on arbitrary hemoglobin levels [38]. Most patients can probably tolerate a hemoglobin as low as 70 g/L but individual patient assessment is needed [39,40]. With the lack of data showing efficacy, it is especially important to consider possible adverse consequences of transfusions, which include immunosuppression, disease transmission, and minor or major transfusion reactions.

Pulmonary edema due to volume load

Hepatitis

Immunosuppression

HIV

Transfusion reaction

Capillary plugging (?)

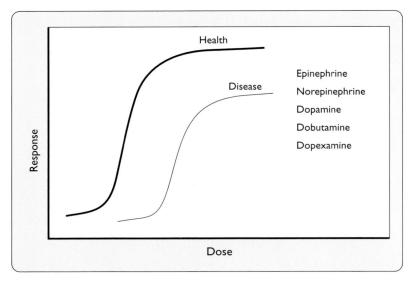

Health

Disease

Epinephrine

Norepinephrine

Dopamine

Dobutamine

Dopexamine

Response

Dose

Figure 25-19.
Vasoactive agents. In addition to improving contractility and stroke volume with adequate preload, vasoactive therapy may be used to lower afterload or directly increase contractility. There are no randomized studies that demonstrate the efficacy of individual vasoactive drugs or compare them with each other. The literature on these drugs has been reviewed [41]. An important point to remember when using these drugs is that sensitivity can vary among patients. As shown in the figure, large shifts in the dose-response curve can occur. Therefore, the drugs should be titrated to the desired response rather than to a preset dose.

RELATIVE ACTIVITY OF SYMPATHETIC DRUGS

Drug	α	β_1	β_2	Dopaminergic
Dobutamine	+	++++	++	0
Dopamine	+ / ++	++++	++	++++
Dopexamine	0	+	++++	++
Epinephrine	++++	++++	+++	0
Norepinephrine	+++	+++	++	0
Phenylephrine	+++	0	0	0

Figure 25-20.
Relative activity of sympathomimetic drugs. The figure shows the relative activity of the various sympathomimetic drugs that are clinically available. Activation of α receptors causes primarily vasoconstriction, activation of β_1 receptors increases myocardial contractility, and β_2–receptor stimulation causes vasodilation. Dopaminergic activity may selectively dilate renal and splanchnic arterioles. Dobutamine has been used in most randomized clinical trials of goal-directed therapy. The usual dose range is 5 to 20 µg/kg/min. It has primarily β-adrenergic activity, but also acts at α_2 receptors. Norepinephrine is useful in patients who remain hypotensive despite fluid therapy [42,43] or who have acute respiratory distress syndrome for whom excessive fluid may be detrimental [35]. Dopamine has never been proven to have any benefit in critically ill patients. Even in a recent study [44], a renal protective effect was not shown. An animal study [45] and a human study [46] showed adverse effects on gut perfusion. Dopexamine is available in Europe. It has dopaminergic and β-adrenergic activity, so it improves cardiac output primarily by reducing afterload. It may have favorable effects on blood flow distribution and was used in one of the clinical trials of goal-directed therapy that proved to be beneficial [17].

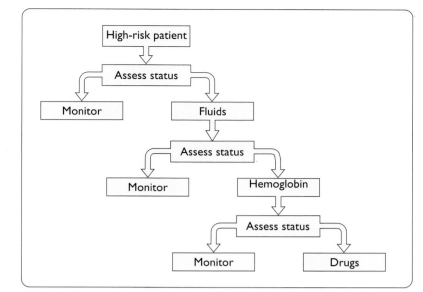

Figure 25-21.

Postoperative management of hemodynamics. Appropriate hemodynamic management may prevent multiple organ dysfunction syndrome in postoperative patients. The role of goal-directed hemodynamic therapy in patients with sepsis and established organ dysfunction is less clear. The approach appears to be safe, if applied with appropriate consideration to the patient's requirements. The first step is to resuscitate the patient with fluids until the pulmonary wedge pressure is at least 12 to 15 mm Hg. Higher values may be appropriate in patients with underlying cardiac dysfunction. A combination of crystalloid and colloid should probably be used, although the evidence needed to produce firm guidelines is lacking. The response to this treatment should be monitored by assessing clinical signs and lactate levels and by using a pulmonary artery catheter. If further resuscitation is needed, the patient should be transfused with erythrocytes until the hemoglobin is 100 to 110 g/L. If the cardiac index or blood pressure remains low, pharmacologic therapy should be started. Norepinephrine should be used if the blood pressure is low; dobutamine or dopexamine should be used if the cardiac index is low. This treatment should be monitored frequently by assessing clinical signs and measuring cardiac output, mixed venous saturation, and lactate.

REFERENCES

1. Abraham E, Bland RD, Cobo JC, Shoemaker WC: Sequential cardiorespiratory patterns associated with outcome in septic shock. *Chest* 1984, 85:75–80.

2. Martin CM, Sibbald WJ: Oxygen delivery in critically ill patients. *Curr Opin Crit Care* 1996, 2:386–390.

3. Heyland DK, Cook DJ, King G, et al.: Maximizing oxygen delivery in critically ill patients: a methodologic appraisal of the evidence. *Crit Care Med* 1996, 24:517–524.

4. Dorinsky PM, Gadek JE: Mechanisms of multiple nonpulmonary organ failure in ARDS. *Chest* 1989, 96:885–892.

5. Martin CM, Yagchi A, Sibbald WJ, et al.: Differential impairment of vascular reactivity of small pulmonary and systemic arteries in hyperdynamic sepsis. *Am Rev Respir Dis* 1993, 148:164–172.

6. Lam C, Tyml K, Martin CM, Sibbald WJ: The skeletal muscle microcirculation in a rat model of normotensive sepsis. *J Clin Invest* 1994, 94:2077–2038.

7. Chung TW, O'Rear EA, Whitsett TL, et al.: Survival factors in a canine septic shock model. *Circ Shock* 1991, 33:178–182.

8. Langenfeld JE, Livingston DH, Machiedo GW: Red cell deformability is an early indicator of infection. *Surgery* 1991, 110:398–404.

9. Langenfeld JE, Machiedo GW, Lyons M, et al.: Correlation between red blood cell deformability and changes in hemodynamic function. *Surgery* 1994, 116:859–867.

10. Flamand F, Sibbald WJ, Girotti MJ, Martin CM: Pentoxifylline does not prevent microvascular injury in normotensive, septic rats. *Crit Care Med* 1995, 23:119–124.

11. Morisaki H, Bloos F, Keys J, et al.: Compared to crystalloid, colloid therapy slows the progression of extrapulmonary tissue injury in septic sheep. *J Appl Physiol* 1994, 77:1507–1518.

12. Bone RC: The pathogenesis of sepsis. *Ann Intern Med* 1991, 115:457–469.

13. Ronco JJ, Fenwick JC, Wiggs BR, et al.: Oxygen consumption is independent of increases in oxygen delivery by dobutamine in septic patients who have normal or increased plasma lactate. *Am Rev Respir Dis* 1993, 147:25–31.

14. Ronco JJ, Phang PT, Walley KR, et al.: Oxygen consumption is independent of changes in oxygen delivery in severe adult respiratory distress syndrome. *Am Rev Respir Dis* 1991, 143:1267–1273.

15. Piiper J, Haab P: Oxygen supply and uptake in tissue models with unequal distribution of blood flow and shunt. *Respir Physiol* 1991, 84:261–271.

16. Walley KR: Heterogeneity of oxygen delivery impairs oxygen extraction by peripheral tissues—theory. *J Appl Physiol* 1996, 81:885–894.

17. Boyd O, Grounds RM, Bennet ED: A randomized clinical trial of the effect of deliberate perioperative increase of oxygen delivery on mortality in high-risk surgical patients. *J Am Med Assoc* 1993, 270:2699–2707.

18. Yu M, Levy MM, Smith P, et al.: Effect of maximizing oxygen delivery on morbidity and mortality rates in critically ill patients: A prospective, randomized, controlled study. *Crit Care Med* 1993, 21:830–838.

19. Tuchschmidt J, Fried J, Astiz M, Rackow E: Elevation of cardiac output and oxygen delivery improves outcome in septic shock. *Chest* 1992, 102:216–220.

20. Shoemaker WC, Appel PL, Kram HB, et al.: Prospective trial of supranormal values of survivors as therapeutic goals in high risk surgical patients. *Chest* 1988, 94:1176–1186.

21. Gattinoni L, Brazzi L, Pelosi P, et al.: A trial of goal-oriented hemodynamic therapy in critically ill patients. SvO$_2$ Collaborative Group. *N Engl J Med* 1995, 333:1025–1032.

22. Yu M, Takanishi D, Myers SA, et al.: Frequency of mortality and myocardial infarction during maximizing oxygen delivery: a prospective, randomized trial. *Crit Care Med* 1995, 23:1025–1032.

23. Hayes MA, Timmins AC, Yau EH, et al.: Elevation of systemic oxygen delivery in the treatment of critically ill patients. *N Engl J Med* 1994, 330:1717–1722.

24. Fleming A, Bishop M, Shoemaker WC, et al.: Prospective trial of supranormal values as goals of resuscitation in severe trauma. *Arch Surg* 1992, 127:1175–1181.

25. Gutierrez G, Palizas F, Doglio G, Wainsztein N: Gastric intramucosal pH as a therapeutic index of tissue oxygenation in critically ill patients. *Lancet* 1992, 339:195–199.

26. Yu M, Burchell S, Nahidh WMA, et al.: Relationship of mortality to increasing oxygen delivery in patients ≥50 years of age: a prospective, randomized trial. *Crit Care Med* 1998, 26:1011–1019.

27. Lobo SMA, Salgado PF, Castillo VGT, et al.: Effects of maximizing oxygen delivery on morbidity and mortality in high-risk surgical patients. *Crit Care Med* 2000, 28:3396–3404.

28. Marik PE, Sibbald WJ: Effect of stored-blood transfusion on oxygen delivery in patients with sepsis. *J Am Med Assoc* 1993, 269:3024–3029.

29. Moss GS, Gould SA: Plasma expanders: an update. *Am J Surg* 1988, 155:425–433.

30. Velanovich V: Crystalloid versus colloid fluid resuscitation: a meta-analysis of mortality. *Surgery* 1989, 105:65–71.

31. Hebert PC, Wells G, Blajchman MA, et al.: A multicenter, randomized, controlled clinical trial of transfusion requirements in critical care. *N Engl J Med* 1999, 340:409–417.

32. Cochrane Injuries Group Albumin Reviewers: Human albumin administration in critically ill patients: systematic review of randomized controlled trials. *BMJ* 1998, 317:235–240.

33. Simmons RS, Berdine GG, Seidenfeld JJ, et al.: Fluid balance and the adult respiratory distress syndrome. *Am Rev Respir Dis* 1987, 135:924–929.

34. Humphrey H, Hall J, Sznajder I, et al.: Improved survival in ARDS patients associated with a reduction in pulmonary capillary wedge pressure. *Chest* 1990, 97:1176–1180.

35. Mitchell JP, Schuller D, Calandrino FS, Schuster DP: Improved outcome based on fluid management in critically ill patients requiring pulmonary artery catheterization. *Am Rev Respir Dis* 1992, 145:990–998.

36. Brigham KL, Woolverton WC, Blake LH, Staub NC: Increased sheep lung vascular permeability caused by pseudomonas bacteremia. *J Clin Invest* 1974, 54:792–804.

37. Silverman JJ, Tuma P: Gastric tonometry in patients with sepsis. Effects of dobutamine infusions and packed red blood cell transfusions. *Chest* 1992, 102:184–188.

38. Choi PTL, Yip G, Quinonez LG, *et al.*: Crystalloid vs. colloids in fluid resuscitation: a systematic review. *Crit Care Med* 1999, 27:200–210.

39. American College of Physicians: Practice strategies for elective red blood cell transfusion. *Ann Intern Med* 1992, 116:403–406.

40. National Institutes of Health: Perioperative red blood cell transfusion. *J Am Med Assoc* 1988, 260:2700–2703.

41. Rudis MI, Basha MA, Zarowitz BJ: Is it time to reposition vasopressors and inotropes in sepsis? *Crit Care Med* 1996, 24:525–537.

42. Martin C, Papazian L, Perrin G, *et al.*: Norepinephrine or dopamine for the treatment of hyperdynamic septic shock? *Chest* 1993, 101:1826–1831.

43. Marik PE, Mohedin M: The contrasting effects of dopamine and norepinephrine on systemic and splanchnic oxygen utilization in hyperdynamic sepsis. *J Am Med Assoc* 1994, 272:1354–1357.

44. Lherm T, Troche G, Rossignol M, *et al.*: Renal effects of low-dose dopamine in patients with sepsis syndrome or septic shock treated with catecholamines. *Int Care Med* 1996, 22:213–219.

45. Segal JM, Phang PT, Walley KR: Low-dose dopamine hastens onset of gut ischemia in a porcine model of hemorrhagic shock. *J Appl Physiol* 1992, 73:1159–1164.

46. Maynard ND, Bihari DJ, Dalton RN, *et al.*: Increasing splanchnic blood flow in the critically ill. *Chest* 1995, 108:1648–1654.

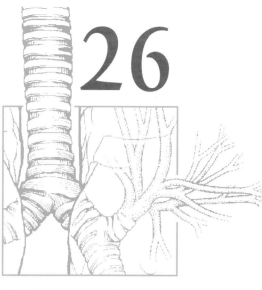
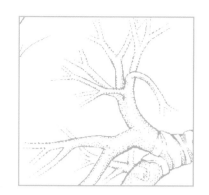
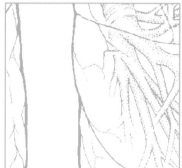

NUTRITION

Barbara Tribl &
William J. Sibbald

Malnutrition in a patient can be present at admission into the intensive care unit (ICU) and can develop during the course of critical illness because of hypermetabolism and lack of oral food intake. The metabolic response to illness and injury differs significantly from that of starvation. In malnutrition caused by starvation, the body attempts to adapt by decreasing its metabolic rate. Glycogen stores are depleted within the first 24 hours, and fat becomes the main source of energy. During starvation, proteins are saved for later. In contrast, during sepsis and after trauma, there is accelerated protein catabolism. When caloric intake is inadequate, energy is derived from protein breakdown and gluconeogenesis. Muscle and visceral proteins are depleted and eventually lead to reduced organ function and increased mortality.

Reduced body weight and anthropometric indices, decreases in hepatic protein levels (albumin, transferrin, retinol-binding protein, and prealbumin), and changes in creatinine can be used to assess nutritional status in critical illness. However, all these tests have limitations because there are many factors at work. In critically ill patients, changes in body weight tend to reflect changes in fluid balance more than in lean body mass. The need for aggressive fluid resuscitation (and the ensuing subcutaneous edema) also limits the use of anthropometric tests. Fluid resuscitation, changes in protein synthesis, catabolism, renal losses, and additional decreases in protein synthesis in the liver, interfere with serum levels of albumin, transferrin, retinol binding protein, and prealbumin. The most reliable tool for the assessment of nutritional status in critically ill patients is a thorough nutritional history.

A. EVIDENCE OF EFFICACY OF NUTRITIONAL THERAPY IN CRITICALLY ILL PATIENTS

Total parenteral nutrition versus standard therapy

A systematic review on the effect of total parenteral nutrition (TPN) in critically ill and surgical patients was done in 1998 [1]. The authors included 26 prospective randomized controlled trials comparing TPN with standard care (oral diet and intravenous dextrose) in surgical patients and critically ill patients. (Trials comparing TPN and enteral nutrition were excluded from this meta-analysis.) Patients receiving TPN tended to have lower complication rates, but this was not statistically significant. The complication rates seemed to be reduced particularly in malnourished patients. TPN had no significant effect on overall mortality. In three of the trials in critically ill, nonsurgical patients, mortality was significantly worse in TPN recipients. There was also a trend for such patients to have higher morbidity. Results of this meta-analysis do not support the use of TPN in critically ill patients.

Enteral nutrition versus parenteral nutrition

Animal studies show that, compared to TPN, enteral nutrition (EN) has the benefit of preserving gut integrity [2], immunologic function of the intestine [3], and results in less bacterial translocation from the gut into systemic circulation [4]. EN also had lower mortality after animals were induced with sepsis [5] or hemorrhage [6].

Trials in humans undergoing laparotomy for blunt trauma, report a significantly lower incidence of major septic complications in enterally fed patients compared to those fed with TPN [7–9]. Starting EN as early as possible seems to be particularly important. Animal studies indicate that an early start (<24 hours) compared with a delayed start (>72 hours) is associated with a reduced postoperative hypermetabolic and catabolic response [10] and less bacterial translocation [11].

Immunonutrition in critical illness

Certain dietary compounds modulate a variety of inflammatory, metabolic, and immune responses when ingested in excess of the normal daily requirements. L-arginine and L-glutamine can stimulate a variety of host defenses [12,13], increase wound healing [14], and reduce nitrogen losses after trauma [15]. L-glutamine may also have beneficial effects in maintaining the integrity of the intestinal barrier function, thus preventing translocation of bacteria and endotoxins from the bowel lumen into the systemic circulation. Nucleic acids enhance a variety of host defenses in patients with cancer [16]. ω-3 essentially fatty acids inhibit cellular and humoral host defense mechanisms [17]. Commercially available enteral nutritional formulas usually contain combinations of immune-enhancing compounds. Meta-analyses of randomized controlled trials comparing the effect of standard enteral nutrition with immunonutrition in critically ill patients stated significant reductions in infection rates and hospital length of stay in the immunonutrition group [18,19].

B. EVIDENCE OF EFFICACY OF PROMOTILITY AGENTS IN CRITICALLY ILL PATIENTS

Agent	Study	No. of patients	Method/parameter	Design	Gut motility	Aspiration
Erythromycin	Chapman [21]	20	Gastric residuals	PRCT	Increased	No data
Erythromycin	Dive [22]	10	Acetaminophen absorption, manometry	2-day crossover	Increased	No data
Erythromycin	Kalliafas [23]	57	Feeding tube migration	PRCT	Increased	No data
Erythromycin	Griffith [24]	36	Feeding tube migration	PRCT	Increased	No data
Metoclopramide	Jooste [25]	10	Acetaminophen absorption	2-day crossover	Increased	No data
Metoclopramide	Whatley [26]	10	Feeding tube migration	PRCT	Increased	No data
Metoclopramide	Heiselman [27]	105	Feeding tube migration	PRCT	No effect	No data
Metoclopramide	Yavaga [28]	305	Frequency of pneumonia	PRCT	No data	No effect

Open questions

Erythromycin as continuous therapy or as a single dose?
What is the effectiveness of erythromycin in the prevention of aspiration/ pneumonia?

Figure 26-1.
A, Evidence of efficacy for nutritional therapy in critically ill patients. **B**, Evidence of efficacy of promotility agents in critically ill patients.

Energy requirement: 25 kcal/kg body weight/day

Measurement of energy expenditure with indirect calorimetry is the most reliable method to examine nutritional requirement. This method is time-consuming and therefore restricted to scientific purpose.

Harris-Benedict equation allows calculation of energy expenditure.

Harris-Benedict equation for:

Female: BEE = 655 + (9.6 x weight in kg) + (1.8 x height in cm) - (4.7 x age in years)

Male: BEE = 66 + (13.7 x weight in kg) + (5 x height in cm) - (6.8 x age in years)

Volume: In general, 1 mL of water/kilocalorie

Fluid restriction may be necessary in cardiac, pulmonary, postoperative, and renal patients in the ICU.

Macronutrients:

	Total calories/d, *g/kg/bw*	Total calories/d, %	Dose adjustment
Glucose	2–5	30–70	blood glucose > 225 mg/dL
Protein	1.2–1.5	15–20	BUN > 100 mg/dL
Fats	0.5–1	15–30	TG > 400 mg/dL

Micronutrients:

Vitamins and trace elements are usually administered as components of TPN and EN.

	Units	Normal	Deficient
Retinol	µg/dL	10–100	<10
25-Hydrxy D	µg/dL	0.8–5.5	<0.7
1,25-Dihydrxy D	ng/dL	2.6–6.5	—
α-Tocopherol	µg/dL	7.0–20.0	<5
Blood thiamine	µg/dL	2.5–7.5	<1.7
Blood riboflavin	µg/dL	10–50	<10
Serum niacin	µg/dL	300–600	<300
Ascorbic acid	mg/mL	0.4–1.5	<0.3
Plasma biotin	ng/dL	30–74	—
Carotenoids	µg/dL	80–400	—
Vitamin B12	pg/mL	205–867	<140
Folic acid	ng/mL	3.3–20	<2.5

Figure 26-2.
General principles of nutritional support. (*Adapted from* The American College of Chest Physicans [20].)

ENTERAL NUTRITION

ROUTE OF ADMINISTRATION OF NUTRITION

Enteral route is preferred because of	Parenteral route is recommended when
Preservation of gut integrity	Enteral route is inaccessible or unusable
Gut barrier function	
Gut immune function	
Reductions in infectious complications	As an additional route when enteral feeding
Lower costs	cannot meet energetic requirements

Figure 26-3.
Route of administration of nutrition. Rationale for choosing a specific route of nutrition in critically ill patients.

COMPLICATIONS AND RECOMMENDATIONS

Complications	Risk for	Recommendation
Gastric residuals >150 mL Vomiting	Aspiration	Small bowel feeding ± simultaneous naso-gastric decompression
		Semirecumbent patient position (45°)
		Metoclopramide, erythromycin
		TPN
Constipation Abdominal distention	Ileus	Bowel sounds, passage of flatus or stool are unnecessary for initiation of EN
Diarrhea	Excessive fluid loss	If >1000 mL/d; evaluation of infectious diarrhea; reduce volume of EN
Sinusitis	Septic focus	Access through PEG or PEJ

Figure 26-4.
Enteral route. Complications and recommendations. Enteral feeding may be associated with complications, as listed in this table. Recommendations for minimizing the occurrence of complications are presented.

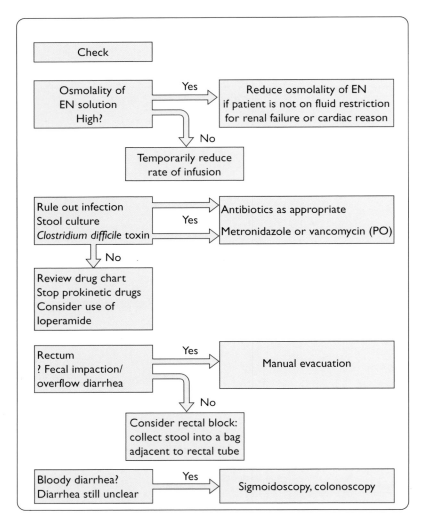

Figure 26-5.
Diarrhea with more than 1000 mL per 24 hours. Diarrhea may occur in critically ill patients when they are receiving enteral feeding. It is often difficult to ignore the potential association. This figure outlines different causes of diarrhea in critically ill patients, in addition to enteral feeding.

Figure 26-6.
Access through the nasogastric or nasoduodenal feeding tube.

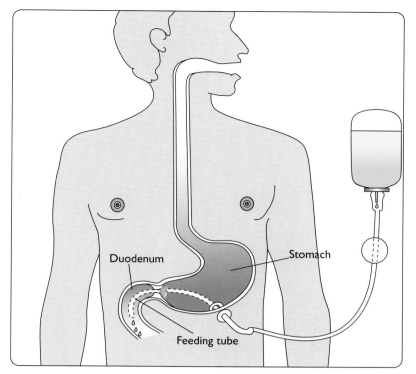

Figure 26-7.
Access through percutaneous gastrostomy (PEG) or percutaneous jejunostomy (PEJ).

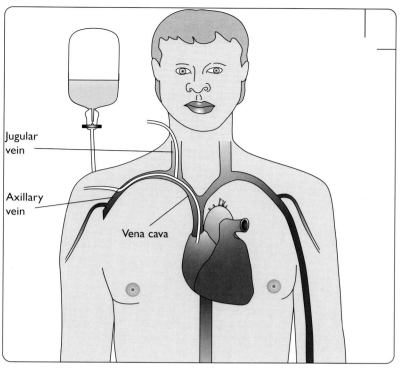

Figure 26-8.
Central venous catheter insertion through the jugular or axillary vein.

PARENTERAL NUTRITION

COMPLICATIONS AND RECOMMENDATIONS

Complication	Risk for	Recommendation
Catheter-related	Infections/sepsis	Sterile insertion
		Regular maintenance
	Line blockage	Regular maintenance
		Catheter removal
	Pneumothorax	Chest radiograph after insertion, thoracostomy
	Brachial-plexus injury	
	Arterial insertion	Surgical removal of catheter
	Venous thrombosis and/or pulmonary embolism	
Metabolic overfeeding	Hyperglycemia	Metabolic surveillance
	Increased RQ	Dosage adjustment
	Hypertriglyceridemia	
	Azotemia	
	Hypertonic dehydration	
	Metabolic acidosis	
	Liver cholestasis	
Refeeding syndrome in low BMI	Hypophosphatemia	Gradual introduction of TPN
	Hypokalemia	
	Hypomagnesemia	Metabolic surveillance
	Volume overload	
	Congestive heart failure	

Figure 26-9.
Parenteral route. Complications and recommendations. This figure lists the complications associated with parenteral nutrition, including recommendations to minimize their occurrence.

SPECIAL CONSIDERATIONS

SIRS with or without MODS

Caloric requirements may need to be increased 10% to 20%. Hyperglycemia is often present. When blood glucose level exceeds 225 mg/dL, glucose load must be reduced and/or regular insulin must be added. The increased protein catabolism necessitates increased protein administration (1.5–2 g/kg body weight/day). If hypertriglyceridemia occurs, total calories and triglyceride load should be reduced, and/or fat should be excluded until triglyceride intolerance has abated.

Renal failure

Renal failure is accompanied by intolerance to fluids and an increase in potassium, magnesium, and phosphate levels. In acute renal failure, there is no need to alter the amount and composition of protein and amino acids of nutrition formulas. The use of dialysis and ultrafiltration leads to losses of nutrients, which need consideration when adjusting the amount of protein administered. In chronic renal failure, a protein dose of 0.5 to 0.8 g/kg body weight/day was associated with preservation of renal function.

Liver failure

If hepatic encephalopathy is present, a reduced protein dose (1.0–1.3 g/kg body weight/day) is recommended. Specifically designed preparations for isolated liver failure are usually used. These products contain an increased amount of branched chain amino acids and a reduced amount of aromatic amino acids.

Respiratory failure

Most patients with respiratory failure can be treated by applying the general principles for nutrition support. In case of difficulties weaning a patient from the ventilator, reduction of the R/Q by applying a high-fat, low carbohydrate formula can be helpful.

Figure 26-10.
Special considerations. This figure lists the special considerations that should be given to patients admitted to the critical care unit with a specific syndrome or disease.

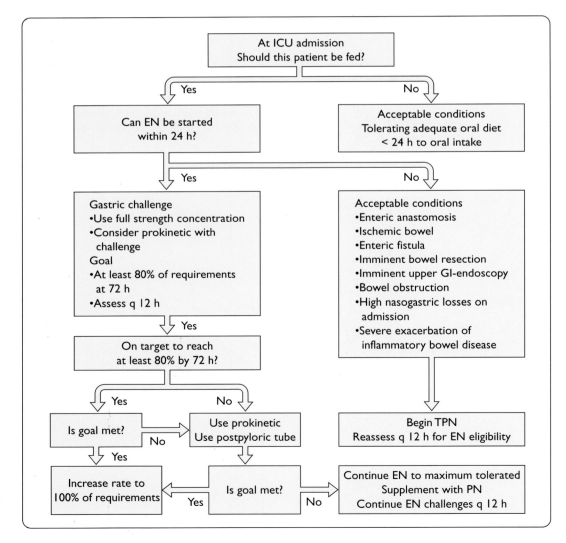

Figure 26-11.
Algorithm for nutrition in the intensive care unit (ICU).

REFERENCES

1. Heyland DK, MacDonald S, Keefe L, Drover JW: Total parenteral nutrition in the critically ill patient: a meta-analysis. *JAMA* 1998, 280:2013–2019.

2. Saito H, Trocki O, Alexander JW, et al.: Effects of route of administration on the nutritional state, catabolic hormone secretion and gut mucosal integrity after burn injury. *JPEN* 1987, 11:1–7.

3. Alverdy J, Chi HS, Sheldon G: The effect of parenteral nutrition on gastrintestinal immunity: the importance of gastrointestinal immunity. *Ann Surg* 1985, 202:681–684.

4. Alverdy JC, Aoys E, Moss GS: TPN promotes bacterial translocation from the gut. *Surgery* 1988, 104:185–190.

5. Kudsk KA, Stone JM, Carpenter G, Sheldon GF: Enteral and parenteral feeding influences mortality after hemoglobin *E. coli* peritonitis in normal rats. *J Trauma* 1983, 23:605–609.

6. Zaloga GP, Knowles R, Black KW, Prielipp R: Total parenteral nutrition increases mortality after hemorrhage. *Crit Care Med* 1990, 19:54–59.

7. Moore FA, Moore EE, Jones TN, McCroskey BL, Petersen VM: TEN versus TPN following major abdominal trauma-reduced septic morbidity. *J Trauma* 1989, 29:916–923.

8. Moore FA, Feliciano DV, Andrassy RJ, et al.: Early enteral feeding, compared with parenteral, reduces septic complications—the results of a meta-analysis. *Ann Surg* 1992, 216:172–183.

9. Kudsk KA, Croce MA, Fabian TC, et al.: Enteral versus parenteral feeding. *Ann Surg* 1992, 215:503–513.

10. Mochizuki H, Trocki O, Dominioni L, Brackett KA, Joffe SN, Alexander JW: Mechanism of prevention of postburn hypermetabolism and catabolism by early enteral feeding. *Ann Surg* 1984, 200:297–308.

11. Inoue S, Epstein MD, Alexander JW, et al.: Prevention of yeast translocation across the gut by a single enteral feeding after burn injury. *JPEN* 1989, 13:565–571.

12. Brittenden J, Park KGM, Heys SD, et al.: L-Arginine stimulates host defenses in patients with breast cancer. *Surgery* 1994, 114:205–212.

13. O'Riordain MG, Fearon KCH, Ross JA, et al.: Glutamine-supplemented total parenteral-nutrition enhances T-lymphocyte response in surgical patients undergoing colorectal resection. *Ann Surg* 1994, 220:212–221.

14. Barbul A, Lazarou SA, Efron DT, Wasserkrug HL, Efron G: Arginine enhances wound healing and lymphocyte immune responses in humans. *Surgery* 1990, 108:331–337.

15. Stehle P, Mertes N, Puchstein C, et al.: Effect of parenteral glutamine peptide supplements on muscle glutamine loss and nitrogen balance after major surgery. *Lancet* 1989, 1:231–233.

16. Khan AL, Richardson S, Drew J, et al.: Polyadenylic polyuridylic acid (PAPU) enhances natural cell-mediated cytotoxicity in patients with breast cancer undergoing mastectomy. *Surgery* 1995, 118:531–538.

17. Purasiri P, McKechnie A, Heys SD, Eremin O: Modulation in vitro of human natural cytotoxicity, lymphocyte proliferative response to mitogens and cytokine production by essential fatty acids. *Immunology* 1997, 92:166–172.

18. Beale RJ, Bryg DJ, Bihari DJ: Immunonutrition in critically ill: a systematic review of clinical outcome. *Crit Care Med* 1999, 27:2799–2805.

19. Heys SD, Walker LG, Smith I, Eremin O: Enteral nutritional supplementation with key nutrients in patients with critical illness and cancer. *Ann Surg* 1999, 229:467–477.

20. American College of Chest Physicians: Consensus Statement of the American College of Chest Physicans. *Chest* 1997, 111:769–778.

21. Chapman MJ, Fraser RJ, Kluger MT, Buist MD, De Nichilo DJ: Erythromycin improves gastric emptying in critically ill patients intolerant of nasogastric feeding. *Crit Care Med* 2000, 28:2334–2337.

22. Dive A, Miesse C, Galanti L, et al.: Effect of erythromycin on gastric motility in mechanically ventilated critically ill patients: a double-blind, randomized, placebo-controlled study. *Crit Care Med* 1995, 23:1356–1362.

23. Kalliafas S, Choban PS, Ziegler D, Drago S, Flancbaum L: Erythromycin facilitates postpyloric placement of nasoduodenal feeding tubes in intensive care unit patients: randomized, double-blinded, placebo-controlled trial. *JPEN* 1996, 20:385–388.

24. Griffith DP, McNally RN, Battey CH, et al.: Efficacy of erythromycin for small intestinal feeding tube placementin ICU patients: a double-blind, randomized, placebo controlled study [abstract]. *JPEN* 1997, 21:S3.

25. Jooste CA, Mustoe J, Collee G: Metoclopramide improves gastric motility in critically ill patients. *Intensive Care Med* 1999, 25:464–468.

26. Whatley K, Turner WW, Dey M, Leonard J, Guthrie M: When does metoclopramide facilitate transpyloric intubation? *JPEN* 1984;8:679–681.

27. Heiselmann DE, Hofer T, Vidovich RR: Enteral feeding tube placement success with intravenous metoclopramide administration in ICU patients. *Chest* 1995, 107:1686–1688.

28. Yavagal DR, Karnad DR, Oak JL: Metoclopramide for preventing pneumonia incritically ill patients receiving enteral tube feeding: a randomized controlled trial. *Crit Care Med* 2000, 28:1408–1411.

INDEX

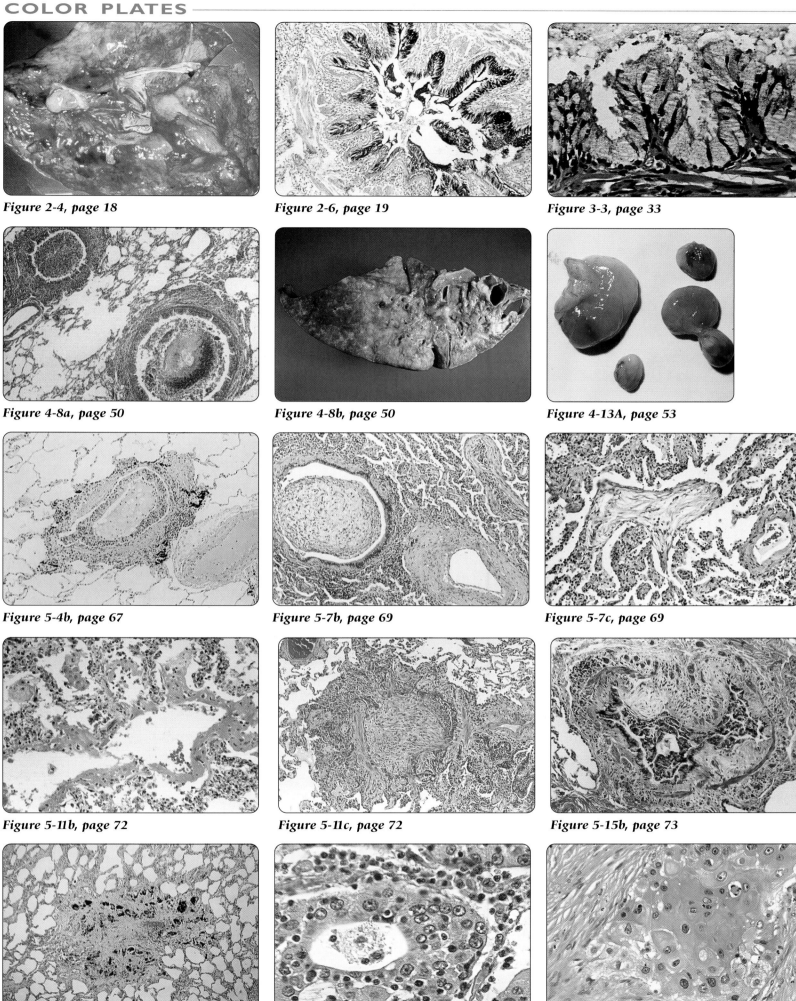

Figure 2-4, page 18

Figure 2-6, page 19

Figure 3-3, page 33

Figure 4-8a, page 50

Figure 4-8b, page 50

Figure 4-13A, page 53

Figure 5-4b, page 67

Figure 5-7b, page 69

Figure 5-7c, page 69

Figure 5-11b, page 72

Figure 5-11c, page 72

Figure 5-15b, page 73

Figure 5-17b, page 75

Figure 7-3a, page 93

Figure 7-3b, page 93

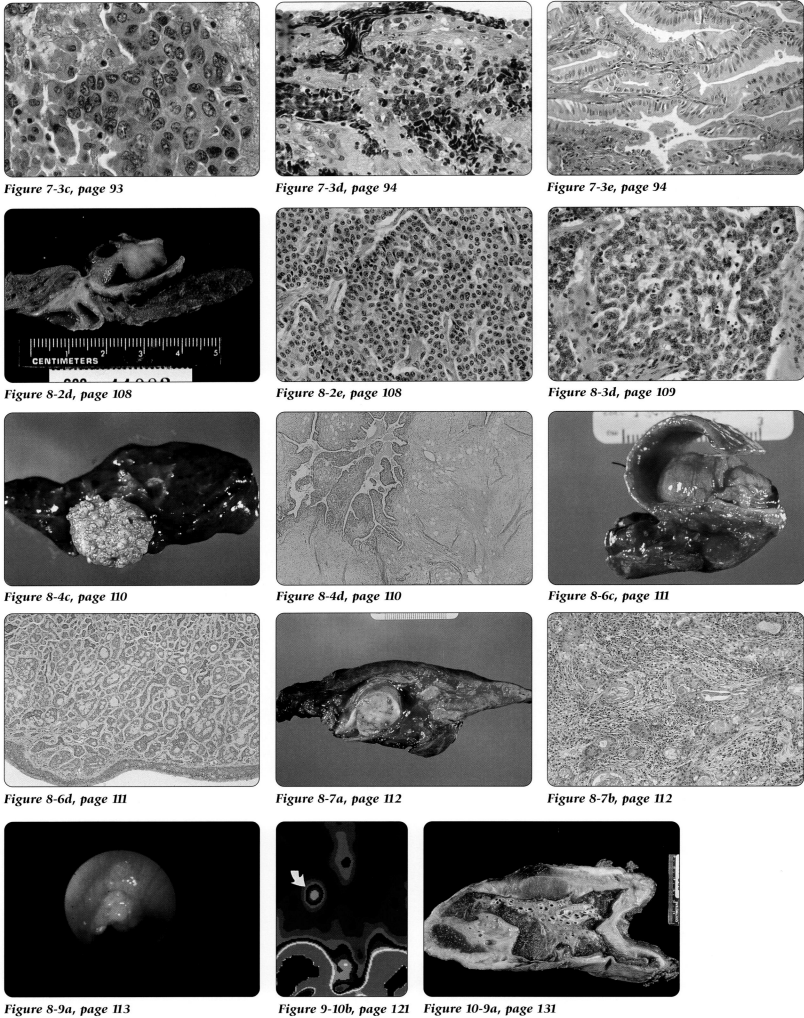

Figure 7-3c, page 93

Figure 7-3d, page 94

Figure 7-3e, page 94

Figure 8-2d, page 108

Figure 8-2e, page 108

Figure 8-3d, page 109

Figure 8-4c, page 110

Figure 8-4d, page 110

Figure 8-6c, page 111

Figure 8-6d, page 111

Figure 8-7a, page 112

Figure 8-7b, page 112

Figure 8-9a, page 113

Figure 9-10b, page 121

Figure 10-9a, page 131

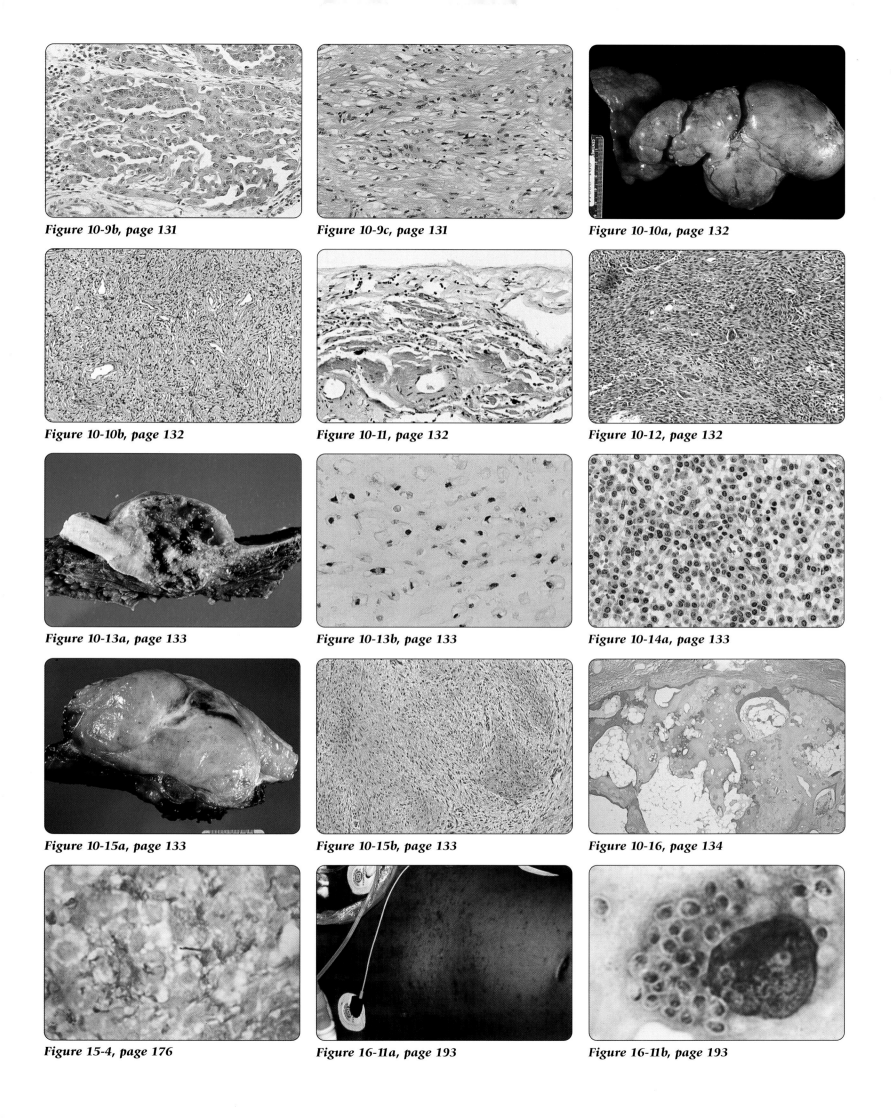

Figure 10-9b, page 131

Figure 10-9c, page 131

Figure 10-10a, page 132

Figure 10-10b, page 132

Figure 10-11, page 132

Figure 10-12, page 132

Figure 10-13a, page 133

Figure 10-13b, page 133

Figure 10-14a, page 133

Figure 10-15a, page 133

Figure 10-15b, page 133

Figure 10-16, page 134

Figure 15-4, page 176

Figure 16-11a, page 193

Figure 16-11b, page 193

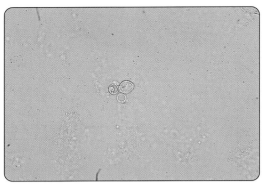
Figure 16-14c, page 194

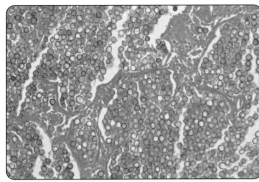
Figure 16-14d, page 194

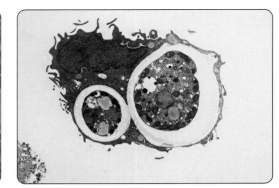
Figure 16-14e, page 194

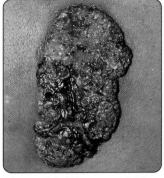
Figure 16-17a, page 196

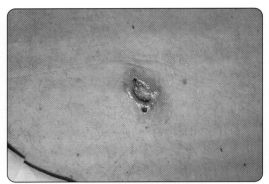
Figure 16-17b, page 196

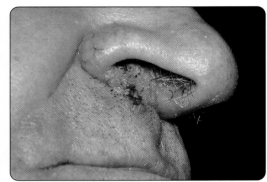
Figure 16-18a, page 196

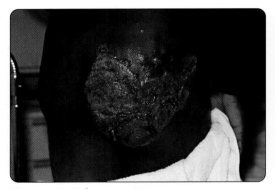
Figure 16-18b, page 196

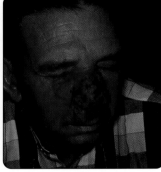
Figure 16-18c, page 196

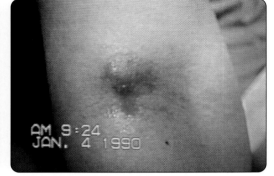
Figure 16-19a, page 197

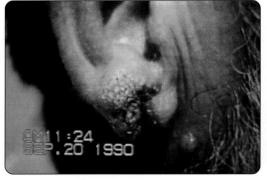
Figure 16-19b, page 197

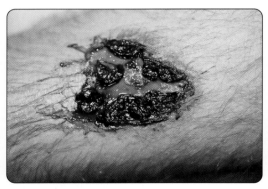
Figure 16-20a, page 197

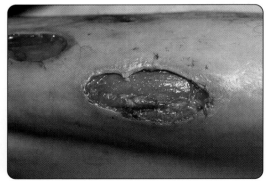
Figure 16-20b, page 197

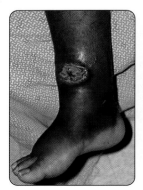
Figure 16-21a, page 197

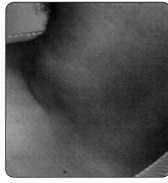
Figure 16-24a, page 199

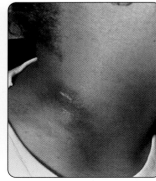
Figure 16-24b, page 199

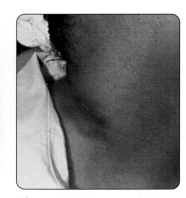
Figure 16-24c, page 199

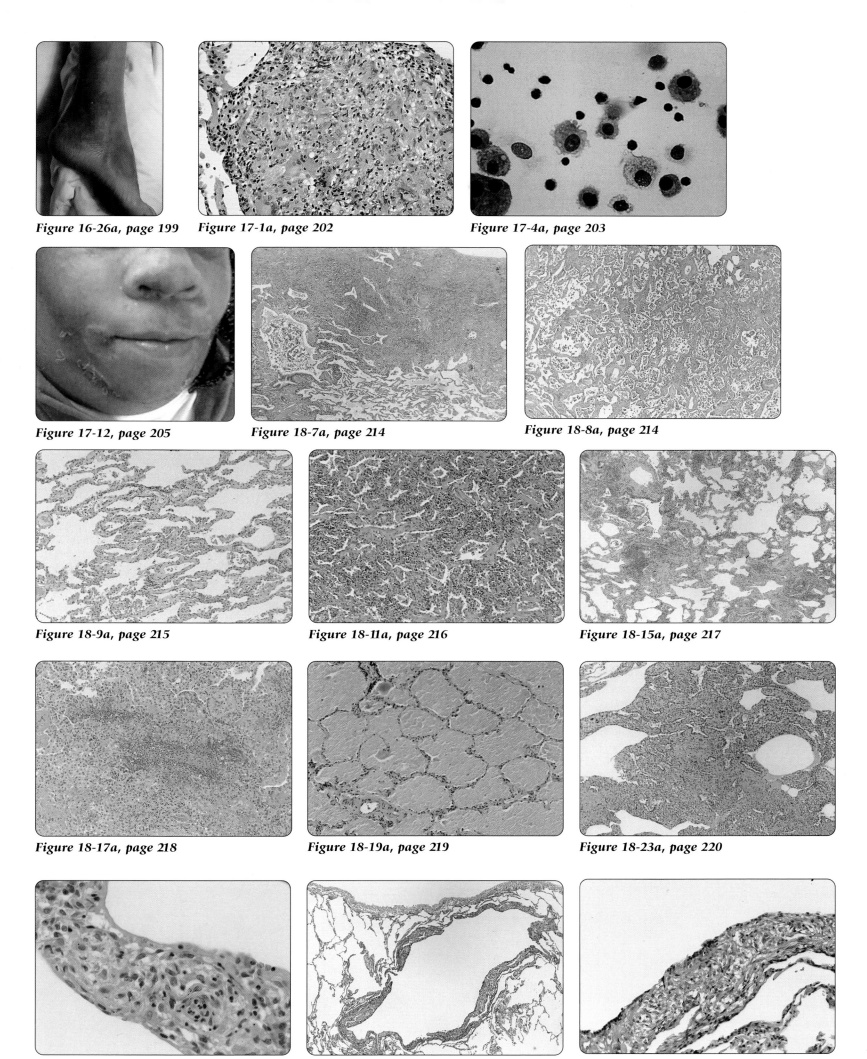

Figure 16-26a, page 199

Figure 17-1a, page 202

Figure 17-4a, page 203

Figure 17-12, page 205

Figure 18-7a, page 214

Figure 18-8a, page 214

Figure 18-9a, page 215

Figure 18-11a, page 216

Figure 18-15a, page 217

Figure 18-17a, page 218

Figure 18-19a, page 219

Figure 18-23a, page 220

Figure 18-23b, page 220

Figure 18-25a, page 221

Figure 18-25b, page 221

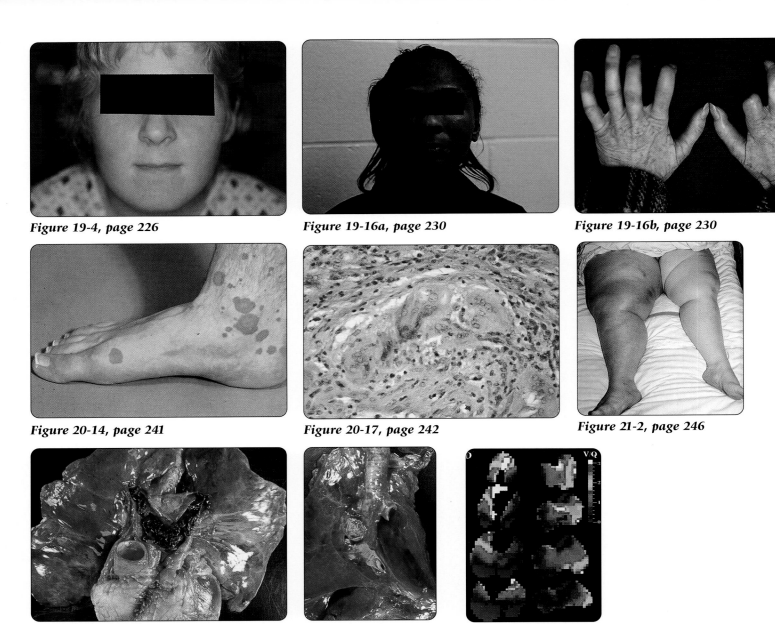

Figure 19-4, page 226

Figure 19-16a, page 230

Figure 19-16b, page 230

Figure 20-14, page 241

Figure 20-17, page 242

Figure 21-2, page 246

Figure 21-3, page 246

Figure 21-30b, page 257

Figure 24-19, page 295